Functional Imaging in Movement Disorders

Editor

W. R. Wayne Martin

Associate Professor
Department of Medicine
University of British Columbia
Health Science Centre Hospital
Vancouver, British Columbia, Canada

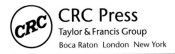

CRC Press
Taylor & Francis Group
Boca Raton London New York

CRC Press is an imprint of the
Taylor & Francis Group, an **informa** business

CRC Press
Taylor & Francis Group
6000 Broken Sound Parkway NW, Suite 300
Boca Raton, FL 33487-2742

Reissued 2019 by CRC Press

© 1990 by Taylor & Francis Group, LLC
CRC Press is an imprint of Taylor & Francis Group, an Informa business

No claim to original U.S. Government works

This book contains information obtained from authentic and highly regarded sources. Reasonable efforts have been made to publish reliable data and information, but the author and publisher cannot assume responsibility for the validity of all materials or the consequences of their use. The authors and publishers have attempted to trace the copyright holders of all material reproduced in this publication and apologize to copyright holders if permission to publish in this form has not been obtained. If any copyright material has not been acknowledged please write and let us know so we may rectify in any future reprint.

Except as permitted under U.S. Copyright Law, no part of this book may be reprinted, reproduced, transmitted, or utilized in any form by any electronic, mechanical, or other means, now known or hereafter invented, including photocopying, microfilming, and recording, or in any information storage or retrieval system, without written permission from the publishers.

For permission to photocopy or use material electronically from this work, please access www.copyright.com (http://www.copyright.com/) or contact the Copyright Clearance Center, Inc. (CCC), 222 Rosewood Drive, Danvers, MA 01923, 978-750-8400. CCC is a not-for-profit organization that provides licenses and registration for a variety of users. For organizations that have been granted a photocopy license by the CCC, a separate system of payment has been arranged.

Trademark Notice: Product or corporate names may be trademarks or registered trademarks, and are used only for identification and explanation without intent to infringe.

A Library of Congress record exists under LC control number:

Publisher's Note
The publisher has gone to great lengths to ensure the quality of this reprint but points out that some imperfections in the original copies may be apparent.

Disclaimer
The publisher has made every effort to trace copyright holders and welcomes correspondence from those they have been unable to contact.

ISBN 13: 978-0-367-24780-5 (hbk)
ISBN 13: 978-0-367-24783-6 (pbk)
ISBN 13: 978-0-429-28435-9 (ebk)

Visit the Taylor & Francis Web site at http://www.taylorandfrancis.com and the
CRC Press Web site at http://www.crcpress.com

PREFACE

One of the most impressive developments to have taken place in clinical neuroscience in the last decade is the rapid implementation of new techniques for imaging the central nervous system. These techniques have not only revolutionized the clinical management of patients with neurological disorders, but have also advanced our understanding of the underlying mechanism of many disorders which affect the brain. While traditional concepts of imaging have focused on the depiction of anatomical details of the brain, the development of "functional imaging" has more recently made possible the *in vivo* study of cerebral physiology in human subjects.

This new field of functional imaging has found particularly fertile ground in the study of movement disorders since these disorders have prominent and often disabling clinical symptomatology implying a significant abnormality of brain function, yet for the most part are characterized by the absence of major structural changes in the brain. The ability to demonstrate abnormalities of regional metabolism and hemodynamics in some of these disorders has not only helped elucidate their pathophysiology but has also helped to clarify some of the normal functional relationships between various components of the brain. The mechanism underlying many of the movement disorders may relate to dysfunction within specific neuronal systems leading to impaired presynaptic neurotransmitter synthesis and/or release, or to abnormal postsynaptic neuroreceptor function. In the past, it has not been possible to directly assess these processes in human subjects *in vivo*. Functional imaging with positron emission tomography (PET), however, has provided the capability to shed further light on transmitter/receptor function and its relationship to these disease processes.

The present volume brings together authoritative, up-to-date, critical accounts of the present status of PET in the study of movement disorders both in terms of the basic science relevant to PET and the clinical science related to the study of specific disease processes. Because an understanding of the methodology itself and its limitations is essential to properly interpret results obtained in clinical studies, a review of the basic principles of PET and tracer kinetics is included. The neurotransmitters and receptors in the basal ganglia which are of relevance to movement disorders are discussed as is the current status of PET in the study of receptor kinetics. Clinical studies concerning presynaptic nigrostriatal function and cerebral energy metabolism in Parkinson's disease and in MPTP-induced parkinsonism are reviewed. Discussions of some of the less common movement disorders such as progressive supranuclear palsy, olivopontocerebellar atrophy, and dystonia are included. Huntington's disease and the potential role of PET in clinical management receives particular attention. Since many of the movement disorders are associated with the eventual development of dementia, a chapter dealing specifically with this component is included. As with any rapidly advancing field, controversies exist and these are dealt with within the relevant chapters.

The primary objectives underlying the production of this volume have been to provide adequate background knowledge for the uninitiated to understand the potentials and pitfalls of the PET/tracer kinetic technique, to provide a critical review of the current status of PET in movement disorders, and to provide a perspective concerning the degree to which PET studies have advanced knowledge and the future role anticipated for PET. It is hoped that these objectives have been met and that this volume will provide a useful guide to this complex and exciting field.

W. R. Wayne Martin
Vancouver, October 1989

THE EDITOR

W. R. Wayne Martin, M. D., F.R.C.P.C. is an Associate Professor, Department of Medicine (Neurology) at the University of British Columbia, Vancouver, B. C., Canada and Associate Director (Medical Research), University of British Columbia/TRIUMF Positron Emission Tomography Program.

Dr. Martin obtained his training at the University of Alberta, Edmonton, Alberta, receiving a B.Med.Sci. degree in 1973 and a M.D. degree in 1975. He completed his neurology training at the University of British Columbia in 1980 followed by a research fellowship in positron emission tomography at Washington University, St. Louis.

Dr. Martin is a member of the Canadian Neurological Society, the American Academy of Neurology, the International Society of Cerebral Blood Flow and Metabolism, the Movement Disorder Society, and the Society of Nuclear Medicine. He is a fellow of the Royal College of Physicians and Surgeons of Canada and has been a scholar of the Medical Research Council of Canada. He has been the recipient of research grants from the Medical Research Council of Canada, the British Columbia Health Care Research Foundation, and the Parkinson's Disease Foundation of Canada.

Dr. Martin has published over 60 publications relating primarily to positron emission tomography and movement disorders and has presented many invited lectures at international meetings. His current major research interests include the role of the basal ganglia in the control of movement and in cognitive function and the use of positron emission tomography in the study of presynaptic and postsynaptic function in movement disorders.

CONTRIBUTORS

Yves Agid, M.D., Ph.D.
Professor, Director of Research
Nouvelle Pharmacie
INSERM U 289
Hopital de la Salepetriere
Paris, France

Walter Ammann, M.D, F.R.C.P.C.
Head, Division of Radiology and
  Nuclear Medicine
University Hospital
University of British Columbia
Vancouver, British Columbia, Canada

Jean-Claude Baron, M.D.
Director of Research
Department of Biology
Service Hopitalier F. Juliet
Hopital d'Orsay
Orsay, France

Jerôme Blin, M.D.
Neurologist
Department of Biology
Service Hopitalier F. Joliot
Hopital d'Orsay
Orsay, France

**Donald B. Calne, F.R.C.P.,
  F.R.C.P.C.**
Head, Division of Neurology
Department of Medicine
University of British Columbia
Vancouver, British Columbia, Canada

Norman L. Foster, M.D.
Assistant Professor of Neurology
Director, Cognitive Disorders Clinic
Department of Neurology
University of Michigan Medical Center
Ann Arbor, Michigan

Albert Gjedde, M.D. D.Sc.
Chief, Positron Imaging Laboratories
Professor of Neurology and Neurosurgery
McConnell Brain Imaging Center
Montreal Neurological Institute
Montreal, Quebec, Canada

Sid Gilman, M.D.
Professor and Chairman
Department of Neurology
University of Michigan Medical Center
Ann Arbor, Michigan

Mark Guttman, M.D., F.R.C.P.C.
Assistant Professor
Department of Neurology and
  Neurosurgery
Montreal Neurological Institute
McGill University
Montreal, Quebec, Canada

**Michael R. Hayden, M.B., Ch.B.,
  Ph.D., D.Ch., F.R.C.P.C.**
Associate Professor
Department of Medical Genetics
University Hospital
University of British Columbia
Vancouver, British Columbia, Canada

Peter Herscovitch, B. Eng., M.D.
Chief, PET Section
NIH Clinical Center
National Institutes of Health
Bethesda, Maryland

Klaus L. Leenders, M.D.
Head, Clinical PET Program
PET Group
Paul Scherrer Institute
Villigen, Switzerland

**W.R. Wayne Martin, M.D.,
  F.R.C.P.C.**
Associate Professor
Department of Medicine
University of British Columbia
Health Science Centre Hospital
Vancouver, British Columbia, Canada

John C. Mazziotta, M.D., Ph.D.
Professor
Departments of Neurology and
  Radiological Sciences
UCLA School of Medicine
Los Angeles, California

John B. Penney, Jr., M.D.
Associate Professor
Department of Neurology
University of Michigan
Ann Arbor, Michigan

Joel S. Perlmutter, M.D.
Assistant Professor of Neurology
  and Radiology
Washington University School
  of Medicine
St. Louis, Missouri

G. Frederick Wooten, M.D.
Professor and Chairman
Department of Neurology
University of Virginia
Charlottesville, Virginia

Anne B. Young, M.D., Ph.D.
Professor
Department of Neurology
University of Michigan
Ann Arbor, Michigan

TABLE OF CONTENTS

Chapter 1

PRINCIPLES OF POSITRON EMISSION TOMOGRAPHY

Peter Herscovitch

TABLE OF CONTENTS

I. INTRODUCTION

The past three decades have seen considerable advances in the methods available for measuring brain blood flow, metabolism, and biochemistry. These advances have culminated in the development of positron emission tomography (PET). To help put the advantages of PET into perspective, the methods that were previously available will be briefly described. The pioneering work of Kety and Schmidt in the 1940s resulted in the development of the nitrous oxide method for measuring hemispheric cerebral blood flow (CBF).[1] These CBF measurements, when combined with measurements of brain arterial-venous differences for glucose and oxygen, permitted the determination of cerebral metabolism as well. The Kety-Schmidt technique, however, did not provide measurements on a regional basis. The desire to obtain regional rather than global data led to the development of methods to measure CBF with radioactive tracers and external probe systems incorporating multiple radiation detectors placed over the head. They were used to measure the clearance from different brain regions of freely diffusible radioactive gases, such as xenon-133, that were administered either by injection into the internal carotid artery or by inhalation.[2,3] Subsequently, external probe techniques using intracarotid injection of tracers labeled with positron-emitting radionuclides were developed for the measurement not only of CBF, but also of cerebral blood volume and metabolism.[4]

These techniques, however, have several drawbacks. The variety of measurements that can be made is quite restricted. Only global measurements of cerebral metabolism can be obtained unless invasive intracarotid artery injections are used. The external detectors employed to obtain regional measurements of CBF have limitations. They record radioactivity from a volume of brain tissue extending a variable depth beneath the probe. Their field of view and sensitivity varies with depth. Radioactivity measurements from heterogeneous tissue elements are superimposed, and the presence of underperfused tissue in the field of view may not be detected. Also, measurements cannot be made from deeper structures such as the basal ganglia.

These limitations provided the impetus for the development of PET, a technique for measuring the absolute concentration of radioactive tracers in the body. From these measurements, the values of physiologic parameters such as blood flow can be calculated on a regional basis. There are three components necessary for the application of PET: (1) tracer compounds of physiologic interest that are labeled with positron-emitting radionuclides; (2) a positron emission tomograph to provide images from which one can accurately measure the amount of positron-emitting radioactivity and thus the amount of tracer compound throughout the brain; and (3) a mathematical model that describes the *in vivo* behavior of the specific radiotracer used, so that the physiologic process under study can be quantitated from the tomographic measurements of regional radioactivity. The first tomograph to be used in this manner was developed at Washington University in St. Louis by Ter-Pogossian and colleagues in the mid 1970s.[5] Subsequently, there has been considerable growth in the field. The design of tomographs has become more sophisticated and radiotracer techniques to perform a wide variety of measurements have been developed. These have been applied to the study of both the normal brain and neuropsychiatric disease.[6,7] In addition, PET has been used in other organ systems, including the heart and lung.[8-10]

The capabilities of PET are particularly relevant to the study of movement disorders. PET permits quantitative measurements to be made from structures such as basal ganglia and cerebellum that were inaccessible by earlier methods. In addition, several radiotracer methods have been developed to study neurotransmitter-neuroreceptor systems. Previously, it was possible to study these systems only by using post-mortem tissue or indirect approaches, such as monitoring the clinical response to pharmacologic interventions.

By reviewing the principles of PET, this chapter provides a basis for the subsequent sections of this volume. The basic components of PET — instrumentation, radiotracer synthesis, and mathematical modeling — will be discussed. Methods for measuring regional cerebral blood flow, blood volume, and metabolism of oxygen and glucose will be described in detail, and issues related to the analysis and interpretation of PET data will be reviewed. Techniques for studying pre- and postsynaptic dopaminergic neurotransmission are dealt with in later chapters.

II. PET INSTRUMENTATION

A. FORMATION OF THE PET IMAGE

PET is a technique for measuring the regional concentration of positron-emitting radio-nuclides in the body. It permits absolute quantitation of the *in vivo* distribution of positron-emitting radioactivity by means of radiation detectors arrayed around the body. The measurements are presented in the form of a gray scale image of a cross-section through the body. The intensity of each point or pixel in the image is proportional to the amount of radioactivity at the corresponding position in the body.

PET depends upon the special nature of a type of radioactive decay. Certain radionuclides decay by the emission of a positron, which is a subatomic particle with the same mass as an electron, but a positive charge. After its emission from the nucleus, the positron travels a few millimeters in tissue, losing its kinetic energy. When almost at rest, it interacts with an electron, resulting in the annihilation of both positron and electron. Their combined mass is converted into energy in the form of electromagnetic radiation. This consists of two high-energy (511 keV) photons that travel in opposite directions away from the annihilation site at the speed of light. Detection of these annihilation photon pairs (one pair per radioactive decay event) is used to measure both the amount and the location of radioactivity. The two annihilation photons can be detected by two radiation detectors that are connected by an electronic coincidence circuit (Figure 1A). The circuit records a decay event only when both detectors sense the arrival of the photons almost simultaneously. A very short time window for photon arrival, typically 5 to 20 ns, called the coincidence resolving time, is allowed for registration of a coincidence event. This coincidence requirement for photon detection localizes the site of the decay event to the volume of space between the pair of detectors.

In practice, a ring of radiation detectors connected in pairs by coincidence circuits is used to surround the distribution of positron-emitting radioactivity in the body. With each decay event, the two annihilation photons are detected as a coincidence line, so that the number of coincidence lines recorded by any pair of detectors is proportional to the amount of radioactivity between them. An image of the distribution of radioactivity is then reconstructed from the coincidence lines (Figure 2). These lines are sorted into parallel groups, each group representing a profile or projection of the radioactivity distribution viewed from a different angle. The profiles are then combined by application of the same mathematical principles used in X-ray computed tomography[11] to obtain the PET image.

The reconstruction process requires a correction for the absorption or attenuation of annihilation photons that occurs within the tissue. This correction is substantial, as much as a factor of 5 to 6 in the center of the head. Estimates of the amount of radiation attenuated by the tissue between detector pairs can be calculated from outlines of the head circumference and an assumed value for the attenuating properties of tissue and bone. Actual measurement of attenuation is more accurate, however.[12] Prior to the emission scan, a separate transmission scan is performed with a source of positron-emitting radioactivity between the subject's head and the detector ring. A measurement is also made without the head in place. The ratio of the two measurements gives the amount of photon attenuation by tissue between each opposing detector pair and is used in the image reconstruction process to correct for attenuation.

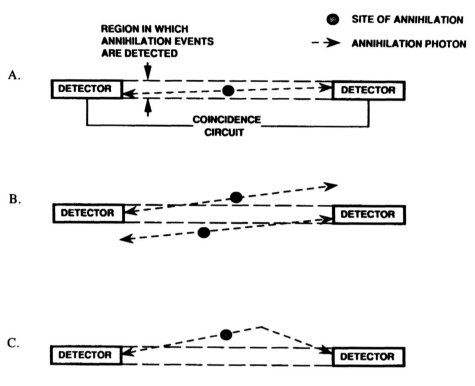

FIGURE 1.   (A) Detection of annihilation photons by two radiation detectors that are connected by a coincidence circuit. A decay event is recorded only when both photons are detected almost simultaneously. This coincidence requirement localizes the site of the annihilation to the volume of space between the detectors. (B) A random coincidence occurs when two photons from two *different* positron annihilations are sensed by a detector pair within the coincidence resolving time. (C) A scattered coincidence occurs when an annihilation photon travelling in tissue is deflected, so that its direction changes. This results in incorrect positioning of the coincidence line.

The intensity of any point in the PET image is proportional to the amount of radioactivity in the corresponding tissue region.[13] To calibrate the PET system to obtain *absolute* radioactivity measurements, a container holding a uniform solution of radioactivity is imaged. The radioactivity in an aliquot of the solution is then measured with a calibrated well counter, and the scanner calibration factor is calculated. The PET image is then scaled to represent absolute amount of radioactivity. To obtain a measurement of local radioactivity, a region of interest is defined on the image with an interactive computer program that computes the average radioactivity value within the region.

A PET system consists of many components. There are several rings of radiation detectors mounted on a gantry. Each detector consists of a small scintillation crystal which gives off light when energy from an annihilation photon is deposited in it. A photomultiplier tube converts the light pulse to an electrical signal which is fed into the electronic coincidence circuitry. Current scanners typically have from 4 to 8 rings, each containing several hundred detectors, although other designs exist.[14] A tomographic image that slices through the body is provided by each ring. In addition, "cross-slices" are derived from coincidences between detectors in adjacent rings. These planes are located halfway between the detector rings. Therefore, up to 15 contiguous tomographic slices can be obtained simultaneously by an eight-ring system. The subject rests on a special couch fitted with a head holder to restrain head movement during the scanning procedure. A computer records the coincidence events and is used to reconstruct and display the tomographic images of radioactivity.

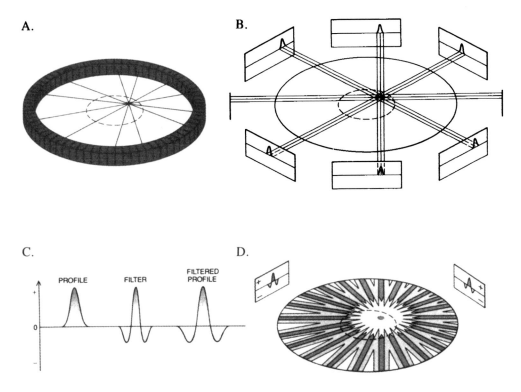

FIGURE 2.   The PET reconstruction process can be explained with reference to this schematic diagram which depicts the imaging of a small uniform region of radioactivity. (A) Multiple coincidence lines are recorded by opposing detectors in the ring. Each line results from a positron emission and annihilation. (B) The lines are sorted into parallel groups. Each group represents the profile or projection of the radioactivity in the field of view viewed from a different angle. (C) Each projection is then mathematically processed by means of a filter function. (D) The modified projections are then combined by "back-projection" to reconstruct an image of the distribution of radioactivity in the field of view of the scanner. (From Ter-Pogossian, M. M. et al., *Sci. Am.*, October, 1980. With permission.)

The engineering design of PET imaging systems involves many factors including selection of the size, shape, and material for the scintillation crystals, the arrangement of the crystals and photomultiplier tubes in the gantry, the design of coincidence electronic circuitry, and the mathematical methods used to reconstruct the tomographic image. All of these factors affect the performance of the tomograph. Detailed reviews of tomograph design have been presented elsewhere.[15-20] Performance characteristics that have a major impact on the quality or interpretation of the physiologic measurements made with PET will be reviewed here. These include image noise, count rate performance, and spatial resolution.

B. PERFORMANCE CHARACTERISTICS OF PET SCANNERS
Statistical noise occurs in the PET image because of the random nature of radioactive decay. The disintegration rate of a radioactive sample undergoes moment-to-moment variation that can be described by a Poisson statistical distribution. The resultant uncertainty in the measurement of the amount of radioactivity, expressed as a fraction of the number of counts recorded, N, is proportional to $1/\sqrt{N}$. Thus, counting noise decreases as N increases. Similarly, the statistical reliability of a local radioactivity measurement depends upon the number of counts recorded. The situation is more complex, however, than the simple Poisson prediction. This is because the measurement of radioactivity in any small brain region is obtained from an image reconstructed from multiple views or projections of the radioactivity distribution throughout the brain slice. Thus, the measurement noise in any individual brain

region is affected by noise in other brain regions. The resultant image noise is greater than would be predicted by Poisson statistics[21] although it still can be reduced by increasing the number of counts (Figure 3). The number of counts collected depends upon the system's sensitivity, that is, the number of counts detected per unit amount of radioactivity in the field of view. Sensitivity is determined by design features of the scanner, such as the nature of the scintillation crystals and their geometrical arrangement in the gantry. Administering more radioactivity to the subject will, of course, increase image counts. This approach is limited, however, not only by considerations of radiation safety, but also by the limitations of the tomograph to measure radioactivity accurately at high count rates. This count rate limitation results from system deadtime losses, and also from increasing image noise due to random coincidence counts.

Deadtime loss refers to the decreasing ability of the scanner to register counts as the count rate increases, because of the time required to handle each count. The main source of deadtime is the electronic circuitry used to process information from the detectors. The count loss due to deadtime can be predicted for a given count rate, and a correction factor applied to the data to compensate for the underestimation of counts. Beyond a certain count rate, however, this correction may break down. Deadtime correction, no matter how accurate, does not compensate for the loss in statistical accuracy that occurs because fewer counts were actually collected.

Another limitation to high count rate performance is the occurrence of random coincidences. These occur when two photons from two *different* positron annihilations are sensed by a detector pair within the coincidence resolving time (Figure 1B). Thus, a false coincidence line will be generated and a false or random count collected. The number of such counts is proportional to the coincidence resolving time of the scanner and to the square of the amount of radioactivity in the scanner field of view. The coincidence resolving time for a given scanner depends upon the design of its detectors and electronic circuits. Because random coincidences increase with the square of the radioactivity, but true coincidences increase only linearly, the fraction of total coincidences recorded that are randoms increases linearly with the radioactivity. Random coincidences add noisy background to the image. Although corrections can be made to subtract this background, the contribution to the image noise persists.[22] Thus, for any given tomograph, the amount of radioactivity administered must be carefully selected to balance the competing effects of the improvement in counting statistics with the "diminishing returns" due to deadtime and random coincidences.

Another source of background noise in the image is scatter. Scatter occurs when an annihilation photon traveling in tissue is deflected by an electron, so that its direction changes. This results in incorrect positioning of the coincidence line (Figure 1C). The effect is to add a background of counts over the image. This leads to an overestimation of radioactivity in the image, especially in those areas containing less radioactivity. This can be important when measuring neuroreceptor binding with PET, if the radioactivity in brain regions devoid of receptor is used to measure the degree of nonspecific binding of tracer in tissue.[23] Because the radioactivity in tissue due to nonspecific binding is small, scatter can result in substantial overestimation of nonspecific binding. Although methods exist to correct for scatter, they vary in their complexity and effectiveness.[19,24]

Spatial resolution has a critical role in determining the accuracy of radioactivity measurements made with PET. The resolution of a scanner can be measured by imaging a narrow line source of positron-emitting radioactivity (Figure 4). Because of the limited resolution of PET, the dot-like image that would be expected appears blurred or spread out. The resulting distribution, the line-spread function, approximates a Gaussian or bell-shaped curve. The width of the line spread function at one half of its maximum amplitude (the full width at half maximum, or FWHM) is a parameter used to quantify scanner resolution. One interpretation of resolution is that it is the distance that two small points of radioactivity must be separated so that they are perceived separately in the reconstructed image.

7

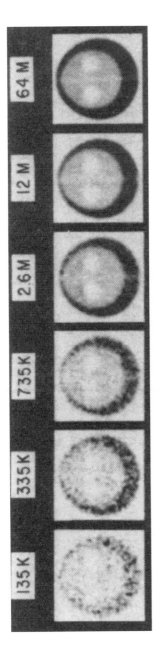

FIGURE 3. Effect of varying counts on image noise. The images are of a cylindrical container or phantom with chambers holding different radiotracer concentrations. With increasing counts (towards the right), the noise in the image decreases. (From Phelps, M. E., *IEEE Trans. Nucl. Sci.*, NS-26, 2746, 1979. With permission.)

PETT

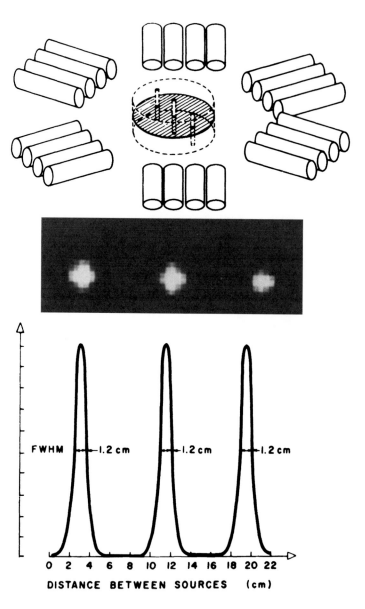

FIGURE 4.   Definition and measurement of the resolution of a PET scanner. Images are obtained by scanning line sources of positron-emitting radioactivity (upper panel). Rather than appearing in the reconstructed image as points, the radioactivity in each source appears spread over a larger area because of limited image resolution (middle panel). Resolution is defined in terms of the amount of spreading that occurs. A plot of the image intensity (lower panel) shows that this spreading takes the form of a Gaussian-like curve, called the spread line function. The width of the line spread function at one half of its maximum amplitude (termed the full width at half maximum, FWHM) is used to quantify scanner resolution. Here the resolution is 1.2 cm (From Ter-Pogossian, M. M. et al., *Radiology* 114, 89, 1975. With permission.)

Factors that limit resolution include the physics of the positron annihilation process and the design of the detectors. The annihilation photons detected by the tomograph do not originate in the radioactive nucleus, the location of which one wishes to measure. Rather they are produced only after the positron has traveled an unknown distance from the nucleus. The average range the positron travels before annihilation depends on its energy and varies with the specific radionuclide involved (e.g., 1.1 mm for ^{11}C, 2.5 mm for ^{15}O).[25] This limits the accuracy with which the location of the radionuclide can be determined. A second physical factor limiting resolution is the noncolinearity of the annihilation photons. Because of residual kinetic energy of the positron at the time of annihilation, the angle between the two photons deviates slightly from 180° resulting in a slight misplacement of the coincidence line with respect to the site of the annihilation. The combined effect of positron range and noncolinearity results in a loss of resolution of about 1 to 3 mm.[26] It is the design of the tomograph, however, that limits the resolution of current PET systems. The size and shape of the radiation detectors determine how accurately the positions of the coincidence lines are recorded, with smaller crystals providing better resolution. The resolution of currently available tomographs is approximately 5 to 6 mm, although a single-ring tomograph with a resolution of 3 mm has been constructed.[27]

The effect of limited resolution is visually apparent as a blurring of the PET image (Figure 5). More important is its effect on the accuracy of measurements of regional radioactivity.[28,29] The radioactivity in a brain region appears blurred, i.e., spread out over a larger area. The worse the resolution, the greater this effect. Thus, in the reconstructed image, a brain region contains only a portion of the radioactivity that was in the corresponding brain structure. In addition, some of the radioactivity in surrounding brain regions appears to be spread into the region of interest. As a result of this effect, called partial volume averaging, a regional measurement will contain a contribution from the radioactivity in the structure of interest, as well as from surrounding structures. In an area of high radioactivity surrounded by low levels of radioactivity, the radioactivity measurement will be underestimated, while in a low-radioactivity area surrounded by high activity, it will be overestimated. These errors are less when the size of the region or structure of interest is large with respect to the scanner resolution. In a circular structure that is 2 × FWHM in diameter and in which the radioactivity concentration is uniform, the radioactivity will be accurately represented in its center. However, statistical considerations limit obtaining a radioactivity measurement from such a small region of interest. Also, the radioactivity in some relatively large structures, such as the thalamus, may not be uniform because of local physiological differences within the structure. In general, it is not possible to obtain measurements that reflect pure gray matter radioactivity, especially in cortical regions. In addition, because of partial volume averaging, PET measurements will frequently include contributions from metabolically inactive cerebrospinal fluid in sulci or ventricles. This will lead to an underestimation of radioactivity, and therefore of tissue blood flow and metabolism.[30]

Axial resolution is also an important scanner design feature because partial volume averaging also occurs in the axial direction.[31] Axial resolution is measured perpendicular to the tomographic plane. It is determined primarily by the thickness of the detectors in the axial direction. The trend in current tomographs is towards a smaller detector axial thickness, so that axial and transverse resolutions are approximately equivalent.[20]

In summary, a variety of features characterize the performance of a PET scanner. These include sensitivity, axial and transverse resolution, and accuracy of corrections for attenuation, random counts, deadtime, and scatter. All of these factors affect the ability to perform accurate measurements of regional radioactivity. Formal procedures have been devised to test each of these factors in a quantitative fashion.[32] These tests should be performed when a scanner is accepted from the manufacturer to determine the limits of operation of the device and repeated at regular intervals to verify that the scanner continues to operate within these specifications.

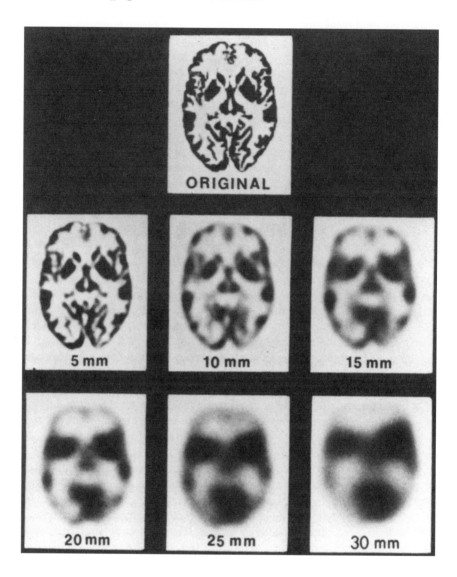

FIGURE 5.   Simulation of the effect of scanner resolution on image quality. At the upper center is an original brain image. Subsequent images simulate the effect of scanning this image with tomographs of varying resolution, from 5 to 30 mm FWHM. Note the apparent spreading or redistribution of radioactivity in the reconstructed images. This effect increases as the scanner resolution worsens (From Mazziotta, J. L. et al., *J. Comput. Assist. Tomogr.* 5, 734, 1981. With permission.)

III. RADIOTRACERS FOR PET

The second requirement for PET is a radiotracer of physiologic importance that has been labeled with a positron-emitting radionuclide. A radiotracer can be a naturally occurring compound in which one of the atoms is replaced with a radionuclide or a labeled analog that has behavior similar to the natural substance. Alternatively, it can be a synthetic substance, such as a radiolabeled drug, which interacts with a specific biologic system. A key requirement is that it should be possible to use the tracer effectively without affecting the physiologic process that is being studied. A wide variety of radiotracers has been synthesized for use with PET. These permit not only the measurement of CBF and the metabolic rate

TABLE 1
Positron-Emitting Nuclides and Representative Radiotracers

Nuclide[a]	Half-life (min)	Radiotracer	Application
Rubidium-82 (^{82}Rb)	1.25	^{82}RbCl	Blood-brain barrier permeability
Oxygen-15 (^{15}O)	2.05	$C^{15}O$	Cerebral blood volume
		$^{15}O_2$	Cerebral oxygen metabolism
		$H_2^{15}O$	Cerebral blood flow
		$C^{15}O_2$	Cerebral blood flow
Nitrogen-13 (^{13}N)	10.0	^{13}N-BCNU	Tissue and tumor drug levels
		^{13}N amino acids	Amino acid transport
Carbon-11 (^{11}C)	20.4	^{11}CO	Cerebral blood volume
		^{11}C-butanol	Cerebral blood flow
		$^{11}CO_2$	Tissue pH
		^{11}C-deoxyglucose	Cerebral glucose metabolism
		^{11}C-3-O-methylglucose	Glucose transport
		^{11}C-N-methylspiperone	Dopamine receptor ligand
		^{11}C-raclopride	Dopamine receptor ligand
		^{11}C-nomifensine	Presynaptic dopamine uptake sites
		^{11}C-carfentanil	Opiate receptor ligand
		^{11}C-deprenyl	Monomine oxidase distribution
Gallium-68 (^{68}Ga)	68.1	^{68}Ga-EDTA	Blood-brain barrier permeability
Fluorine-18 (^{18}F)	110	^{18}F-fluorodeoxyglucose	Cerebral glucose metabolism
		^{18}F-fluoromethane	Cerebral blood flow
		^{18}F-spiperone	Dopamine receptor ligand
		^{18}F-fluoro-dopa	Presynaptic dopaminergic function
		^{18}F-cyclofoxy	Opiate receptor ligand
		^{18}F-fluoroestradiol	Estrogen receptor ligand
		^{18}F-setoperone	Serotonin S_2 receptor ligand

[a] The standard abbreviation for the radionuclide listed is shown in parentheses.

of glucose and oxygen, but also the study of neuroreceptors, neurotransmitters, tissue pH, blood-brain barrier permeability, and drug kinetics.

In Table 1 are listed the most commonly-used positron-emitting radionuclides: ^{15}O, ^{11}C, and ^{18}F are particularly important. Radionuclide half-lives and examples of applications in specific radiotracers are also tabulated. The chemical nature of ^{15}O, ^{13}N, and ^{11}C is identical to that of the nonradioactive counterparts, which are basic constituents of living matter and most drugs. Thus, they can be incorporated into radiotracers that have the same biochemical behavior as the corresponding nonradioactive compound. Although ^{18}F and ^{68}Ga are not nuclides of biologically significant elements, they can be used to label a variety of compounds of physiologic interest. For example, ^{18}F is used as a substitute for hydrogen or hydroxyl groups to synthesize analogs with characteristics similar to those of the unsubstituted compound. Some drugs naturally contain fluorine, and therefore can be labeled with ^{18}F. The half-lives of these positron-emitting radionuclides are short, e.g., 2 min for ^{15}O, 110 min for ^{18}F. Thus, relatively large amounts of radioactivity can be administered to human subjects (e.g., 5 mCi of ^{18}F, 30 mCi of ^{11}C) to obtain tomographic images of good statistical quality, while maintaining radiation exposure within acceptable limits. Also, the short half-life of some of these nuclides, especially ^{15}O, permits repeat studies in the same subject in one experimental session, because of rapid decay of the radiotracer after each administration.

The preparation of radiotracers for PET is complicated, however, because of these short half-lives. On-site preparation of the positron-emitting radionuclides is required, usually with a cyclotron to produce ^{15}O, ^{11}C, ^{13}N, and ^{18}F.[33] The cyclotron is an instrument that accelerates ions (Figure 6). The resultant beam of high-energy particles is deflected onto a target containing stable atoms of a specific element, producing a nuclear reaction in which

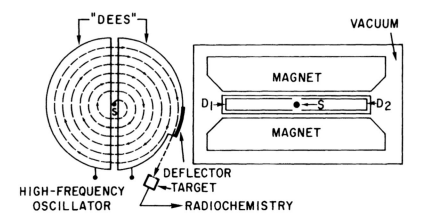

FIGURE 6.   Simplified schematic diagram of a cyclotron; top (left) and side (right) views. The ion source (S) provides the particles which are accelerated. A high-frequency oscillating source supplies the voltage to two "dees" which accelerate the ions in a vacuum chamber. The magnetic field controls the position of the ions in the dees. The deflector allows the extraction of the beam of high-energy particles, which interact in the target with stable atoms to produce positron-emitting nuclides. (From Sorenson, J. A. and Phelps, M. E., *Physics in Nuclear Medicine*, 2nd ed., Grune & Stratton, Orlando, FL, 1987. With permission.)

positron-emitting nuclides are formed. ^{11}C is formed when nitrogen is bombarded with protons, ^{18}F when neon gas is bombarded with deuterons. The targetry is often designed to produce a labeled precursor compound which is then used in the synthesis of a desired radiotracer. For example, the precursor $^{11}CO_2$ can be produced in the target box. Simple chemical reactions convert $^{11}CO_2$ to the synthetic precursor methyl iodide, which can then be used to produce ^{11}C-labeled tracers such as ^{11}C-*N*-methylspiperone, ^{11}C-*N*-6-methyl-bromocriptine, and ^{11}C-*N*-methyl-diazepam. Recent advances in cyclotron design include computer control, automated target changers, and built-in shielding ("self-shielding") to reduce the amount of shielding required to surround the cyclotron itself. In contrast to cyclotrons, generator systems are relatively simple and inexpensive. They contain a nuclide with a relatively long half-life, which decays continuously to form the nuclide of interest. Unfortunately, generator-produced nuclides for PET are rather limited, consisting in practice of ^{68}Ga and ^{82}Rb.

The synthesis of radiotracers for PET is demanding, not only because of the short half-lives of the radionuclides, but also because they must be safe for use in humans. Rapid techniques must be devised for radiochemical synthesis and purification, and for quality control. These must yield radiotracers that are sterile, nontoxic, and apyrogenic. The synthetic product must be chemically and radiochemically pure. Most or all of the positron-emitting radioactivity in the product should be attached to the radiotracer compound. The presence of other labeled products that behave differently from the desired product would confound the use of the corresponding tracer kinetic model. A critical issue in the synthesis of radiotracers is specific activity, i.e., the amount of radioactivity present per unit mass of compound. For ^{15}O, ^{11}C, and ^{13}N, it is not possible to remove traces of the stable element from the target material. Therefore, during the synthesis of the radiotracer, some of the compound of interest is also produced in its nonradioactive form, lowering the specific activity. This is less of a problem with ^{18}F, so that higher specific activity compounds can be produced. Radiotracers must be of high enough specific activity so that their administration will result in levels of tissue radioactivity sufficient to be measured with PET but without any concomitant physiologic or pharmacologic effects. Specific activity requirements depend upon the potential for the compound to produce such effects. Therefore, specific activity is not critical with ^{15}O-labeled water, but is important for ^{15}O- or ^{11}C-labeled carbon monoxide. It is also important for neuroreceptor ligands, for which central pharmacologic effects of the tracer must be avoided. In spite of the difficulties involved, a wide variety of positron-emitting radiopharmaceuticals has been synthesized.[34-47]

It should be emphasized that the selection and development of new PET radiotracers for human use is a complex process, especially for tracers intended to study neuroreceptors.[38] Several factors must be considered. In addition to the issues related to radiochemical synthesis noted above, the tracer must have the appropriate *in vivo* properties to permit the desired PET measurement to be made. The ability of the tracer to cross the blood-brain barrier, the formation and behavior of labeled metabolites in both blood and tissue, the ability to develop a mathematical model which describes the behavior of the tracer, and for neuroreceptor ligands, the binding characteristics must all be addressed. The requirements for neuroreceptor ligands, especially for the study of dopamine receptors with PET, are discussed in later chapters in this volume. The *in vivo* behavior of a compound can be substantially altered by what appears to be a modest change in molecular structure required by the labeling process. Rather than developing a positron-emitting tracer directly for human use, extensive preliminary studies are often undertaken. These may use tracers labeled with long-lived nuclides such as ^{3}H and ^{14}C, tissue sampling or autoradiography in animal models, and PET studies in animals with the positron-emitting radiotracer.

Although the short half-life of PET radionuclides limits the radiation exposure to subjects who are scanned, this exposure is not negligible. The radiation dosimetry is an important consideration, given the public's sensitivity to issues relating to radiation and the fact that subjects who are scanned are either normal volunteers or patients who are studied for research purposes rather than as part of their medical care.[39,40] The potential risks associated with these low levels of radiation are carcinogenesis and genetic effects in future generations.[41] Although the risk is very low and the exact magnitude controversial, it is agreed that the least amount of radiotracer necessary to perform an adequate PET study should be administered.

Methods have been developed to determine the radiation exposure from radiopharmaceuticals, including PET radiotracers.[42-43] The biodistribution kinetics of the specific radiotracer, i.e., a description of the distribution of the tracer in the body as a function of time following its administration is first determined from measurements made in a small group of human subjects,[44,45] from extrapolation of measurements obtained in animals,[46] or from calculations that are based on physiologic models of *in vivo* tracer behavior. Then, for a given radionuclide, the radiation exposure to each organ in the body is calculated. Limits on radiation exposure to subjects participating in research studies are set by various regulatory bodies, such as the U.S. Food and Drug Administration, and also by institutional human studies committees. Radiation exposures for typical PET studies, as well as for certain diagnostic procedures, are listed in Table 2.

IV. RADIOTRACER TECHNIQUES

A. GENERAL PRINCIPLES

The critical step in the application of PET is the employment of a model that describes the *in vivo* behavior of the radiotracer being used. The model is a mathematical description of the relationship over time between the amount of tracer presented to a brain region in its arterial input and the amount of radiotracer in the region. By means of a model, one can calculate the value of a specific biological variable, such as CBF, from tomographic measurements of local brain radiotracer concentration and from measurements of the radiotracer concentration in blood. The use of such models allows PET to be a quantitative physiological and biochemical technique rather than only an imaging method.

TABLE 2
Radiation Dosimetry of Commonly Used PET Radiotracers and Selected Nuclear Medicine Diagnostic Procedures

Radiotracer (method of administration)	Critical organ[a]	Administered activity (mCi)[b]	Radiation exposure (rem)[c]
PET studies			
[18]F-fluorodeoxyglucose (intravenous)[44,45]	Bladder	5	1.05 (voiding 1 h post-injection)
$C^{15}O_2$ (continuous inhalation)[47]	Lung	50	1.22
[82]Rb (intravenous)[48]	Kidney	100	1.9
[18]F-spiperone (intravenous)[46]	Bladder	4	5.2
[18]F-fluoro-dopa (intravenous)[49]	Bladder	2	5.2 (voiding 2 h post-injection)
Nuclear Medicine Procedures			
[133]Xe (inhalation, lung ventilation scan)[43]	Lung	18	2
[201]Tl (intravenous, heart scan)[43]	Kidney	3	3.5

[a]   The critical organ is that organ which receives the greatest radiation exposure following the administration radiotracer. Note that it is usually not the organ of physiologic interest in the study.
[b]   The amount of radioactivity administered for a given radiotracer may vary among investigators.
[c]   The figures listed depend upon biodistribution data and/or specific assumptions in the dosimetry calculations, and may vary among authors.

Two general approaches to modeling can be used, compartmental or distributed. Because of their relative mathematical simplicity, virtually all models used in PET are compartmental. These models assume that there are compartments in which the radiotracer concentration is uniform at any instant in time. Each compartment has uniform physiological and biochemical properties with respect to the tracer. The compartments can be physical spaces, such as the extravascular space, or biochemical entities, such as specific neuroreceptor binding sites. Rate constants describe the movement of tracer between compartments. The amount of tracer that leaves a compartment is proportional to the amount that is in the compartment; the rate constant is the constant of proportionality. It equals the fraction of the total tracer amount in the compartment that leaves per unit time and has units of inverse time. Thus, a rate constant of 0.02/min means that 2% of the tracer in the compartment leaves per minute. This basic concept can be expressed mathematically as

$$\frac{dA}{dt} = - k A \tag{1}$$

where k is the rate constant, A is the amount of tracer in the compartment, and the time-derivative equals the rate of change of A. (Note that because PET measures the amount of tracer per unit volume of tissue, model equations are often presented in terms of tracer *concentration* rather than *amount*.) There is usually more than one compartment in a tracer model, with separate rate constants for the movement of tracer in each direction between communicating compartments. The model also incorporates a term for the radiotracer input, i.e., the arterial time-activity curve. The modeling process results in a set of differential equations containing rate constants and time derivatives of radiotracer amount or concentration in each compartment. The unknowns in the model, e.g., rate constants or the size of a compartment, are calculated from PET measurements of local brain radotracer concentration and the arterial time-activity curve. Applications of these principles will be discussed in more detail in this chapter and in later chapters which deal with PET studies of neuroreceptors. More extensive treatments can be found in texts dealing with tracer kinetic methods.[50-53]

Distributed models differ from compartmental ones in that they take into account the presence of time-varying concentration gradients of radiotracer in blood and tissue. For example, radiotracer concentration can vary along the length of a capillary because of movement of tracer into and out of the capillary along its length. Although distributed models may provide a more accurate description of radiotracer behavior,[54,55] their greater mathematical complexity has limited their use in PET.

An alternative approach to analyzing tracer-kinetic data, called graphical analysis, has been used in certain circumstances.[56-58] The method assumes that one is studying a homogeneous tissue region which is perfused by blood containing a varying but known concentration of tracer. The tissue region may consist of several compartments that communicate reversibly with the blood, either directly or through intermediary compartments. In addition, there must be at least one other compartment that the tracer enters in an irreversible manner. A graph is constructed in which the ordinate is the ratio of the tissue tracer concentration at the times of measurement [A(T)] to the plasma tracer concentration [C_p(T)] at the same times, and the abscissa is the ratio of the time-integral of plasma tracer concentration to C_p(T). If the tissue studied does have unidirectional, irreversible uptake of the tracer into a compartment, then this graph will result in a curve that becomes linear, with a slope K_i that equals the influx rate constant for the irreversible uptake process. The equation for the linear part of the curve is

$$\frac{A(T)}{C_p(T)} = K_i \frac{\int_0^T C_p(t)\, dt}{C_p(T)} - B \tag{2}$$

where B is a constant. This approach has been used to determine the presence of irreversible uptake and the value of the uptake rate constant for dopamine receptor ligands such as ^{11}C-N-methylspiperone,[59] and for ^{18}F-fluorodopa, a tracer used to study presynaptic dopaminergic function.[60]

Several factors must be considered in the development and use of tracer models. The selection of the number and nature of the compartments in a model is based on an *a priori* knowledge of the structure of the system being studied. Issues that must be considered include the local delivery of tracer by arterial blood to the tissue, the transport of tracer across the blood-brain barrier, the behavior of the tracer and any of its labeled metabolites in brain, the presence of tracer in the vascular space of the brain rather than in tissue, the recirculation of any labeled metabolites from the rest of the body to the brain, and the potential for alterations in radiotracer behavior in the presence of local pathology. The issue of labeled metabolites is an important consideration, especially for many of the tracers used to study neuroreceptor systems. In general, it is preferable that no labeled metabolites be formed. If they are formed in brain, one must take into account whether they remain in the tissue. The contribution of labeled metabolites in blood to the arterial time-activity curve must be determined. If labeled metabolites in blood can cross the blood-brain barrier, the modeling process may be substantially complicated, as one must account for their behavior in tissue as well as the behavior of the original radiotracer. With PET, one measures the total amount of radioactivity in a brain region. The measurement does not distinguish among the various compartments in which the tracer may be resident, e.g., intravascular vs. extravascular, or receptor-bound vs. free. In addition, there is no distinction between the radiotracer and any of its radioactive metabolites which may be present. The tracer model must also incorporate corrections for physical decay of the radiotracer,[61] since the half-lives of the radionuclides used are comparable to the duration of the study. This differs from tissue autoradiographic measurements of CBF and metabolism in laboratory animals that use long-lived isotopes such as [14]C. Finally, in all PET tracer models, it is assumed that a physiologic steady-state exists with respect to the variable being measured. This is an important consideration when designing and using models to measure variables which can change very rapidly, such as CBF.

The number of unknown variables in the model cannot be so large that it is impossible to solve the model accurately from the scan data. In some cases, there is a single unknown that can be expressed in terms of measurable or known terms, so that its calculation is straightforward. Often, though, there are many unknowns, and parameter estimation techniques must be used to determine their values. This is done by means of numerical search procedures, in which the values of the unknown parameters are adjusted in a stepwise manner until the response predicted by the model best fits the measured scan data. Simplifying assumptions may be required in the process of model development to limit the number of compartments and thus the number of unknown variables. The accuracy with which a physiologic variable can be estimated depends upon the statistical accuracy of the PET image, i.e., the number of counts. Factors which limit the number of counts that can be collected include the radiation exposure to the subject, the count rate at which the tomograph can operate accurately, the amount of radiotracer that enters brain tissue, and the time available for data collection. This time depends upon the physical half-life of the tracer, the requirement for a physiologic steady-state during the scan period, and patient comfort and cooperation.

Two important components of the modeling process are error analysis and model validation. Error analysis consists of mathematical simulations of the performance of the model. A variety of potential sources of error in the calculated parameters can be examined. These include the effects of deviations from model assumptions such as uniformity of a compartment, and the effects of local pathology which may invalidate certain model assumptions. In addition, the effects of errors or statistical uncertainties in the measurement of tissue radioactivity and arterial time-activity curves can be examined. Several approaches can be used to validate a model and demonstrate that it provides correct measurements. A preliminary step is to examine the ability of the model to fit the experimental data, i.e., when model parameters are estimated and inserted into the model, they should predict the observed tissue radioactivity measurements. Specific experiments designed to validate the model can also be performed. With indirect validation, the experimental environment is manipulated and one determines whether the measured parameters vary in the manner expected. For example, the ability of a CBF measurement technique to follow changes in flow produced by alterations in arterial pCO_2 can be studied. Direct validation experiments consist of comparing the measured parameter to the same physiologic variable determined in an independent fashion. For example, one can compare a method to measure blood flow with PET to measurements made in the same animals with radiolabeled microspheres and tissue sampling.

Tracer kinetic models have been developed to perform a wide variety of measurements with PET. To date most studies of movement disorders and other neurologic diseases with PET have used methods to measure cerebral blood volume, blood flow, and metabolism of glucose and oxygen. These techniques will be described below. PET methods used to study pre- and postsynaptic dopaminergic function will be discussed in later chapters.

B. CEREBRAL BLOOD VOLUME

The measurement of regional cerebral blood volume (rCBV), one of the earliest PET techniques to be implemented, is relatively simple. Carbon monoxide, labeled with either

[11]C[63,64] or ^{15}O,[65,66] is administered in trace amounts by inhalation. The labeled carbon monoxide binds avidly to hemoglobin in red blood cells, and is thus confined to the intra-vascular space. The local radioactivity recorded from brain is directly proportional to the local red cell volume. Therefor, rCBV can be calculated from the ratio of the radioactivity concentration in brain to that in peripheral whole blood. Due to the behavior of blood in the microvasculature of the brain, however, the concentration of red cells in blood, i.e., the hematocrit, is less in brain than in peripheral large vessels. To correct for this difference, in the calculation of rCBV a parameter (R) is incorporated which equals the ratio of the cerebral hematocrit to peripheral, large vessel hematocrit.

After inhalation of labeled CO, scanning is begun when labeled carboxyhemoglobin has equilibrated throughout the blood pool of the body, which takes approximately 2 min.[66] rCBV, in units of milliliters of blood per 100 g of brain, is calculated from the tissue radiotracer concentration C_t (counts/sec-g) and the average blood radiotracer concentration C_{bl} (counts/sec-ml) as follows:

$$rCBV = \frac{C_t \cdot 100}{C_{bl} \cdot R} \qquad (3)*$$

A representative image of rCBV is shown in Figure 7a. A value of 0.85 has been used for R, based on an average of values obtained in both animal and human studies.[63,64] Recent tomographic studies in which cerebral hematocrit was calculated from measurements of both plasma volume and red cell volume indicate, however, that the routine use of this single value may be incorrect. This ratio was found to be 0.69,[67] and to vary in different phys-iological conditions, such as during carbon dioxide inhalation.[68]

Although the same tracer model applies to both [11]CO and C[15]O, the use of [15]O has certain practical advantages. First, the shorter half-live of [15]O results in rapid decay of the radioactive background following the rCBV measurement, so that other PET determinations, some of which may require the use of longer-lived nuclides, such as ^{11}C or ^{18}F, can be made. Second, the use of [15]O results in lower radiation exposure to the subject.[69] Finally, the rCBV determination is often made in conjunction with measurements of cerebral blood flow and oxygen metabolism that use [15]O. The utilization of [15]O for the rCBV measurement as well avoids changing the cyclotron targetry that is used for radionuclide production during the study. [11]CO may be preferable, however, when a tomograph with few slices is used. Multiple tomographic images covering the whole brain can be obtained sequentially following single administration of the longer-lived tracer by repositioning the subject in the axial direction within the tomograph. In addition, in order to collect sufficient counts with C[15]O during the relatively short time period available, a relatively large amount of radiotracer must be initially administered. If the tomograph is unable to handle the resulting high count rates, [11]CO would be the preferable tracer.

The measurement of rCBV is of physiologic interest since it may reflect local vasodilation of the cerebral vasculature in response to decreased perfusion pressure, for example distal to a narrowed internal carotid artery.[70] In addition, determination of rCBV is often an important component of other PET measurements. rCBV data may be required to correct measurements of local radiotracer concentration for radiotracer located in the intravascular

---

* Note that PET measurements of tissue radioactivity are made per unit volume of tissue, i.e., counts/sec-ml. However, by convention, units of cerebral blood volume, blood flow, and metabolism are usually quoted per 100 g of tissue. Therefore, it is necessary to divide measured tissue radioactivity concentration by the density of brain, 1.05 g/ml. For simplicity, this will not be shown explicitly in the tracer equations in this chapter. In addition, appropriate corrections must be made for the physical decay of both blood and tissue radioactivity that occurs during the course of a PET study.[61] Again for clarity, these will not be shown in the tracer equations presented.

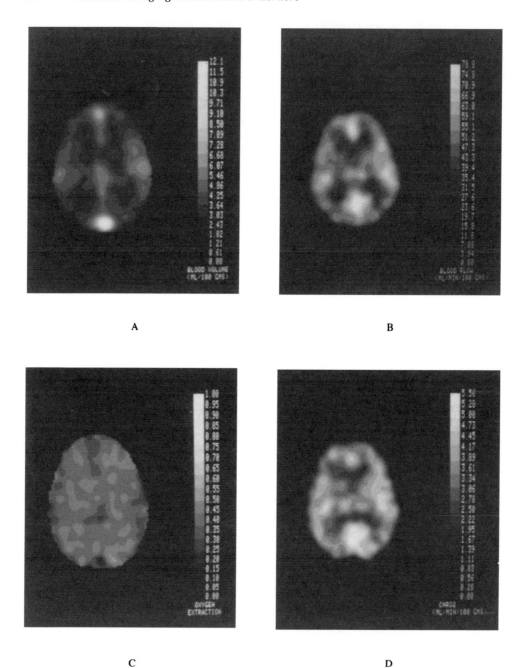

FIGURE 7. Quantitative PET images obtained with ^{15}O-labeled tracers and the PETT VI tomograph in a normal human subject. These are horizontal slices at the level of the thalamus, oriented such that anterior is up and left is to the reader's left. (A) Cerebral blood volume measured following C^{15}O inhalation. The superior sagittal sinus is seen anteriorly and posteriorly, and differences in vascular density between gray and white matter are delineated. (B) Image of rCBF obtained following bolus intravenous injection of H$_2$^{15}O. (C) Image of cerebral oxygen extraction fraction calculated from scan data obtained following the brief inhalation of ^{15}O$_2$. The image is relatively uniform throughout the brain because oxygen metabolism and blood flow are matched throughout the brain in the resting state. (D) Image of the cerebral metabolic rate for oxygen.

space of the brain, so as to determine the amount of radiotracer that actually enters brain tissue (see below).

C. CEREBRAL BLOOD FLOW

1. Background

Methods for measuring rCBF with PET are based upon a model developed by Kety and colleagues. It describes the *in vivo* behavior of inert tracers that can diffuse freely between blood and tissue.[71-74] The tracer is introduced into the circulation by intravenous injection. Subsequently, the rate of change of tracer concentration in a tissue region is equal to the difference in the rate at which the tracer is transported to the tissue in arterial blood and the rate at which it is washed out from the tissue in its venous drainage. This concept, known as the Fick principle, can be expressed mathematically as

$$\frac{dC_t}{dt} = fC_a - fC_v \tag{4}$$

where f is the tissue blood flow (ml/min-g), C_t is the tissue radiotracer concentration (cps/g), and C_a and C_v are the respective tracer concentrations (cps/ml) in the arterial input and venous drainage. Since C_v cannot be measured on a regional basis, Kety[71,72] introduced the substitution $C_v = C_t/\lambda$, where λ is the brain-blood partition coefficient for the tracer. It is defined as the ratio between the tissue and blood radiotracer concentrations at equilibrium. λ can be determined from independent experiments based on this definition, or it can be calculated as the ratio of the solubilities of the tracer in brain and blood.[71,72,75] When there is no limitation to diffusion of the tracer across the blood-brain barrier, venous radiotracer remains in equilibrium with radiotracer in tissue, so that C_v in Equation 4 can be replaced by C_t/λ:

$$\frac{dC_t}{dt} = f(C_a - C_t/\lambda) \tag{5}$$

This equation, originally developed to measure rCBF in laboratory animals with tissue autoradiography, is the basis for tracer models used to measure rCBF with PET.

^{15}O-labeled water ($H_2^{15}O$) is a commonly employed tracer for measuring rCBF with PET. It has several useful characteristics for this application. Water is a biologically inert, chemically stable compound that occurs naturally in the body and has no undesirable physiologic or pharmacologic effects. $H_2^{15}O$ is easily synthesized in large quantities.[76] Because of the short half-life of ^{15}O, relatively large amounts of radioactivity can be administered to obtain satisfactory PET images over brief time periods with an acceptable radiation exposure to the subject. In addition, rapid decay of the radioactive background permits other PET measurements to be performed with little delay.

2. Steady-State Method

The most widely used method for measuring rCBF with PET is the steady-state inhalation technique.[12,77,78] rCBF is measured during the continuous inhalation of trace amounts of $C^{15}O_2$. The catalytic action of carbonic anhydrase in red blood cells in the pulmonary vasculature results in rapid transfer of the ^{15}O label to water. Therefore, $H_2^{15}O$ is constantly generated in the lungs and circulates throughout the body. After approximately 10 min of inhalation, a steady-state is reached in which the amount of radioactivity delivered to a brain region in its arterial input equals that leaving the region by the combined processes of radioactive decay and washout into the venous circulation. The distribution of radioactivity in the brain remains constant, and because the rate of change of regional radioactivity is zero, Equation 5 may be reformulated as:

$$\frac{dC_t}{dt} = f(C_a - C_t/\lambda) - \alpha\, C_t = 0 \tag{6}$$

where α is the decay constant of ^{15}O, i.e., ln 2/half-life of ^{15}O. The value of λ, 0.91 ml/ g, is calculated from the ratio of the water contents of brain and blood, which is equivalent to ratio of the solubility of $H_2{}^{15}O$ in brain and in blood.[75] Solving Equation 6 for flow gives:

$$f = \frac{\alpha}{C_a/C_t - 1/\lambda} \tag{7}$$

C_a is determined by sampling arterial blood and C_t is measured with PET. The steady-state method is applicable with all tomographs, but is particularly suited to those that operate accurately only at a low count rate. The rate of delivery of radiotracer can be adjusted to suit the count rate capability of the tomograph and scan data sufficient to reconstruct the image can be accumulated over several minutes of $C^{15}O_2$ inhalation. The method was especially convenient for use with the early, single-ring tomographs, since multiple tomographic slices could be obtained by repositioning the patient during a prolonged period of tracer inhalation. Only a few samples of arterial blood are required, and the timing of these samples is not critical. rCBF measured with this technique in experimental animals changed appropriately in response to variations in arterial pCO_2,[79,80] and in a baboon, measured rCBF was similar to that obtained in the same animal with a reference microsphere technique.[81]

The advantages and limitations of steady-state rCBF method have been extensively analyzed.[47,82-86] Most of its limitations arise from the nonlinear relationship between rCBF and measured tissue radiotracer concentration (Equation 7 and Figure 8). At higher flow levels, a large change in rCBF produces a relatively smaller change in brain ^{15}O concentration. Thus, errors in measurement of tissue radioactivity produce proportionately larger errors in flow measurement. Calculated flow values are also sensitive to errors in the measurement of C_a and to any difference between the value of λ used in Equation 7 and its true value, which may vary in pathological conditions due to changes in brain water content.[75] Another limitation resulting from the nonlinearity of the model relates to its behavior in heterogeneous tissue regions (Figure 8). With this technique, as well as with all other PET tracer methods, it is assumed that the region-of-interest in which the measurement is made is uniform. However, because of the limited spatial resolution of PET, a region will receive tissue count contributions from both gray and white matter.[29] Due to the nonlinear nature of Equation 7, the flow measured in a heterogeneous region underestimates the true weighted regional flow by up to 20%. Deviation from the steady-state requirement of constant arterial radiotracer concentration, caused either by fluctuation in cyclotron delivery of $C^{15}O_2$, or by variation in the patient's respiratory pattern, has been a matter of concern.[87-89] It has been demonstrated, however, that the effect of such variations can be minimized if the average tracer concentration from multiple arterial samples is used.

Jones and colleagues[90] modified the steady-state method by using continuous intravenous administration of $H_2{}^{15}O$. The advantages of this approach include lower radiation dose to the lungs and trachea, reduced radioactivity in the nasopharynx (which decreases random coincidence counts), and ease of tracer administration in patients unable to maintain a regular respiratory rate. The operational equation was also modified so that scanning can begin at the onset of radiotracer administration, before equilibrium is reached. Thus, more counts are collected with the same radiation dose. This method also produces a more linear relationship between brain radiotracer concentration and flow.

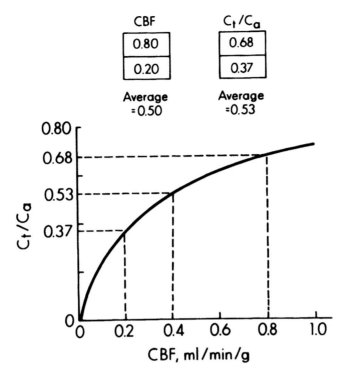

FIGURE 8.   Effect of nonlinearity of the steady state operational equation on the accuracy of rCBF calculation in a heterogeneous tissue region. The relationship between local CBF and tissue radioactivity concentration C_t (expressed as a fraction of arterial concentration C_a) is illustrated. Because this relationship is nonlinear, CBF in a heterogeneous ROI is underestimated. Consider a region of interest (upper left) in which 50% of tissue has a flow of 80 ml/min-100 g and 50% has a flow of 20m/min-100 g, so that the average flow is 50 ml/min-100 g. Radioactivity concentrations corresponding to these flows are 0.68 and 0.37, respectively. The average radioactivity concentration is 0.53, which corresponds to a flow of 40 ml/min-100 g, substantially lower than the true average flow. (From Herscovitch, P. and Raichle, M. E., *J. Cereb. Blood Flow Metab.*, 3, 407, 1983. With permission.)

3. PET/Autoradiographic Method

An alternative approach to measuring rCBF with $H_2^{15}O$ is the adaptation to PET[91-93] of Kety's tissue autoradiographic method[72-74] for measuring rCBF in laboratory animals. With Kety's technique, a biologically inert, freely diffusible radiotracer is infused for a brief time period T, and the animal is then decapitated. The behavior of the radiotracer is described by Equation 5, which can be integrated and rearranged to give

$$C_t(T) = f \int_0^T C_a(t) \exp[-f/\lambda(T-t)] \, dt$$

$$= f \, C_a(t) * \exp(-ft/\lambda) \tag{8}$$

where * denotes the mathematical operation of convolution. Equation 8 indicates that at any time T following onset of tracer administration, the local brain radiotracer concentration $C_t(T)$ depends upon the blood flow f, the arterial time-activity curve $C_a(t)$, and the partition coefficient λ, which is a measure of the relative solubility of the tracer in brain and blood.

This equation is solved for flow, using $C_t(T)$ as measured by quantitative tissue autoradiography, and $C_a(t)$, which is obtained by frequent blood sampling. The method cannot be used in this form in PET, however, because tomographs cannot measure the instantaneous brain radiotracer concentration $C_t(T)$ due to their limited temporal resolution. Therefore, the tissue autoradiographic equation (Equation 6) was modified[91,92] for PET by an integration of the instantaneous count rate, $C_t(T)$, over the scan time, T_1 to T_2, to correspond to the summing process of tomographic data collection:

$$C = \int_{T_1}^{T_2} C_t(T) \, dT$$

$$= f \int_{T_1}^{T_2} C_a(t) * \exp(-ft/\lambda) \, dT \qquad (9)$$

where C is the local number of counts per unit weight of tissue recorded by the tomograph. To implement this approach,[91] $H_2{}^{15}O$ is administered by bolus intravenous injection, and a 40-sec scan is obtained following arrival of radiotracer in the head (Figure 7b). Blood is sampled every 4 to 5 sec via an indwelling arterial catheter. Once a value for λ is specified,[75] Equation 9 can be solved numerically for flow. rCBF measurements with this technique have been validated in the baboon by direct comparison to flow measured in the same animals by intracarotid injection of radiotracer and external residue detection.[92] In order to obtain statistically adequate images, a relatively large amount of radioactivity must be administered and the scanner must be able to operate accurately at the resulting high count rates. In addition, a multislice scanner is preferable, so that a large portion of the brain can be imaged following a single radiotracer injection.

The relationship between tissue counts, C, and rCBF for the PET-autoradiographic approach is almost linear. This has several advantageous consequences.[91] Errors in measurement of tissue radioactivity result in approximately equivalent errors in rCBF. There is no amplification of error at high flows, as occurs with the steady-state technique. The method works well in the unavoidable situation of tissue heterogeneity; in a mixed gray matter—white matter brain region, the measured flow is approximately equal to the true weighted flow. In addition, inaccuracy in the value of λ used in Equation 8 results in minimal error in flow. The tomographic image of tissue counts closely reflects relative differences in flow in different brain regions. Thus, in functional mapping studies of the brain, in which local CBF responses to neurobehavioral tasks are examined, relative changes in rCBF can be determined from the images alone and arterial sampling to provide absolute flow measurements is not required.[91,94-96] A relative disadvantage of the technique is the need for frequent, accurately timed, arterial blood samples. The peripheral arterial time-activity curve is assumed to be equal to the arterial input to the brain. If this is not true, inaccuracy will occur in the calculation of rCBF. In fact, the bolus of radioactivity arrives at the radial artery sampling site several seconds later than in the brain, because the distance between heart and artery is greater than that between heart and brain. This time difference can be measured and the arterial curve appropriately shifted in time.[92,97] In addition, dispersion or smearing of the arterial curve occurs while the tracer bolus traverses the arterial system.[98] Because of the difference in the distance traveled to brain and to radial artery, somewhat more dispersion may occur in the sampled arterial curve.

Recently, automated blood withdrawal and counting systems have been developed.[98-100] These make it possible to obtain a more finely sampled blood curve, and also have the advantage of reducing radiation exposure to investigators that occurs during blood sampling.

4. Other Methods for Measuring rCBF

Several other approaches have been described to measure rCBF. These methods are also derived from the Kety model described above.

Huang and colleagues have described a technique which uses $H_2^{15}O$.[101,102] Following bolus intravenous administration of $H_2^{15}O$, scan data are collected over a 10-min period, and arterial sampling is performed. Two image sets are reconstructed, using decay-corrected and non-decay-corrected scan data, respectively. The operational equations for this method, derived from the basic Kety formulation, permit the estimation of both rCBF and λ for $H_2^{15}O$. The values for λ obtained in humans by this method were about 15% lower than would be expected based on the known water content of brain. A potential explanation for this discrepancy is that not all water in cerebral tissue is freely exchangeable with water in blood. Further studies are required to clarify this issue. Simulation studies of this approach have shown that the error in rCBF measurement in heterogeneous tissue is quite small, and that propagation of error in tissue count measurement is not excessive.

Alpert[103] and Carson[104] have described variations of this technique of using scan data in two different forms. Their approaches both involve multiplying the terms in the basic Kety equation (Equation 3 or 6) by two different, time-dependent weighting functions. The resultant two equations are then solved for both rCBF and λ. The mathematical form of the weighting functions can be selected to minimize the effect of statistical noise in the tomographic measurements on the flow calculation.[104] Another approach involves collecting scan data in the form of sequential, brief frames after bolus intravenous administration of tracer.[105] Equation 7 is used to describe the relationship between local tissue counts and flow for each of these images. Parameter estimation techniques are used to calculate both rCBF and λ from scan data and measurements of arterial radioactivity. These methods that use bolus intravenous administration of radiotracer all require accurately timed arterial blood samples and shifting of the arterial blood curve to account for differences in arrival time of tracer between brain and arterial sampling site.

In all of these methods, it is assumed that the tracer is freely diffusible across the blood-brain barrier, so that for any specific arterial time-activity curve, the amount of tracer entering tissue depends only upon the local flow. However, $H_2^{15}O$ does not exhibit this ideal behavior. At higher flow levels, there is a progressive decline in the extraction of $H_2^{15}O$ from blood by brain.[106] This results in less tracer entering tissue than would be predicted and leads to an underestimation of rCBF. This has been experimentally demonstrated in baboons with the PET-autoradiographic method[92] and would be expected to occur with the other methods using $H_2^{15}O$ as well.[83] A recent study[107] using the PET-autoradiographic method has compared flow measurements obtained in the same subjects using both $H_2^{15}O$ and ^{11}C-butanol, a flow tracer that is not diffusion limited. In comparison to ^{11}C-butanol, $H_2^{15}O$ was found to underestimate rCBF by approximately 15%, presumably because of its diffusion limitation. Although ^{11}C-butanol provides more accurate estimates of rCBF, its relatively long half-life and more complex synthesis make it a much less convenient flow tracer to use. This is especially so when the experimental protocol requires multiple measurements of rCBF or measurement of regional oxygen metabolism as well.

Another radiopharmaceutical that has been used to measure rCBF is ^{18}F-labeled fluoromethane, an inert gas administered by inhalation.[108] Scan data are collected in the form of sequential 1-min images. rCBF and λ are calculated from scan data and measurements of arterial radioactivity using parameter estimation techniques. Koeppe and colleagues[109] described a modification of this technique that uses measurements of radioactivity in expired air and venous blood to replace measurement of the arterial time-activity curve. This approach is limited, however, because it does not permit other PET measurements that require arterial sampling to be made in conjunction with the flow determination. Preliminary data obtained in isolated dog brain indicate that fluoromethane is freely diffusible at average whole brain flows of up to 70 ml/ (min-100 g).[108] More recently, fluoromethane has been labeled with

[11]C rather than [18]F.[110] Using ^{11}C rather than ^{18}F may be more convenient if it is difficult to produce the large amounts of ^{18}F that are required or if the rCBF measurements are to be combined with the use of other ^{11}C-labeled tracers. Potential disadvantages of fluoromethane as a CBF tracer include the relatively long time interval required for its clearance from the body via the lungs before another PET study can be performed (at least 30 min) and the more cumbersome inhalation mode of administration.

D. CEREBRAL OXYGEN METABOLISM
1. Background

Two methods have been developed to measure the regional cerebral metabolic rate for oxygen ($rCMRO_2$) with PET. One uses continuous inhalation of ^{15}O-labeled oxygen ([15]O_2) and was developed in conjunction with the steady-state technique for measuring rCBF.[12,78] The other, which uses a brief inhalation of [15]O_2, is a companion method to the PET-autoradiographic method.[65] The principles underlying these methods are the same. A fraction of the oxygen (approximately 0.40) that is delivered to the brain is extracted and used in the oxidative metabolism of glucose. Both methods measure this regional oxygen extraction fraction (rOEF). The rate of oxygen utilization is determined from the product of rOEF and the rate of oxygen delivery which equals rCBF multipled by arterial oxygen content.

Strategies that use [15]O_2 to measure rOEF and $rCMRO_2$ must adequately describe the fate of the [15]O label following [15]O_2 inhalation. [15]O_2 that is extracted from arterial blood into tissue is converted to ^{15}O-labeled water of metabolism, which is then washed out of the brain in the venous circulation. Labeled water of metabolism, rapidly produced by both brain and the rest of the body, recirculates to brain via its arterial input and diffuses into and out of the tissue. The tracer model must take into account the various sources from which the measured [15]O activity in brain arises: [15]O_2 in incoming arterial blood; extracted [15]O_2 that is converted to ^{15}O-water of metabolism and washed out of the brain; unextracted [15]O_2 in the capillary and venous circulation of the brain; and recirculating ^{15}O-water of metabolism that washes into and out of brain tissue. The radioactivity measured in whole blood following [15]O_2 inhalation consists of [15]O_2 bound to hemoglobin and H_2[15]O in both plasma and red cells. Separate measurements of plasma radioactivity are made to calculate the amount of radioactivity in blood due to H_2[15]O. The radioactivity in blood due to [15]O_2 in red cells can then be obtained by subtraction.

2. Steady-State Method

With the steady-state method, rCBF is determined using C[15]O_2 inhalation. Scanning is also performed during the continuous inhalation of [15]O_2. Arterial blood samples are obtained to measure the radioactivity in both whole blood and plasma. rOEF is computed from the ratio of tissue counts during the [15]O_2 and C[15]O_2 inhalations and from the measurements of blood radioactivity (Figure 9).[12,78] As originally formulated, the model did not include a term to account for intravascular [15]O_2. This led to an overestimation of both rOEF and $rCMRO_2$ because it was assumed that the total measured radioactivity in brain was only from tissue when in fact there was a contribution from the intravascular compartment as well.[83] A technique for correcting for intravascular [15]O_2 has been developed and implemented using data from a separate measurement of rCBV with labeled CO.[111-114]

The steady-state measurement of $rCMRO_2$ has the same practical features as the C[15]O_2 flow technique. It is particularly suited to tomographs requiring low count rates and to tomographs with few slices. When rOEF measurements were compared to direct measurements of the cerebral arterial-venous oxygen difference in baboons,[79] 13% overestimation of rOEF was observed, most likely because there was no correction for intravascular tracer. In indirect validation experiments, rCBF was changed by manipulating the arterial pCO_2. With increasing pCO_2, rCBF increased and rOEF decreased while $CMRO_2$ remained constant,

(a) rOEF Calculation Without Blood Volume Correction

$$r\,OEF' = \frac{\dfrac{C_O}{C_W}\dfrac{A_W}{P_O} - \dfrac{A_W}{P_W}}{\dfrac{A_O}{P_O} - \dfrac{A_W}{P_W}}$$

where

A_W, P_W, C_W = arterial blood, plasma, and tissue radioactivity concentrations, respectively, during $C^{15}O_2$ inhalation

A_O, P_O, C_O = arterial blood, plasma, and tissue radioactivity concentrations, respectively, during $^{15}O_2$ inhalation

(b) rOEF Calculation With Blood Volume Correction

$$r\,OEF = \frac{rOEF' - X}{1 - X}$$

where

$$X = \frac{rCBF/100 + \alpha}{rCBF/(R \cdot rCBV) + \alpha}$$

R = ratio of cerebral-to-large vessel hematocrit

α = decay constant of ^{15}O

(c) rCMRO$_2$ Calculation

$rCMRO_2 = rCBF \cdot rOEF \cdot$ arterial oxygen content

FIGURE 9. Calculation of regional oxygen extraction fraction (rOEF) with the steady-state method. (a) The equation for calculating rOEF from scan and blood radioactivity measurements, without a correction for intravascular $^{15}O_2$.[12,78] (b) Calculation of rOEF with a correction for intravascular $^{15}O_2$.[111-114] A correction factor X, which includes the value of the local CBV, is applied to the rOEF' calculated in (a). (c) rCMRO$_2$ is the product of rCBF, the arterial oxygen content (the product of these two factors equals the amount of oxygen delivered per minute per gram of tissue), and rOEF.

as would be expected.[80] Several error analyses of the steady-state method for measuring rOEF and CMRO$_2$ have been performed, including studies of the accuracy of the measurements in relation to tomographic counting statistics.[83,84,88,111,115,116] Tissue heterogeneity has a small effect on the accuracy of the rOEF calculation, but a large effect on CMRO$_2$ values, because it is calculated from rCBF. Instability of arterial radiotracer concentration, caused either by fluctuation in cyclotron delivery of ^{15}O-labeled gases, or by variation in the subject's respiratory pattern, results in inaccuracies in the calculation of rCMRO$_2$.[88] These inaccuracies can be decreased by the use of multiple arterial samples and by a modification of the tracer model that does not assume equilibrium.[89]

$$\text{rOEF} = \frac{C - \text{rCBF} \int_{T_1}^{T_2} C_a^{H_2^{15}O}(t) * e^{-Kt} dt - \text{rCBV} \int_{T_1}^{T_2} C_a^{15O_2}(t) dt}{\text{rCBF} \int_{T_1}^{T_2} C_a^{15O_2}(t) * e^{-Kt} dt - 0.835 \, \text{rCBV} \int_{T_1}^{T_2} C_a^{15O_2}(t) dt}$$

where $K = $ rCBF / Partition coefficient of water

$C_a^{H_2^{15}O}(t), \; C_a^{15O_2}(t) = $ arterial time-activity curves for $H_2^{15}O$, $^{15}O_2$, respectively

$$\text{rOEF} = \frac{\begin{array}{c}\text{Local tissue radioactivity}\\ \text{measured with PET}\end{array} - \begin{array}{c}\text{Correction for recirculating,}\\ \text{labelled water of metabolism}\end{array} - \begin{array}{c}\text{Correction for } ^{15}O_2\\ \text{intravascular radioactivity}\end{array}}{\begin{array}{c}\text{Theoretical local radioactivity}\\ \text{if oxygen extraction was 100\%}\end{array} - \begin{array}{c}\text{Correction for } ^{15}O_2\\ \text{intravascular radioactivity}\end{array}}$$

$\text{rCMRO}_2 = \text{rCBF} \cdot \text{rOEF} \cdot$ arterial oxygen content

FIGURE 10.   Calculation of regional oxygen extraction fraction with the brief inhalation technique.[65] The meaning of each term in the equation is given in the equation in word form. Note that the ratio of the first terms in the numerator and denominator would be equal to the rOEF, if no corrections for intravascular $^{15}O_2$ and recirculating labeled water were needed. A simplified form of this equation has been developed which facilitates the calculation of rOEF.[117]

3. Brief Inhalation Method

Mintun and colleagues[65] described an alternative method for measuring rOEF and rCMRO_2 that uses scan data obtained following brief inhalation of $^{15}O_2$. The method also involves measurement of rCBF with $H_2^{15}O$ and the PET-autoradiographic approach, and of rCBV with $C^{15}O$. A two-compartment model is used to analyze the scan data. It accounts for the production and egress of water of metabolism in the tissue, recirculating water of metabolism, and the arterial, venous, and capillary contents of $^{15}O_2$ in the brain. To implement this technique, a 40 sec emission scan is obtained following brief inhalation of $^{15}O_2$, and frequent arterial blood samples are obtained for measurements of blood radioactivity. rOEF and rCMRO_2 are calculated as indicated in Figure 10. Representative images are shown in Figures 7 c and d.

As with the PET-autoradiographic technique for measuring rCBF, this method also requires a tomograph capable of operating at high count rates. Although the equation for the calculation of rOEF from the measured data is mathematically complex (Figure 10), an accurate simplification of the equation facilitates this calculation.[117] The brief inhalation technique was validated in baboons by direct comparison of rOEF measured with PET to OEF measured by intracarotid injection of $^{15}O_2$ in the same animals.[65] Simulation studies of this method have demonstrated that measurement errors in rCBV or rCBF cause approximately equivalent percent errors in rOEF and rCMRO_2 determinations at high or normal levels of rCMRO_2, although errors are amplified at low metabolic rates. Tissue heterogeneity has a small effect on the accuracy of the rOEF and rCMRO_2 calculations.[115]

Both the steady-state and the brief inhalation methods for measuring rOEF and $rCMRO_2$ require the combination of tomographic data from three separate emission scans obtained over a 30 to 60 min period. It is assumed that during this time, there is a physiologic steady state with respect to cerebral blood flow, blood volume, and metabolism. In addition, it is important that the subject's head remains in a constant position throughout the scans so that proper registration of the three images will be maintained. For the steady-state method, only a few millimeters of head movement can result in large errors in calculated $CMRO_2$.[116] To overcome these difficulties, methods have been sought in which $CMRO_2$ can be estimated from scan data obtained following a single administration of $^{15}O_2$. Because such data contain information about not only $CMRO_2$, but also CBF and CBV, it has been hypothesized that it may be possible to estimate all three parameters from sequential scan frames collected after a single $^{15}O_2$ inhalation.[118] Experimental data show that while this may not be feasible, estimates of $CMRO_2$ alone obtained from a single scan are similar to those obtained with the three-scan, brief inhalation method.[119]

E. CEREBRAL GLUCOSE METABOLISM

1. Deoxyglucose Method

The most widely used PET technique, the ^{18}F-deoxyglucose method to measure regional cerebral glucose metabolism (rCMRGlu), is based on the deoxyglucose method developed by Sokoloff to measure rCMRGlu in laboratory animals.[120,121] Sokoloff's technique uses 2-deoxy-D-[^{14}C]glucose (DG) as the metabolic tracer and tissue autoradiography to determine local brain radioactivity. DG is an analogue of glucose and differs only by the substitution of a hydrogen atom for the hydroxyl group on the second carbon atom. It is transported bidirectionally across the blood-brain barrier by the same carrier-mediated transport system as glucose. In tissue, DG is phosphorylated, as is glucose, by hexokinase, so that ^{14}C-deoxyglucose-6-phosphate (DG-6-P) is formed. Because of its anomalous structure, however, DG-6-P is not metabolized further through the glycolytic pathway. Also, there is little dephosphorylation of DG-6-P back to DG due to the low activity of glucose-6-phosphatase in brain. As a result of this "metabolic trapping" of DG-6-P and its low membrane permeability, there is negligible loss of DG-6-P from tissue over the time course of the experiment. Because metabolized tracer is retained in brain, the calculation of rCMRGlu from measurements of local tissue radioactivity is greatly facilitated.

Sokoloff and colleagues developed a three-compartment model to describe the *in vivo* behavior of DG (Figure 11). These compartments, in part physical, in part biochemical, consist of (1) DG in plasma in brain capillaries; (2) free DG in tissue; and (3) DG-6-P in tissue. Three first-order rate constants are used to describe the movement of tracer between these compartments, k_1^* for the transport of DG from plasma to tissue across the blood-brain barrier, k_2^* for the transport of DG back from tissue to plasma, and k_3^* for the phosphorylation of DG to DG-6-P. An operational equation was developed to calculate rCMRGlu based on several assumptions: (1) the rate of local glucose utilization and the plasma glucose concentration are constant during the experiment; (2) the concentrations of glucose and DG in the capillary plasma can be represented by their arterial plasma concentrations; and (3) compartmental assumptions (described above) hold and DG is present in tracer quantities. The operational equation and its interpretation are shown in Figure 12a. It permits calculation of rCMRGlu from a single autoradiographic measurement of total tissue radiotracer concentration (i.e., DG and DG-6-P), arterial plasma concentration of DG measured as a function of time, and the plasma glucose concentration. In addition to values for the rate constants, an additional factor, the lumped constant (LC), must be specified. The LC is a multiplicative term in the operational equation that is required to correct for the fact that a glucose analog, DG, rather than glucose, is used as the tracer. The LC accounts for differences between glucose and DG in transport across the blood-brain barrier and in phosphorylation.

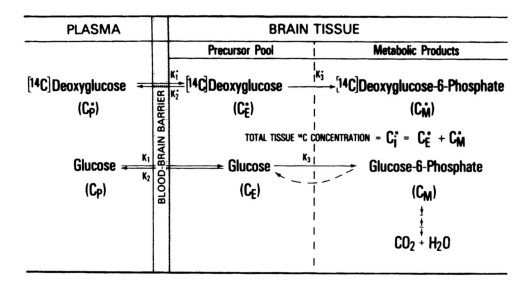

FIGURE 11.   Diagrammatic representation of Sokoloff's three-compartment model used to measure regional cerebral glucose metabolism with ^{14}C-deoxyglucose (DG). The compartments consist of DG in the plasma in brain capillaries, DG in brain tissue, and DG-6-P in tissue. The lower portion of the figure shows the metabolic fate of glucose; the upper portion, that of DG. In the adaption of this model to PET, ^{18}F-labeled DG is used. In addition, a fourth rate constant, k_4^*, is added to account for dephosphorylation of DG-6-P back to DG (From Sokoloff, L. et al., *J. Neurochem.*, 28, 897, 1977. With permission.)

   Neither the rate constants nor the LC can be determined in each experimental animal or condition. Calculation of the rate constants requires multiple autoradiographic measurements of tissue radioactivity following intravenous injection of DG. Therefore, their values were determined in a separate group of animals, by means of the equation shown in Figure 12b. The rate constant values were found to be uniform in gray matter and also in white matter. Thus, mean values for gray and white matter are used in the operational equation. Note that the rate constants can vary as a function of experimental condition, e.g., species, local pathology. In fact, the value of k_3^*, which is related to the phosphorylation rate, depends upon the local CMRGlu. A strategy was developed to minimize the error associated with the use of standard values for the rate constants, based on the observation that the terms containing them in the operational equation approach zero with increasing time. A 45-min time interval between DG injection and animal sacrifice was chosen to minimize error associated with uncertainty in the rate constants. A longer period was avoided to minimize potential loss of DG-6-P from tissue, due to the small amount of glucose-6-phosphatase activity in brain, and because of the difficulty in maintaining a physiological steady state during very long experimental periods.
   The measurement of the LC in animals on a regional basis would be very difficult. Theoretical arguments were developed, however, to demonstrate that the LC should be relatively uniform throughout the brain and constant in value under normal physiological conditions. Therefore, a method was developed to measure the LC of the whole brain. This measurement is based on the mathematical demonstration that the LC is equivalent to the ratio of the whole brain arterial-venous extraction fraction of DG to that of glucose, measured under steady-state conditions.

2. Adaptation of the DG Method to PET
   The DG method was subsequently adapted for use with PET in humans.[122-124] DG was labeled with ^{18}F to produce ^{18}F-2-fluoro-2-deoxy-D-glucose (FDG). The behavior of FDG is similar to that of DG (Figure 12). It is phosphorylated to FDG-6-P, which is metabolically

(a) Operational Equation of the Deoxyglucose Method

$$rCMRGlu = \frac{C_p}{LC} \cdot \frac{C(T) - k_1^* \exp[-(k_2^* + k_3^*)T] \int_0^T C_p^*(t) \exp[(k_2^* + k_3^*)t]\, dt}{\int_0^T C_p^*(t)\, dt - \exp[-(k_2^* + k_3^*)T] \int_0^T C_p^*(t) \exp[(k_2^* + k_3^*)t]\, dt}$$

$$= \frac{\text{plasma glucose}}{\text{lumped constant}} \cdot \frac{\text{tissue radioactivity} - \text{concentration of free DG in tissue at time T}}{\text{total amount of DG entering tissue}}$$

(b) Expression for the Total Radioactivity in Tissue at Time T

$$C(T) = k_1^* \exp[-(k_2^* + k_3^*)T] \int_0^T C_p^*(t) \exp[(k_2^* + k_3^*)t]\, dt$$

$$+ k_1^* k_3^* \int_0^T \left\{ \exp[-(k_2^* + k_3^*)\tau] \int_0^\tau C_p^*(t) \exp[(k_2^* + k_3^*)t]\, dt \right\} d\tau$$

FIGURE 12.   (a) Operational equation of the deoxyglucose (DG) method of Sokoloff used to measure the cerebral metabolic rate for glucose. The simplified form of the equation (expressed in word form) aids in understanding the model. C(T) is the local radioactivity concentration in tissue measured at time T. The concentration of free DG in tissue at time T is calculated from the plasma concentration of DG over time $[C_p^*(t)]$ and the rate constants. The difference between these two terms in the numerator equals the local concentration of DG-6-P that has been formed. The denominator essentially represents the total amount of DG delivered to tissue. Therefore, the ratio on the right-hand side of the equation represents the fractional rate of phosphorylation of DG. Multiplying this by the plasma glucose concentration (C_p) would give the rate of glucose phosphorylation if DG and glucose had the same behavior. This is not the case, and to account for this difference, an additional term, the lumped constant (LC), is included. In the adaptation of this model to PET, a fourth rate constant, k_4^*, is included to account for dephosphorylation of DG-6-P, and the resultant operational equation is more complex.[124] (b) Equation used to estimate the value of the rate constants k_1^*, k_2^*, and k_3^* from C(T) and $C_p^*(t)$. Measurements of C(T) are made at multiple time points, and a parameter estimation technique is used to determine the values of the rate constants.

trapped in the tissue. In order to obtain the PET image, it is necessary to scan beyond the 45 min that is used between tracer administration and animal sacrifice in tissue autoradiography. Dephosphorylation of FDG-6-P, although small, becomes more important. To account for this, a fourth rate constant, k_4^*, was added to the model. The four rate constants were calculated for a group of normal subjects from regional radioactivity measurements in serial PET scans obtained over several hours following FDG administration. Average gray and white matter values were computed for use in the operational equation. Originally, the value for the LC in humans was not explicitly measured. Rather, its value (0.42) was selected so that the average value for whole brain CMRGlu measured with FDG in normal subjects would equal that determined by earlier investigators with the more invasive Kety-Schmidt technique.[123]

To implement the FDG method, PET images are obtained starting about 45 min after intravenous injection of 5 to 10 mCi of tracer. Blood samples are collected from the time of injection to the end of scanning to measure the concentration of glucose and FDG in plasma as a function of time. Peripheral arterial blood is sampled through an indwelling arterial catheter or by venous sampling from a hand heated to 44°C to "arterialize" venous blood by the production of arterial-venous shunts. With multislice tomographs, the subject is often repositioned in the axial direction by a fraction of the slice thickness (e.g., one half) to further increase axial sampling. Scan duration is typically 5 to 10 min to collect sufficient counts for accurate reconstruction. Local CMRGlu is calculated from the image of tissue counts and blood measurements by means of the operational equation, and the standard values for the four rate constants and LC. Note that the tracer model assumes that carbohydrate metabolism in the brain is a steady state from the time of FDG administration to the end of scanning. Should this not be the case, for example with a seizure, the measured rCMRGlu is approximately a weighted average of the metabolic values during the experiment, with the weightings proportional to the plasma FDG concentration at the corresponding times.[125] Thus rCMRGlu during the early part of the uptake period is predominantly reflected.

The accuracy of the DG method and its extension to PET has been the subject of considerable analysis and discussion.[126] The major issue is the appropriateness of using standard values for the rate constants and LC in both normal and pathological conditions. The originators of the DG method indicated that the value of these parameters may vary in abnormal or pathological conditions.[120-122] Recent work with FDG has included studies of the impact of using incorrect rate constant values, the development of more accurate methods for measuring the rate constants and CMRGlu, and the measurement of the LC in humans on both a global and regional basis.

The mathematical form of the operational equation lessens the impact of errors in the values of the rate constants on calculated rCMRGlu when the uptake period is relatively long, i.e., 45 min or greater. In pathological conditions, however, such as ischemia when rCMRGlu deviates considerably from normal, the use of standard rate constants can result in substantial error.[125,127,128] Several investigators have suggested alternative formulations of the operational equation to decrease its sensitivity to differences between the actual and standard rate constant values.[128-131] In addition, methods used to calculate the rate constants from sequential tomographic images have been refined and applied in both normal and pathological conditions.[131-135] Note that the ability of PET to provide multiple measurements of tissue radioactivity over time in the same subject makes such determinations much easier than in tissue autoradiography where multiple animals must be sacrificed to obtain data for each time point. For accurate measurement of rate constants, it is necessary to include a term for the amount of FDG that is present in the intravascular space of the brain. This amount is initially high in relation to that present within the tissue and neglecting its contribution to measured radioactivity leads to errors in the values of the rate constants and rCMRGlu.

The value of the LC for whole brain in normal humans has been measured from determinations of steady-state arterial and internal-jugular venous concentrations of FDG and glucose.[136] The measured value, 0.52, was substantially higher than the previously calculated one of 0.42.[123] Data obtained in animal studies and more recently in humans indicate that the LC varies from its normal value in pathological states, such as hyperglycemia, ischemia, and seizures.[121,137] In acute cerebral ischemia in the cat, the LC was found to increase by a factor of up to 2.4.[138,139] Gjedde and colleagues[140] have developed a method to measure the LC regionally in humans with PET using FDG and 3-O-^{11}C-methylglucose. The latter tracer is transported bidirectionally across the blood-brain barrier, but is not metabolized. Its distribution in brain is used to calculate the local glucose content and then the value of the LC. Although the LC was found to be relatively uniform throughout normal brain, in some regions of recent cerebral infarction its value was increased three- to sixfold. Finally, the effect of aging on the LC in rats has been studied.[141] A 17% decline in its value between rats 3 and 24 months of age was observed. Since the calculated rCMRGlu is inversely proportional to the value of the LC, the use of a standard value for the LC in conditions where it may vary leads to a corresponding error in rCMRGlu calculation. Thus, in pathological conditions, it is necessary to redetermine the values of both the LC and the rate constants to avoid errors in the measurement of rCMRGlu.

Several years after the FDG technique was developed, it was observed that some of the syntheses used result in a product consisting of not only FDG, but also 5 to 50% ^{18}F-labeled deoxymannose.[136,142] This compound behaves differently *in vivo* from FDG[143] and its presence may lead to errors in the calculation of rate constants and rCMRGlu, the magnitude of which depend upon the extent of contamination. This problem highlights the importance of ensuring that radiopharmaceuticals used in PET are pure.

Reivich and colleagues[136,144] applied the DG method with PET using ^{11}C rather than ^{18}F as the positron emitter. The shorter half-life of ^{11}C results in more rapid decay of the radioactive background so that a repeat scan can be performed in the same subject approximately 2 h later. This facilitates experimental designs in which a subject is used as his or her own control, for example studies of the effects of neurobehavioral tasks on rCMRGlu. More recently, an approach to performing repeat measurements of CMRGlu involving sequential injections of FDG has been proposed.[145-147] These involve two sequential injections of FDG. Scan data used to compute rCMRGlu during the second scan period are corrected for the residual ^{18}F radioactivity remaining from the first procedure.

3. Use of ^{11}C-Glucose

An alternative approach to measuring rCMRGlu involves the use of ^{11}C-labeled glucose.[148,149] ^{11}C-glucose is transported and metabolized in the same fashion and at the same rate as natural glucose. Therefore, a correction factor such as the LC is not required to account for differences between radiotracer and glucose. A disadvantage is that the labeled metabolites of glucose, such as ^{11}CO$_2$, are not all trapped within the tissue. Thus, tracer models must account for the rapid formation and loss of labeled metabolites. A model has been used which consists of four compartments: tracer in plasma, unmetabolized tracer in tissue, ^{11}C-labeled metabolites in tissue, and ^{11}C-labeled metabolites such as ^{11}CO$_2$ that can leave the tissue and enter blood. Several brief, sequential scans are obtained to determine local tissue radioactivity as a function of time and measurements of the concentration of glucose, ^{11}C-glucose, and ^{11}C-CO$_2$ in peripheral arterial blood are made. These data are used in the differential equations of the tracer model to calculate the rate constants and rCMRGlu. The time course of production and loss ^{11}CO$_2$ depends on the position of the ^{11}C label on the glucose molecule.[150] Therefore, the use of glucose labeled in the 6 position, rather than uniformly labeled glucose, may lessen the difficulties in accounting for labeled metabolites.[148] Methods for measuring rCMRGlu with ^{11}C-glucose are at a much earlier stage of development than those using DG, but with further work it may become more widely used, especially in pathological conditions.

V. ANALYSIS AND INTERPRETATION OF PET DATA

Although in some cases visual inspection of PET images may show gross abnormalities, systematic, quantitative data analysis techniques are required to obtain scientifically useful information from a PET study. In fact, the tasks of data reduction, analysis, and interpretation are usually more complex and time consuming than the actual performance of the scan and generation of physiologic images. Some of the difficulties faced include handling large amounts of image data, correlating the regional PET measurements with neuroanatomical information, coping with the variance in PET data, identifying abnormalities or differences among various study groups, and interpreting any changes that are found.

A. IMAGE DISPLAY

After a PET study has been performed, the appropriate tracer model is used to obtain values of the corresponding physiologic variable from measurements of tissue and blood radioactivity. For methods to measure CBF and metabolism, the model is applied to the PET images on a point-by-point basis. In the resultant images, the intensity is directly proportional to the local value of the physiologic variable. A gray (or color) scale is used to indicate the physiologic values that correspond to the levels of image intensity (see Figure 7). For several tracers, the mathematical model is too complex to be applied directly to the PET image. In some cases, model simplifications or computational shortcuts can be used to generate images.[117,151] In other cases, the numerical complexity of the model may preclude its application to the entire PET image, or the statistical noise in the image may require the use of measurements of tissue radioactivity from brain regions larger than a single image pixel. This often arises with neuroreceptor compartmental models, which are solved by means of parameter estimation techniques that use tissue time-activity curves obtained from sequential PET images. Here, the model is solved only for specific brain regions in which the average local radioactivity value from each image is used.[152,153]

The quantitative images obtained from a typical PET study contain a large amount of data. For example, a study of cerebral hemodynamics and oxygen metabolism with ^{15}O-labeled tracers and a tomograph with 7 slices[70] results in a total of 28 images per patient (7 each of regional CBF, CBV, OEF, and $CMRO_2$). New scanners now available provide 15 slices simultaneously,[20] and therefore more data. Analysis of these large data sets is greatly facilitated by the use of specially designed, interactive computer programs. Both regional and global data can be obtained with such programs. Small regions of interest (ROIs) of arbitrary size and shape are placed over selected areas of the image, and the average physiologic variable computed for the region. The location of regions specified on one image, e.g., of CBF, can be stored and used with other physiologic images, e.g., of $CMRO_2$, obtained in the same subject. Two sets of images obtained in a subject under different physiological conditions can be compared, for example, at rest and during a physiologic stimulus,[154] or before and after administration of a drug.[155] This can be accomplished by subtracting the two images to obtain a third image representing the change in local flow or metabolism that occurred between the two scan states. Global measurements can be obtained by averaging over multiple contiguous PET slices[30] or by averaging multiple representative regions.[156]

B. ANATOMIC LOCALIZATION IN PET IMAGES

Regional physiologic data obtained with PET must be related to the corresponding anatomic brain regions. Anatomic localization in PET is a subject of ongoing research[157,158] and many methods have been proposed. Most methods require the use of a special head-holder.[159] There are several methods for immobilizing the head on the support. These include a heat-pliant face mask individually molded to the subject and fixed to the headrest,[160] a polyurethane material that hardens behind the subject's head,[161] cushioned pads held against the face,[162] or a rigid glass fiber mesh surrounding the head.[163] With all such devices, there is a trade off between patient comfort and strict head immobilization. It is important to maintain immobilization to ensure that the transmission scan and all emission images are in registration. Head movement during a scan will also decrease the effective resolution of the images. Head holders can be used to reposition the head for subsequent scan sessions. The degree to which any device holds the head still or succeeds in repositioning has in general not been reported in a quantitative fashion, but preliminary data for a heat-pliant mask indicate that 1 to 2 mm of translational head movement and 2° of head "nodding" can occur during the period of a typical FDG scan.[164] A novel approach for repositioning uses a video system to compare the head position in different scan sessions;[165] it achieved z-axis repositioning accuracy of 1 mm. In addition to the head holder itself, most scanners incorporate a laser positioning device. The projection of the laser line on the subject's head corresponds to the plane of a specific PET slice and is used to position the head in the scanner.

Several methods of anatomic localization have been used. Early techniques involved visual inspection of the PET images. One method is to obtain the images in standard tomographic planes relative to external landmarks, such as the canthomeatal line. The PET images are then visually compared to anatomic brain sections in equivalent planes from a brain atlas and ROIs are manually drawn.[166] The visual approach, however, is subjective and liable to observer bias. The relatively poor resolution of many tomographs limits the amount of detail in the image. More importantly, it cannot be assumed that PET images which are based on physiology delineate the anatomy of the brain, especially in cases of local pathology. In early Huntington's disease,[167] the caudate nucleus is difficult to visualize on FDG images because of its decreased metabolism, although it is still structurally intact. In Parkinson's disease, uptake of ^{18}F-fluorodopa may be decreased in the striatum,[60] and this decrease may be heterogenous. Therefore, manual placement of a ROI over what appears to be an anatomic region in the striatum on the PET image is subject to error.

An alternative approach uses a stereotactic method of anatomical localization.[160] With this technique, a correspondence is established between anatomic regions in a stereotactic brain atlas and specific ROIs on the PET image. At the time of the PET study, a plastic plate with embedded radioopaque wires corresponding to the tomographic slices is attached to the headrest of the scanner and is aligned with the positioning laser line. A lateral skull X-ray records the position of the PET slices, indicated by the wires, in relation to the bony landmarks of the skull. This information is used to set up a transformation between the coordinate system of the stereotactic brain atlas and the coordinate system defining the location of ROIs on the PET slices. ROIs corresponding to specific brain structures can then be placed on the PET images, and conversely, the anatomic location of an ROI selected on the PET image can be determined. This method provides objective and reproducible anatomic localization when brain anatomy is normal.

Other methods are required when there are structural abnormalities in the brain such as cerebral atrophy, or when there is a focal brain lesion for which regional measurements are desired. A general approach useful for both normal and abnormal brain utilizes anatomical images obtained in the same planes as the PET slices. Coplanar PET and X-ray computerized tomograph (CT) images can be obtained by use of a rigid, tightly fitting head holder that can be attached to both the PET and the CT couches.[163] Alternatively, CT scanners can provide a lateral view of the skull in the gantry. If a lateral X-ray is taken at the time of PET to record the location of the reference laser line and corresponding PET slice, these two lateral skull views can be used to angulate the CT gantry to obtain coplanar PET and CT slices.[30] A similar method can be used with magnetic resonance imaging (MRI).[168] A thin tube filled with $CuSO_4$, which is visualized on MRI, is affixed to the head coincident with the reference laser line. This tube appears as a line on a sagittal MRI view and is used as a reference to define transverse MRI planes. A novel method recently described aligns PET and MRI data *after* they have been collected.[169] The external surface of the head is defined from both PET transmission images and anatomic images. The coordinate transformations that bring these models of the surface into three-dimensional congruence are calculated with an iterative mathematical technique. These transformations can then be used to reslice the higher resolution MRI data along the planes of the PET images, to obtain pairs that can be directly compared.

Once anatomic images coplanar with the PET slices are obtained, they can be accessed by a computer image analysis program and ROIs can be transferred between them. ROIs can be drawn on the anatomic image over structures of interest. Alternatively, an atlas of standard ROIs, defined for a representative brain, can be applied to the anatomic image.[168,170,171] Adjustments to specific ROIs can be made to account for individual variations in brain anatomy; areas of focal pathology can be manually outlined and transferred to the PET images.[168]

C. ANALYSIS OF REGIONAL PET DATA

Analysis of regional PET data obtained by the methods described above is complicated by the fact that there are often relatively wide variations in measured values among subjects in a study. This variability can be expressed in terms of the coefficient of variation (COV), i.e., the ratio of the standard deviation to the mean. Values for the COV have been about 15 to 25% for typical PET studies of rCMRGlu with FDG[166,172,173] and of rCBF and rCMRO$_2$ with ^{15}O-labeled tracers.[155] These variations may reflect normal physiologic differences, or may result from methodological errors, such as inaccuracies in scanner calibration and in measurement of the input function. As a result, the absolute measurement in a given region, e.g., the visual cortex, may vary considerably among subjects, although the relative differences measured between two brain regions, e.g., visual cortex and white matter, may be similar in all subjects. Similarly, during a sensory stimulus, a specific brain region may demonstrate increased flow compared to the rest of the brain, but the absolute flow value may be lower than that seen in the same region in the resting state in the same or another subject. Therefore, approaches have been developed to facilitate the detection of regional changes by adjusting for the effect of global variations.

Several methods are used to "normalize" regional data. These include dividing each regional value by the global value;[154,166,175] calculating the ratio of the values for homologous right and left regions of the brain;[155] and calculating the ratio of the measurement in a structure of interest to another structure presumed to be minimally involved in the disease process, for example the ratio of metabolism in the caudate to the lateral cerebral cortex in Huntington's disease.[176] Such techniques, however, could result in a loss of information contained in the absolute values especially if more widespread changes accompany a focal change. If not only the numerator, but also the denominator of the ratio used, differs between groups, erroneous conclusions may be drawn. For example, in dementia of the Alzheimer type, the ratio of caudate to global metabolism is significantly increased.[177] This is, however, because of a greater *decrease* in global metabolism than in caudate metabolism. For some PET tracers, the local radioactivity measurement is proportional or almost proportional to the value of the physiologic variable. This is true for the measurement of rCBV with labelled CO, and for the PET-autoradiographic measurement of rCBF with H$_2$^{15}O, as discussed above.[91] Ratios of tissue count data therefore can provide the same information as normalized physiologic measurements. Thus it is possible to obtain information from the PET images without the use of a model, and blood sampling during the scan is not required. This is of practical importance for rCBF measurements,[96] as it permits mapping the functional responses of the brain during neurobehavioral tasks without the use of an arterial catheter. For many PET tracer-kinetic models, however, the relationship between local radioactivity and the physiologic variable is nonlinear, and images of radioactivity cannot be used to determine relative regional differences.

The standard approach of analyzing PET images is to compare absolute or normalized measurements from specific brain regions between subject groups. Other procedures have been developed, however, to analyze the relationships between multiple regional measurements. One such procedure involves calculating the correlation coefficient between measurements from pairs of brain regions, for many such pairs.[172,178,179] A high correlation coefficient for any two regions has been ascribed to a functional coupling between them. This method has some disadvantages, including the possibility of finding certain correlations by chance because of the large number that are calculated, the possibility of artifactual correlations,[180] and potential difficulty in interpreting a change in the number of regional correlations that may occur in a disease state. Other methods have been developed which attempt to divide the variability in a set of regional measurements into components representing the individual differences in global metabolic rate, a consistent regional pattern in the subject group specific for the disease state, and a residual component, either experimental error or regional differences between individual subjects.[181,182] These methods are at a relatively early stage in their application.

Recently, a powerful metod has been described and applied to detect rCBF changes that accompany the increase in local neuronal activity during neurobehavioral tasks.[183-186] Briefly, the steps include: normalizing each image to an average global CBF; computing a difference image of normalized rCBF changes by subtracting the control image from the image obtained during activation; mapping these difference images into common anatomic format — a system of coordinates defined relative to a stereotactic atlas; averaging the spatially standardized images of CBF change over all subjects; and finally searching this single, averaged, difference image with an automated program to determine the stereotactic location and magnitude of local rCBF changes. This method can be applied to other types of studies to seek state-dependent regional changes in pairs of PET images, for example before and after acute administration of a medication, and also to compare a group of patients to a control group.

D. SUBJECT SELECTION AND CHARACTERIZATION

As part of the initial experimental design, one requires appropriate criteria for selecting subjects and defining experimental conditions. An understanding of these issues is also important during data interpretation so that any changes or abnormalities found in a subject group will be properly ascribed to the biological process being studied. Age, sex, handedness, and condition of health must be considered. With normal aging, several changes occur,[187] such as reduced performance in neuropsychological tests, macroscopic atrophy of gray and white matter, a decrease in neuronal number that is not uniform throughout brain, and biochemical changes in specific neurotransmitter systems. Not surprisingly, age-related changes have been seen with PET. The uptake rate constant of ^{18}F-fluorodopa decreases with age,[60] as does D_2 dopamine receptor level measured with ^{11}C-N-methylspiperone.[152] Several investigators using PET and other methods have observed declines in CBF and metabolism with aging, although others have found no change.[187] The effect of gender has been less well studied. There are some reports of a higher CBF or CMRGlu in females in some[188,189] but not all studies.[190] Handedness is an obvious reflection of lateralization of certain brain functions. In addition to functional asymmetries, there are anatomic asymmetries, such as in the size of the planum temporale.[191] Therefore, it cannot be assumed that regional measurements obtained from homologous right-left brain regions are normally equal. Significant regional asymmetries in CBF, CMRO$_2$[174] and CMRGlu[192] have been reported in normal subjects; these may be due to functional or anatomic asymmetries. The health status of normal controls must be carefully assessed, especially in elderly subjects who may harbor clinically silent vascular or neurological disease. Proper definition of the status of patients being studied is also important. Several factors related to their disease may affect PET measurements, such as the presence and severity of specific manifestations, the duration of the condition, and treatment history. The status of subjects *during* the scan must also be considered. Attention, thought content, and anxiety, all of which may vary among subjects, or even in the same subject during different scans, may affect PET measurements. PET findings may also depend on the presence and severity of disease manifestations, such as tremor, during the scan session. Medications, such as L-dopa, can alter local flow and metabolism.[155] and neuroleptics and anti-Parkinsonian drugs can interfere with measurements of neuroreceptor systems. Appropriate periods of medication withdrawal prior to the PET study are usually required.

E. INTERPRETATION OF CHANGES IN CEREBRAL BLOOD FLOW AND METABOLISM

It has been generally thought that neuronal activity, oxidative energy metabolism, and blood flow are closely coupled, both in the resting brain and during increased local neuronal activity. Furthermore, it has been assumed that the increase in local CBF that would be needed to maintain metabolism (because there are virtually no stores of glucose or oxygen in the brain) occurs via regulatory mechanisms mediated by vasoactive metabolites. Recent observations have lead to a growing understanding of these relationships, but have also challenged some traditional concepts. Because PET measurements of rCBF and metabolism are widely used as indicators of local neuronal function, these observations will be reviewed here.[193-196]

The energy metabolism that supports neuronal activity is required primarily for the maintenance of ionic gradients across cell membranes by the ATP-dependent Na^+/K^+ pump.[193,197] This pump constitutes a major fraction of the brain's energy consumption. The site of largest metabolic demand is not in the neuronal cell body, but in the neuropil where axons terminate and synapse with dendrites.[198,199] This is where neurons have the greatest surface-area to volume ratio, and therefore where ion pumping across cell membranes is the greatest. Furthermore, it has been shown that not only excitatory activity but also inhibitory activity of axon terminals can increase energy consumption in the neuropil.[200] Several investigators have demonstrated that an increase is not necessarily linear over the frequency range studied.[193,201] Other factors, such as electrophysiologic limitations on the ability of neuronal systems to follow the stimulation frequency may be involved.[154,201]

CBF measurements have been widely used as an indirect indicator of changes in both energy metabolism and neuronal activity, based on the assumption that changes in local CBF occur in response to an alteration in oxidative metabolic demand. Recent findings have challenged this assumption. In the resting state in both animals and man, there is a tight correlation between local CBF and local glucose or oxygen metabolism.[194,202] It has been demonstrated with PET, however, that although a transient increase in neural activity induced by somatosensory stimulation produces a large, coupled increase in rCBF and rCMRGlu, there is only a slight increase in $rCMRO_2$.[194,196] Thus, there appears to be mainly nonoxidative consumption of glucose and the acute energy yield would be considerably smaller than expected. This argues against oxidative glucose metabolism as the regulating factor for the acute CBF change. In fact, there is considerable evidence that the classic metabolic candidates for the coupling of flow to metabolism, such as locally increased H^+ or adenosine, or decreased pO_2, are not involved, and the rapid vascular response precedes their appearance, if they are produced at all.[194,195] It has been postulated, therefore, that an intrinsic neural system may regulate acute flow changes. Rather than metabolism determining flow, acute changes in both flow and energy metabolism may be accomplished by different mechanisms that both depend upon neural firing.[195]

These observations have implications for the interpretation of PET studies. Measurement of rCBF with $H_2^{15}O$ and PET remains the most powerful method for mapping the response of the human brain during neurobehavioral tasks. Although the local flow response (as well as glucose metabolism) depends upon the frequency of the stimulus, it may not be proportionally related throughout the entire frequency range.[154] This means that in the design of activation tasks, the stimulus repetition rate or the performance rate for a motor task must be taken into account, because it may affect the degree or even the occurrence of a local CBF or metabolic response. Furthermore, a local response may not necessarily be due to increased local neuronal firing, but more likely may reflect increased activity in neurons which project to the locus, and which may even be inhibitory in nature.

The use of PET to study disease states also requires careful interpretation. PET has been extensively used to study cerebrovascular disease. Here, measurements of rCBF and $rCMRO_2$

relate quite directly to pathophysiology. For example, one can examine the adequacy of substrate delivery, the metabolic requirements for the maintenance of tissue viability, and the hemodynamic and metabolic response of the brain to a decrease in perfusion pressure due to a narrowed or occluded vessel. Measurements of CBF alone, however, are inadequate to characterize a given situation; metabolic data are also needed.[70] In a cerebral infarct, both rCBF and rCMRO$_2$ are decreased. Distal to a severely narrowed or occluded carotid artery, rCBF can also be decreased but rCMRO$_2$ may be relatively well maintained, indicating tissue viability. This is accomplished by two mechanisms available to the brain to compensate for decreased perfusion pressure; local vasodilation which results in increased rCBV, and increased oxygen extraction. Finally, following a subcortical infarct, both cortical rCBF and rCMRO$_2$ may be equally depressed with a normal rOEF, due to an interruption in the afferent projections to the region. In all these cases, a decrease in rCBF is accompanied by different tissue responses that require rCMRO$_2$ measurements to identify.

Measurements of rCBF and metabolism are also performed in psychiatric disease and in neurologic disease other than stroke. In these conditions, flow and metabolism are not primarily involved in the pathophysiology of the disease, and there are several possible interpretations of abnormal findings. There may be a local change in the number of neurons or in the density of axonal terminals projecting to a region. There could be a change in local neuronal activity, or, more likely, a change in the activity of neurons projecting to the region. For example, Wooten and Collins[203] found increased rCMRGlu in the pallidum ipsilateral to a lesioned substantia nigra in the rat. They hypothesized that depletion of striatal dopamine content results in disinhibition of some striatal efferents, which produces increased metabolism in terminal fields within the globus pallidus.

Finally, several technical factors may lead to an artifactual change in measured rCBF or metabolism. Partial volume averaging due to the limited spatial resolution of PET (see Section II) must be taken into account. The concentration of radioactivity in gray matter structures will tend to be underestimated, and therefore so will the physiologic measurements. Also, in two structures with the same shape and local radiotracer concentration but with different sizes, the concentration of radioactivity will be underestimated in the smaller structure.[28] For example, if the caudate nucleus decreases in size, but has an unchanged metabolic rate per gram of tissue, rCMRGlu will be underestimated. Similarly, if a structure is larger, such as the left planum temporale in right-handers, it may appear to have increased metabolism. These effects will be reduced but not eliminated with scanners of better resolution. Cerebral atrophy presents a special problem. In several conditions, including normal aging, and Alzheimer's disease, widespread atrophy can occur. PET measurements can be artifactually reduced, because of partial volume averaging of tissue with the enlarged cerebrospinal fluid spaces. A method has been developed to correct global PET measurements using data from structural CT or MR images.[30] It is more difficult to correct regional data for atrophy, although a strategy for doing this has been described.[204] Head tilt in the lateral direction during the scan can cause an apparent asymmetry in brain structures. The resulting asymmetric partial volume effects in the basal ganglia, for example, may produce an artifactual asymmetry in measurements from these structures.[205] Finally, one must consider the possibility that changes in radiotracer behavior in disease states can cause apparent changes in PET measurements. In cerebral ischemia and brain tumor, changes in the rate constants and lumped constant used in the standard FDG model can lead to erroneous measurements of rCMRGlu. In CBF measurements with H$_2$^{15}O, a local increase in the permeability of the blood-brain barrier to water[107] would result in an apparent increase in flow.

In summary, the interpretation of PET images is a complex process. A complete understanding of the issues involved is required to obtain scientifically useful information.

REFERENCES

1. **Kety, S. S. and Schmidt, C. F.**, The nitrous oxide method for the quantitative determination of cerebral blood flow in man: theory, procedure, and normal values, *J. Clin. Invest.*, 27, 476, 1948.
2. **Obrist, W. D., Thompson, H. K., King, C. H., and Wang, H. S.**, Determination of regional cerebral blood flow by inhalation of xenon-133, *Circ. Res.*, 20, 124, 1967.
3. **Lassen, N. A. and Ingvar, D. H.**, Radioisotopic assessment of regional cerebral blood flow, *Prog. Nucl. Med.*, 1, 376, 1972.
4. **Welch, M. J., Eichling, J. O., Straatman, M. G., Raichle, M. E., and Ter-Pogossian, M. M.**, New short-lived radiopharmaceuticals for CNS studies, in *Noninvasive Brain Imaging: Computed Tomography and Radionuclides*, DeBlanc, H. J., Jr. and Sorenson, J. A., Eds., The Society of Nuclear Medicine, New York, 1975, 25.
5. **Ter-Pogossian, M. M., Phelps, M. E., Hoffman, E. J., and Mullani, N. A.**, A positron-emission transaxial tomograph for nuclear imaging (PETT), *Radiology*, 114, 89, 1975.
6. **Jamieson, D., Alavi, A., Jolles, P., Chawluk, J., and Reivich, M.**, Positron emission tomography in the investigation of central nervous system disorders, *Radiol. Clin. North Am.*, 26, 1075, 1988.
7. Council on Scientific Affairs, Positron emission tomography — a new approach to brain chemistry, *JAMA*, 260, 2704, 1988.
8. **Bergmann, S. R., Fox, K. A. A., Geltman, E. M., and Sobel, B. E.**, Positron emission tomography of the heart, *Semin. Nucl. Med.*, 28, 165, 1985.
9. Council on Scientific Affairs, Positron emission tomography in oncology, *JAMA*, 259, 2126, 1988.
10. **Shuster, D. P.**, Positron emission tomography: theory and its application to the study of lung disease, *Am. Rev. Resp. Dis.*, 139, 818, 1989.
11. **Brooks, R. A. and Di Chiro, G.**, Principles of computer assisted tomography (CAT) in radiographic and radioisotopic imaging, *Phys. Med. Biol.*, 21, 689, 1976.
12. **Frackowiak, R. S. J., Lenzi, G.-L., Jones, T., and Heather, J. D.**, Quantitative measurement of regional cerebral blood flow and oxygen metabolism in man using ^{15}O and positron emission tomography: theory, procedure and normal values, *J. Comput. Assist. Tomogr.*, 4, 727, 1980.
13. **Eichling, J. O., Higgins, C. S., and Ter-Pogossian, M. M.**, Determination of radionuclide concentration with positron CT scanning, *J. Nucl. Med.*, 18, 845, 1977.
14. **Muehllehner, G., Karp, J. S., Mankoff, D. A., Beerbohm, D., and Ordonez, C. E.**, Design and performance of a new positron tomograph, *IEEE Trans. Nucl. Sci.*, 35, 670, 1988.
15. **Ter-Pogossian, M. M.**, Special characteristics and potential for dynamic function studies with PET, *Semin. Nucl. Med.*, 11, 13, 1981.
16. **Brooks, R. A., Sank, V. J., Friauf, W. S., Leighton, S. B., Cascio, H. E., and Di Chiro, G.**, Design considerations for positron emission tomography, *IEEE Trans. Biomed. Eng.*, BME-28, 158, 1981.
17. **Hoffman, E. F.**, Instrumentation for quantitative tomographic determination of concentrations of positron-emitting, receptor binding radiotracers, in *Receptor-Binding Radiotracers*, Vol. II, Eckelman, W. C., Ed., CRC Press, Boca Raton, FL, 1982, 141.
18. **Muehllehner, G. and Karp, J. S.**, Positron emission tomography imaging — technical considerations, *Semin. Nucl. Med.*, 16, 35, 1986.
19. **Hoffman, E. J. and Phelps, M. E.**, Positron emission tomography: principles and quantitation, in *Positron Emission Tomography and Autoradiography*, Phelps, M.E., Mazziotta, J. C., and Schelbert, H. R., Eds., Raven Press, New York, 1986, 237.
20. Council on Scientific Affairs, Instrumentation in positron emission tomography, *JAMA*, 259, 1351, 1988.
21. **Budinger, T. F., Derenzo, S. E., Greenberg, W. L., Gullberg, G. T., and Huesman, R. H.**, Quantitative potentials of dynamic emission computed tomography, *J. Nucl. Med.*, 19, 309, 1978.
22. **Hoffman, E. J., Huang, S.-C., Phelps, M. E., and Kuhl, D. E.**, Quantitation in positron emission computed tomography IV. Effect of accidental coincidences, *J. Comput. Assist. Tomogr.*, 5, 491, 1981.
23. **Mintun, M. A., Raichle, M. E., Kilbourn, M. R., Wooton, G. F., and Welch, M. J.**, A quantitative model for the in vivo assessment of drug binding sites with positron emission tomography, *Ann. Neurol.*, 15, 217, 1984.
24. **Bergström, M., Eriksson, L., Bohm, C., Blomqvist, G., and Litton, J.**, Correction for scattered radiation in a ring detector positron camera by integral transformation of the projections, *J. Comput. Assist. Tomogr.*, 7, 42, 1983.
25. **Phelps, M. E., Hoffman, E. J., Huang, S.-C., and Ter-Pogossian, M. M.**, Effect of positron range on spatial resolution, *J. Nucl. Med.*, 16, 649, 1975.
26. **Phelps, M. E. and Hoffman, E. J.**, Resolution limit of positron cameras, *J. Nucl Med.*, 17, 757, 1976.
27. **Derenzo, S. E., Huesman, R. H., Cahoon, J. L., Geyer, A., Uber, D., Vuletich, T., and Budinger, T. F.**, Initial results from the Donner 600 crystal positron tomograph, *IEEE Trans. Nucl. Sci.*, 34, 321, 1987.

28. **Hoffman, E. J., Huang, S.-C., and Phelps, M. E.,** Quantitation in positron emission computed tomography. I. Effect of object size, *J. Comput. Assist. Tomogr.*, 3, 299, 1979.
29. **Mazziotta, J. C., Phelps, M. E., Plummer, D., and Kuhl, D. E.,** Quantitation in positron computed tomography. V. Physical-anatomical effects, *J. Comput. Assist. Tomogr.*, 5, 734, 1981.
30. **Herscovitch, P., Auchus, A. P., Gado, M., Chi, D., and Raichle, M. E.,** Correction of positron emission tomography data for cerebral atrophy, *J. Cereb. Blood Flow Metab.*, 6, 120, 1986.
31. **Kessler, R. M., Ellis, J. R., Jr., and Eden, M.,** Analysis of emission tomographic scan data: limitations imposed by resolution and background, *J. Comput. Assist. Tomogr.*, 8, 514, 1984.
32. **Daube-Witherspoon, M. E.,** Acceptance testing, maintenance, and quality control of PET instrumentation in *PET/SPECT: Instrumentation, Radiopharmaceuticals, Neurology, and Physiological Measurement,* American College of Nuclear Physicians, Washington, 1988, 60.
33. **Wolf, A.,** Cyclotrons for clinical and biomedical research with PET, in *PET/SPECT: Instrumentation, Radiopharmaceuticals, Neurology, and Physiological Measurement,* American College of Nuclear Physicians, Washington, 1988, 109.
34. **Welch, M. J. and Kilbourn, M. R.,** Positron emitters for imaging, in *Freeman and Johnson's Clinical Radionuclide Imaging,* Freeman L. M., Ed., Grune & Stratton, Orlando, FL, 1984, 181.
35. **Palmer, A. J. and Taylor, D. M.,** Radiopharmaceuticals labeled with halogen isotopes, *Int. J. Appl. Radiat. Isot.*, 37, 645, 1986.
36. **Fowler, J. S. and Wolf, A.,** Positron emitter-labelled compounds: priorities and problems, in *Positron Emission Tomography and Autoradiography,* Phelps, M. E., Mazziotta, J. C., and Schelbert, H. R., Eds., Raven Press, New York, 1986, 391.
37. Council on Scientific Affairs, Cyclotrons and radiopharmaceuticals in positron emission tomography, *JAMA,* 259, 1854, 1988.
38. **Kilbourn, M. R. and Zalutsky, M. R.,** Research and clinical potential of receptor based radiopharmaceuticals, *J. Nucl. Med.*, 26, 655, 1985.
39. **Veatch, R. M.,** The ethics of research involving radiation, *IRB,* 4, 3, 1982.
40. **Huda, W. and Scrimger, J. W.,** Irradiation of volunteers in nuclear medicine, *J. Nucl. Med.*, 30, 260, 1989.
41. **Brill, A. B.,** Biological effects of ionizing radiation, in *Nuclear Medical Physics,* Vol. I, Williams, L. E., Ed., CRC Press, Boca Raton FL, 1988, 163.
42. **Loevinger, R., Budinger, T. F., and Watson, E. E.,** *MIRD Primer for Absorbed Dose Calculations,* The Society of Nuclear Medicine, New York, 1988.
43. **Cloutier, R. J. and Watson, E. E.,** Internal dosimetry — an introduction to the ICRP technique, in *Nuclear Medical Physics,* Vol. I, Williams, L. E., Ed., CRC Press, Boca Raton, FL, 1987, 143.
44. **Jones, S. C., Alavi, A., Christman, D., Montanez, I., Wolf, A. P., and Reivich, M.,** The radiation dosimetry of 2-[F-18]fluoro-2-D-glucose in man, *J. Nucl. Med.*, 23, 613, 1982.
45. **Jones, S.C., Alavi, A., Christman, D., Wolf, A. P., and Reivich, M.,** Re: The radiation dosimetry of 2-[F-18]fluoro-2-D-glucose in man, *J. Nucl. Med.*, 24, 447, 1983.
46. **Welch, M. J., Katzenellenbogen, J. A., Mathias, C. J., Brodack, J. W., Carlson, K. E., Chi, D. Y., Dence, C. S., Kilbourn, M. R., Perlmutter, J. S., Raichle, M. E., and Ter-Pogossian, M. M.,** N-(3-[¹⁸F]fluoropropyl)-spiperone: the preferred ¹⁸F labeled spiperone analog for positron emission tomographic studies of the dopamine receptor, *Nucl. Med. Biol.*, 15, 83, 1988.
47. **Jones, S. C., Greenberg, J. H., and Reivich, M.,** Error analysis for the determination of cerebral blood flow with the continuous inhalation of ¹⁵O-labeled carbon dioxide and positron emission tomography, *J. Comput. Assist. Tomogr.*, 6, 116, 1982.
48. **Kearfott, K. J.,** Radiation absorbed dose estimates for positron emission tomography (PET): K-38, Rb-81, Rb-82, and Cs-130, *J. Nucl. Med.*, 23, 1128, 1982.
49. **Harvey, J., Firnau, G., and Garnett, E. S.,** Estimation of the radiation dose in man due to 6-[¹⁸F]-fluoro-L-Dopa, *J. Nucl. Med.*, 26, 931, 1985.
50. **Riggs, D. S.,** *The Mathematical Approach to Physiological Problems,* MIT Press, Cambridge, MA, 1970.
51. **Shipley, R. A. and Clark, R. E.,** *Tracer Methods for In Vivo Kinetics,* Academic Press, New York, 1972.
52. **Lassen, N. A. and Perl, W.,** *Tracer Kinetic Methods in Medical Physiology,* Raven Press, New York, 1979.
53. **Lambrecht, R. M. and Rescigno, A.,** *Tracer Kinetics and Physiologic Modeling,* Springer-Verlag, Berlin, 1983.
54. **Graham, M. M., Bassingthwaighte, J. B., and Chan, J.,** Validation of compartmental models of deoxyglucose kinetics using data froma distributed model, *J.Cereb. Blood Flow Metab.*, 5 (Suppl. 1), S573, 1985.
55. **Larson, K. B., Markham, J., and Raichle, M. E.,** Tracer-kinetic models for measuring cerebral blood flow using externally detected radiotracers, *J. Cereb. Blood Flow Metab.*, 7, 443, 1987.
56. **Gjedde, A.,** High- and low-affinity transport of D-glucose from blood to brain, *J. Neurochem.*, 36, 1463, 1981.

57. **Patlak, C. S., Blasberg, R. G., and Fenstermacher, J. D.,** Graphical evaluation of blood-to-brain transfer constants from multiple-time uptake data, *J. Cereb. Blood Flow Metab.*, 3, 1, 1983.

58. **Patlak, C. S. and Blasberg, R. G.,** Graphical evaluation of blood-to-brain transfer constants from multiple-time uptake data. Generalizations, *J. Cereb. Blood Flow Metab.*, 5, 584, 1985.

59. **Wong, D. F., Gjedde, A., and Wagner, H. N., Jr.,** Quantification of neuroreceptors in the living human brain. I. Irreversible binding of ligands, *J. Cereb. Blood Flow Metab.*, 6, 137, 1986.

60. **Martin, W. R. W., Palmer, M. R., Patlak, C. S., and Calne, D. B.,** Nigrostriatal function in humans studied with positron emission tomography, *Ann. Neurol.*, 26, 535, 1989.

61. **Videen, T. O., Perlmutter, J. S., Herscovitch, P., and Raichle, M. E.,** Brain blood volume, flow, and oxygen utilization measured with ^{15}O radiotracers and positron emission tomography: revised metabolic computations, *J. Cereb. Blood Flow Metab.*, 7, 513, 1987.

62. **Carson, R. E.,** Parameter estimation in positron emission tomography, in *Positron Emission Tomography and Autoradiography*, Phelps, M. E., Mazziotta, J. C., and Schelbert, H. R., Eds., Raven Press, New York, 1986, 391.

63. **Grubb, R. L., Jr., Raichle, M. E., Higgins, C. S., and Eichling, J. O.,** Measurement of regional cerebral blood volume by emission tomography, *Ann. Neurol.*, 4, 322, 1978.

64. **Phelps, M. E., Huang, S. C., Hoffman, E. J., and Kuhl, D. E.,** Validation of tomographic measurement of cerebral blood volume with C-11-labeled carboxyhemoglobin, *J. Nucl. Med.*, 20, 328, 1979.

65. **Mintun, M. A., Raichle, M. E., Martin, W. R. W., and Herscovitch, P.,** Brain oxygen utilization measured with O-15 radiotracers and positron emission tomography, *J. Nucl. Med.*, 25, 177, 1984.

66. **Martin, W. R. W., Powers, W. J., and Raichle, M. E.,** Cerebral blood volume measured with inhaled $C^{15}O$ and positron emission tomography, *J. Cereb. Blood Flow Metab.*, 7, 421, 1987.

67. **Lammertsma, A. A., Brooks, D. J., Beaney, R. P., Turton, D. R., Kensett, M. J., Heather, J. D., Marshall, J., and Jones, T.,** In vivo measurement of regional cerebral haematocrit using positron emission tomography, *J. Cereb. Blood Flow Metab.*, 4, 317, 1984.

68. **Sakai, F., Nakazawa, K., Tazaki, Y., Ishii, K., Hino, H., Igarushi, H., and Kanda, T.,** Regional cerebral blood volume and hematocrit measured in normal human volunteers by single-photon emission computed tomography, *J. Cereb. Blood Flow Metab.*, 5, 207, 1985.

69. **Kearfott, K. J.,** Absorbed dose estimates for positron emission tomography (PET): $C^{15}O$, ^{11}CO, and $CO^{15}O$, *J. Nucl. Med.*, 23, 1031, 1982.

70. **Powers, W. J.,** Positron emission in tomography in cerebrovascular disease: clinical applications?, in *Clinical Neuroimaging*, Theodore W. H., Ed., Alan R. Liss, New York, 1987, 49.

71. **Kety, S. S.,** The theory and applications of the exchange of inert gas at the lungs and tissues, *Pharmacol. Rev.*, 3, 1, 1951.

72. **Kety, S. S.,** Measurement of local blood flow by the exchange of an inert diffusible substance, *Methods Med. Res.*, 8, 228, 1960.

73. **Landau, W. M., Freygang, W. H., Jr., Rowland, L. P., Sokoloff, L., and Kety, S.,** The local circulation of the living brain; values in the unanesthetized and anesthetized cat, *Trans. Am. Neurol. Assoc.*, 80, 125, 1955.

74. **Sakurada, O., Kennedy, C., Jehle, J., Brown, J. C., Carbon, G. L., and Sokoloff, L.,** Measurement of local cerebral blood flow with iodo[14C]antipyrine, *Am. J. Physiol.*, 234, H59, 1978.

75. **Herscovitch P. and Raichle M. E.,** What is the correct value for the brain-blood partition coefficient for water?, *J. Cereb. Blood Flow Metab.*, 5, 65, 1985.

76. **Welch, M. J. and Kilbourn, M. R.,** A remote system for the routine production of oxygen-15 radiopharmaceuticals, *J. Labeled Compd.*, 22, 1193, 1985.

77. **Jones, T., Chesler, D. A. and Ter-Pogossian, M. M.,** The continuous inhalation of oxygen-15 for assessing regional oxygen extraction in the brain of man, *Br. J. Radiol.*, 49, 339, 1976.

78. **Subramanyam, R., Alpert, N. M., Hoop, B., Jr., Brownell, G. L., and Taveras, J. M.,** A model for regional cerebral oxygen distribution during continuous inhalation of $^{15}O_2$, $C^{15}O$, and $C^{15}O_2$, *J. Nucl. Med.*, 19, 13, 1978.

79. **Baron, J. C., Steinling, M., Tanaka, T., Cavalheiro, E., Soussaline, F., and Collard, P.,** Quantitative measurement of CBF, oxygen extraction fraction (OEF) and $CMRO_2$ with the ^{15}O continuous inhalation technique and positron emission tomography (PET): experimental evidence and normal values in man, *J. Cereb. Blood Flow Metab.*, 1 (Suppl. 1), S5, 1981.

80. **Rhodes, C. G., Lenzi, G. L., Frackowiak, R. S. J., Jones, T., and Pozzilli, C.,** Measurement of CBF and $CMRO_2$ using continuous inhalation of $C^{15}O_2$ and $^{15}O_2$: experimental validation using CO_2 reactivity in the anaesthetised dog, *J. Neurol. Sci.*, 50, 381, 1981.

81. **Steinling, M., Baron, J. C., Maziere, B., Lasjaunias, P., Loch'h, C., Cabanis, E. A., and Guillon, B.,** Tomographic measurement of cerebral blood flow by the ^{68}Ga-labelled-microsphere and continuous-$C^{15}O_2$-inhalation methods, *Eur. J. Nucl. Med.*, 11, 29, 1985.

82. **Huang, S.-C., Phelps, M. E., Hoffman, E. J., and Kuhl, D. E.,** A theoretical study of quantitative flow measurements with constant infusion of short-lived isotopes, *Phys. Med. Biol.*, 24, 1151, 1979.

83. **Lammertsma, A. A., Jones, T., Frackowiak, R. S. J., and Lenzi, G.-L.**, A theoretical study of the steady-state model for measuring regional cerebral blood flow and oxygen utilization using oxygen-15, *J. Comput. Assist. Tomogr.*, 5, 544, 1981.

84. **Lammertsma, A. A., Heather, J. D., Jones, T., Frackowiak, R. S. J., and Lenzi, G.-L.**, A statistical study of the steady state technique for measuring regional cerebral blood flow and oxygen utilization using ^{15}O, *J. Comput. Assist. Tomogr.*, 6, 566, 1982.

85. **Steinling, M. and Baron, J. C.**, Mesure du debit sanguin cerebral local par inhalation continue de $C^{15}O_2$ et tomographie d'emission: etude des limites du modele, *J. Biophys. Med. Nucl.*, 6, 48, 1982.

86. **Herscovitch, P. and Raichle, M. E.**, Effect of tissue heterogeneity on the measurement of cerebral blood flow with the equilibrium $C^{15}O_2$ inhalation technique, *J. Cereb. Blood Flow Metab.*, 3, 407, 1983.

87. **Meyer, E. and Yamamoto, Y. L.**, The requirement for constant arterial radioactivity in the $C^{15}O_2$ steady-state blood-flow model, *J. Nucl. Med.*, 25, 455, 1984.

88. **Lammertsma, A. A., Correia, J. A., and Jones, T.**, Stability of arterial concentrations during continuous inhalation of $C^{15}O_2$ and $^{15}O_2$ and the effects on computed values of CBF and $CMRO_2$, *J. Cereb. Blood Flow Metab.*, 8, 411, 1988.

89. **Senda, M., Buxton, R. B., Alpert, N. M., Correia, J. A., Mackay, B. C., Weise S. B., and Ackerman R. H.**, The ^{15}O steady-state method: correction for variation in arterial concentration, *J. Cereb. Blood Flow Metab.*, 8, 681, 1988.

90. **Jones, S. C., Greenberg, J. H., Dann, R., Robinson, G. D., Jr., Kushner, M., Alavi, A., and Reivich, M.**, Cerebral blood flow with the continuous infusion of oxygen-15 labeled water, *J. Cereb. Blood Flow Metab.*, 5, 566, 1985.

91. **Herscovitch, P., Markham, J., and Raichle, M. E.**, Brain blood flow measured with intravenous $H_2^{15}O$. I. Theory and error analysis, *J. Nucl. Med.*, 24, 782, 1983.

92. **Raichle, M. E., Martin, W. R. W., Herscovitch, P., Mintun, M. A., and Markham, J.**, Brain blood flow measured with intravenous $H_2^{15}O$. II. Implementation and validation, *J. Nucl. Med.*, 24, 790, 1983.

93. **Kanno, I., Iida, H., Miura, S., Murakami, M., Takahashi, K., Sasaki, H., Inugami, A., Shishido, F., and Uemura, K.**, A system for cerebral blood flow measurement using an $H_2^{15}O$ autoradiographic method and positron emission tomography, *J. Cereb. Blood Flow Metab.*, 7, 143, 1987.

94. **Fox, P. T., Mintun, M. A., Raichle, M. E., and Herscovitch, P.**, A noninvasive approach to quantitative functional brain mapping with $H_2^{15}O$ and positron emission tomography, *J. Cereb. Blood Flow Metab.*, 4, 329, 1984.

95. **Mazziotta, J. C., Huang, S.-C., Phelps, M. E., Carson, R. E., MacDonald, N. S., and Mahoney, K.**, A noninvasive positron computed tomography technique using oxygen-15-labeled water for the evaluation of neurobehavioral task batteries, *J. Cereb. Blood Flow Metab.*, 5, 70, 1985.

96. **Fox, P. T. and Mintun, M. A.**, Noninvasive functional brain mapping by change-distribution analysis of averaged PET images of $H_2^{15}O$ tissue activity, *J. Nucl. Med.*, 141, 1989.

97. **Iida, H., Higano, S., Tomura, N., Shishido, F., Kanno I., Miura, S., Murakami, M., Takahashi, K., Sasaki, H., and Uemura, K.**, Evaluation of regional differences of tracer appearance time in cerebral tissues using [^{15}O]water and dynamic positron emission tomography, *J. Cereb Blood Flow Metab.*, 8, 285, 1988.

98. **Iida, H., Kanno, I., Miura, S., Takahashi, K., and Uemura, K.**, Error analysis of a quantitative cerebral blood flow measurement using $H_2^{15}O$ autoradiography and positron emission tomography, with respect to the dispersion of the input function, *J. Cereb. Blood Flow Metab.*, 6, 536, 1986.

99. **Hutchins, G. D., Hichwa, R. D., and Koeppe, R. A.**, A continuous flow input function detector for O-15 H_2O blood flow studies in positron emission tomography, *IEEE Trans. Nucl. Sci.*, NS-33, 546, 1986.

100. **Eriksson, L., Holte, S., Bohm, C., Kesselberg, M., and Hovander, B.**, Automated blood sampling systems for positron emission tomography, *IEEE Trans. Nucl. Sci.*, NS-35,703, 1988.

101. **Huang, S.-C., Carson, R. E., and Phelps, M. E.**, Measurement of local blood flow and distribution volume with short-lived isotopes: a general input technique, *J. Cereb. Blood Flow Metab.*, 2, 99, 1982.

102. **Huang, S.-C., Carson, R. E., Hoffman, E. J., Carson, J., MacDonald, N., Barrio, J. R., and Phelps, M. E.**, Quantitative measurement of local cerebral blood flow in humans by positron computed tomography and ^{15}O-water, *J. Cereb. Blood Flow Metab.*, 3, 141, 1983.

103. **Alpert, N. M., Eriksson, L., Chang, J. Y., Bergstrom, M., Litton, J. E., Correia, J. A., Bohm, C., Ackerman, R. H., and Taveras, J. M.**, Strategy for the measurement of regional cerebral blood flow using short-lived tracers and emission tomography, *J. Cereb. Blood Flow Metab.*, 4, 28, 1984.

104. **Carson, R. E., Huang, C.-C., and Green, M. V.**, Weighted integration method for local cerebral blood flow measurements with positron emission tomography, *J. Cereb. Blood Flow Metab.*, 6, 245, 1986.

105. **Koeppe, R. A., Holden, J. E., and Ip, W. R.**, Performance comparison of parameter estimation techniques for the quantitation of local cerebral blood flow by dynamic positron computed tomography, *J. Cereb. Blood Flow Metab.*, 5, 224, 1985.

106. **Eichling, J. O., Raichle, M. E., Grubb, R. J., Jr., and Ter-Pogossian, M. M.**, Evidence of the limitations of water as a freely diffusible tracer in the brain of the rhesus monkey, *Circ. Res.*, 35, 358, 1974.

107. **Herscovitch, P., Raichle, M. E., Kilbourn, M. R., and Welch, M. J.,** Positron emission tomographic measurements of cerebral blood flow and permeability-surface area product of water using [^{15}O] water and [^{11}C]butanol, *J. Cereb. Blood Flow Metab.*, 7, 527, 1987.

108. **Holden, J. E., Gatley, S. J., Nickles, R. J., Koeppe, R. A., Celesia, G. G., and Polcyn, R. E.,** Regional cerebral blood flow measurement with fluoromethane and positron emission tomography, in *Positron Emission Tomography of the Brain*, Heiss, W.-D. and Phelps, M. E., Eds., Springer-Verlag, Berlin, 1983, 90.

109. **Koeppe, R. A., Holden, J. E., Polcyn, R. E., Nickles, R. J., Hutchins, G. D., and Weese, J. L.,** Quantitation of local cerebral blood flow and partition coefficient without arterial sampling: theory and validation, *J. Cereb. Blood Flow Metab.*, 5, 214, 1985.

110. **Stone-Elander, S., Roland, P., Eriksson, L., Litton, J.-E., and Johnström, P.,** The preparation of ^{11}C-labelled fluoromethane for the study of regional cerebral blood flow using positron emission tomography, *Eur. J. Nucl. Med.*, 12, 236, 1986.

111. **Lammertsma, A. A. and Jones, T.,** Correction for the presence of intravascular oxygen-15 in the steady state technique for measuring regional oxygen extraction ratio in the brain. I. Description of the method, *J. Cereb. Blood Flow Metab.*, 13, 416, 1983.

112. **Lammerstma, A. A., Wise, R. J. S., Heather, J. D., Gibbs, J. M., Leenders, K. L., Frackowiak, R. S. J., Rhodes, C. G., and Jones, T.,** Correction for the presence of intravascular oxygen-15 in the steady-state technique for measuring regional oxygen extraction ratio in the brain: 2. Results in normal subjects and brain tumor and stroke patients, *J. Cereb. Blood Flow Metab.*, 3, 425, 1983.

113. **Pantano, P., Baron, J.-C., Crouzel, C., Collard, P., Sirou, P., and Samson, Y.,** The ^{15}O continuous-inhalation method: correction for intravascular signal using C^{15}O, *Eur. J. Nucl. Med.*, 10, 387, 1985.

114. **Lammertsma, A. A., Baron, J.-C., and Jones, T.,** Correction for intravascular activity in the oxygen-15 steady-state technique is independent of the regional hematocrit, *J. Cereb. Blood Flow Metab.*, 7, 372, 1987.

115. **Herscovitch, P. and Raichle, M. E.,** Effect of tissue heterogeneity on the measurement of regional cerebral oxygen extraction and metabolic rate with positron emission tomography, *J. Cereb. Blood Flow Metab.*, 5(Suppl. 1), S671, 1985.

116. **Correia, J. A., Alpert, N. M., Buxton, R. B., and Ackerman, R. H.,** Analysis of some errors in the measurement of oxygen extraction and oxygen consumption by the equilibrium inhalation method, *J. Cereb. Blood Flow Metab.*, 5, 591, 1985.

117. **Herscovitch, P., Mintun, M. A., and Raichle, M. E.,** Brain oxygen utilization measured with oxygen-15 radiotracers and positron emission tomography: generation of metabolic images, *J. Nucl. Med.*, 26, 416, 1985.

118. **Huang, S.-C., Feng, D., and Phelps, M. E.,** Model dependency and estimation reliability in measurement of cerebral oxygen utilization rate with oxygen-15 and dynamic positron emission tomography, *J. Cereb. Blood Flow Metab.*, 6, 105, 1986.

119. **Meyer, E., Tyler, J. L., Thompson, C. J., Redies, C., Diksic, M., and Hakim, A. M.,** Estimation of cerebral oxygen utilization rate by single-bolus ^{15}O$_2$ inhalation and dynamic positron emission tomography, *J. Cereb. Blood Flow Metab.*, 7, 403, 1987.

120. **Sokoloff, L., Reivich, M., Kennedy, C., Des Rosiers, M. H., Patlak, C. S., Pettigrew, K. D., Sakurada, O., and Shinohara, M.,** The [^{14}C]deoxyglucose method for the measurement of local cerebral glucose utilization: theory, procedure, and normal values in the conscious and anesthetized albino rat, *J. Neurochem.*, 28, 897, 1977.

121. **Sokoloff, L. and Smith, C. B.,** Basic principles underlying radioisotopic methods for assay of biochemical processes in vivo, in *The Metabolism of the Human Brain Studied with Positron Emission Tomography*, Greitz, T., Ingvar, D. H., and Widen, L., Eds., Raven Press, New York, 1985, 123.

122. **Reivich, M., Kuhl, D., Wolf, A., Greenberg, J., Phelps, M., Ido, T., Casella, V., Fowler, J., Hoffman, E., Alavi, A., Som, P., and Sokoloff, L.,** The (^{18}F)-fluorodeoxy-glucose method for the measurement of local cerebral glucose utilization in man, *Circ. Res.*, 44, 127, 1979.

123. **Phelps, M. E., Huang, S.-C., Hoffman, E. J., Selin, C., Sokoloff, L., and Kuhl, D. E.,** Tomographic measurement of local cerebral glucose metabolic rate in humans with (F-18) 2-fluoro-2-deoxy-D-glucose: validation of method, *Ann. Neurol.*, 6, 371, 1979.

124. **Huang, S.-C., Phelps, M. E., Hoffman, E. J., Sideris, K., Selin, C. J., and Kuhl, D. E.,** Non-invasive determination of local cerebral metabolic rate of glucose in man, *Am. J. Physiol.*, 238, E69, 1980.

125. **Huang, S.-C., Phelps, M. E., Hoffman, E. J., and Kuhl, D. E.,** Error sensitivity of fluorodeoxyglucose method for measurement of cerebral metabolic rate of glucose, *J. Cereb. Blood Flow Metab.*, 1, 391, 1981.

126. **Cunningham, V. and Cremer, J. E.,** Current assumptions behind the use of PET scanning for measuring glucose utilization in brain, *Trends Neurosci.*, 8, 96, 1985.

127. **Hawkins, R. A., Phelps, M. E., Huang, S.-C., and Kuhl, D. E.,** Effect of ischemia on quantification of local cerebral glucose metabolic rate in man, *J. Cereb. Blood Flow Metab.*, 1, 37, 1981.

128. **Wienhard, K., Pawlik, G., Herholz, K., Wagner, R., and Heiss, W.-D.,** Estimation of local cerebral glucose utilization by positron emission tomography of {^{18}F}2-fluoro-2-deoxy-D-glucose, A critical appraisal of optimization procedures, *J. Cereb. Blood Flow Metab.*, 5, 115, 1985.

129. **Brooks, R. A.,** Alternative formula for glucose utilization using labeled deoxyglucose, *J. Nucl. Med.*, 23, 538, 1982.

130. **Hutchins, G. D., Holden, J. E., Koeppe, R.A., Halama, J. R., Gatley, S. J., and Nickles, R. J.,** Alternative approach to single-scan estimation of cerebral glucose metabolic rate using glucose analogs, with particular application to ischemia, *J. Cereb. Blood Flow Metab*, 4, 35, 1984.

131. **Lammertsma, A. A., Brooks, D. J., Frackowiak, R. S. J., Beany, R. P., Herold, S., Heather, J. D., Palmer, A. J., and Jones, T.,** Measurement of glucose utilization with [^{18}F]2-fluoro-2-deoxy-D-glucose, a comparison of different analytical methods, *J. Cereb. Blood Flow Metab.*, 7, 161, 1987.

132. **Kato, A., Diksic, M., Yamamoto, Y. L., Strother, S. C., and Feindel, W.,** An improved method for measurement of regional cerebral rate constants in the deoxyglucose method with positron emission tomography, *J. Cereb. Blood Flow Metab.*, 4, 555, 1984.

133. **Hawkins, R. A., Phelps, M. E., and Huang, S.-C.,** Effects of temporal sampling, glucose metabolic rates, and disruptions of the blood-barrier on the FDG model with and without a vascular compartment: studies in human brain tumors with PET, *J. Cereb. Blood Flow Metab.*, 6, 170, 1986.

134. **Sasaki, H., Kanno, I., Murakami, M., Shishido, F., and Uemera, K.,** Tomographic mapping of kinetic rate constants in the fluorodeoxyglucose model using dynamic positron emission tomography, *J. Cereb. Blood Flow Metab.*, 6, 447, 1986.

135. **Evans, A. C., Diksic, M., Yamamoto, Y. L., Kato, A., Dagher, A., Redies, C., and Hakim, A.,** Effect of vascular activity in the determination of rate constants for the uptake of ^{18}F-labeled 2-fluoro-2-deoxy-D-glucose: error analysis and normal values in older subjects, *J. Cereb. Blood Flow Metab.*, 6, 724, 1986.

136. **Reivich, M., Alavi, A., Wolf, A., Greenberg, J. H., Fowler, J., Christman, D., MacGregor, R., and Jones, S. C, London, J., Shiue, C., and Yonekura, Y.,** Use of 2-deoxy-D[1-^{11}C]glucose for the determination of local cerebral glucose metabolism in humans: variation within and between subjects, *J. Cereb. Blood Flow Metab.*, 2, 307, 1982.

137. **Pardridge, W. M., Crane, P. D., Mietus, L. J., and Oldendorf, W. H.,** Kinetics of regional blood-brain barrier transport and brain phosphorylation of glucose and 2-deoxyglucose in the barbituate-anesthetized rat, *J. Neurochem.*, 38,, 560, 1982.

138. **Ginsberg, M. D. and Reivich, M.,** Use of the 2-deoxyglucose method of local cerebral glucose utilization in the abnormal brain: evaluation of the lumped constant during ischemia, *Acta Neurol. Scand.*, 60, (Suppl. 72), 226, 1979.

139. **Nakai, H., Yamamoto, Y. L., Diksic, M., Matsuda, H., Takara, E., Meyer, E. and Redies, C.,** Time-dependent changes of lumped and rate constants in the deoxyglucose method in experimental cerebral ischemia, *J. Cereb. Blood Flow Metab.*, 7, 640, 1987.

140. **Gjedde, A., Wienhard, K., Heiss, W.-D., Kloster, G., Diemer, N. H., Herholz, K., and Pawlik G.,** Comparative regional analysis of 2-fluorodeoxyglucose and methylglucose uptake in brain of four stroke patients. With special reference to the regional estimation of the lumped constant, *J. Cereb. Blood Flow Metab.*, 5, 163, 1985.

141. **Takei, H., Fredericks, W. R., Rapoport, S. I.,** The lumped constant in the deoxyglucose procedure declines with age in Fischer-344 rats, *J. Neurochem.*, 46, 931, 1986.

142. **Bida, G. T., Satyamurthy, N., and Barrio, J. R.,** The synthesis of 2-[F-18]fluoro-2-deoxy-D-glucose using glycals: a reexamination, *J. Nucl. Med.*, 25, 1327, 1984.

143. **Braun, A. R., Carson, R. E., Finn, R. D., Adams, H. R., Francis, B. E., Stein, S., and Packer, M. J.,** Kinetic comparison of F-18 2-fluoro-2-deoxyglucose and F-18 2-fluoro-2-deoxymannose using PET, *J. Nucl. Med.*, 29 (Abstr.), 772, 1988.

144. **Reivich, M., Alavi, A., Wolf, A., Fowler, J., Russell, J., Arnett, C., MacGregor, R. R., Shiue, C. Y., Atkins, H., Anand, A., Dann, R., and Greenberg, J. H.,** Glucose metabolic rate kinetic model parameter determination in humans: the lumped constants and rate constants for [^{18}F]fluorodeoxyglucose and [^{11}C]deoxyglucose, *J. Cereb. Blood Flow Metab.*, 5, 179, 1985.

145. **Brooks, R. A., Di Chiro, G., Zukerberg, B. W., Bairamian, D., and Larson, S. M.,** Test-retest studies of cerebral glucose metabolism using fluorine-18 deoxyglucose: validation of method, *J. Nucl. Med.*, 28, 53, 1987.

146. **Chang, J. Y., Duara, R., Barker, W., Apicella, A., and Finn, R.,** Two behavioral states studied in a single PET/FDG procedure: theory, method, and preliminary results, *J. Nucl. Med.*, 28, 852, 1987.

147. **Chang, J. Y., Duara, R., Barker, W., Apicella, A., Yoshii, F., Kelley, R. E., Ginsberg, M. D., and Boothe, T. E.,** Two behavioral states studied in a single PET/FDG procedure: error analysis, *J. Nucl. Med.*, 30, 93, 1989.

148. **Mintun, M. A., Raichle, M. E., Welch, M. J., and Kilbourn, M. R.,** Brain glucose metabolism measured with PET and U-^{11}C-glucose, *J. Cereb. Blood Flow Metab.*, 5(Suppl. 1), S623, 1985.

149. **Blomqvist, G., Bergstrom, K., Bergstrom, M., Ehrin, E., Eriksson, L., Garmelius, B., Lindberg, B., Lilja, A., Litton, J.-E., Lundmark, L., Lundqvist, H., Malmborg, P., Mostrom, U., Nilsson, L., Stone-Elander, S., and Widen, L.,** Models for ^{11}C-glucose, in *The Metabolism of the Human Brain Studied with Positron Emission Tomography,* Greitz, T., Ingvar, D. H., and Widen, L., Eds., Raven Press, New York, 1985, 185.

150. **Lear, J. L. and Ackermann, R. F.,** Comparison of cerebral glucose metabolic rates measured with fluorodeoxyglucose and glucose labelled in the 1,2,3-4, and 6 positions using double label quantitative digital autoradiography, *J. Cereb. Blood Flow Metab.,* 8, 575, 1988.

151. **Blomqvist, G.,** On the construction of functional maps in positron emission tomography, *J. Cereb. Blood Flow Metab.,* 4, 629, 1984.

152. **Wong, D. F., Wagner, H. N., Jr., Dannals, R. F., Links, J. M., Frost, J. J., Ravert, H. T., Wilson, A. A., Rosenbaum, A. E., Gjedde, A., Douglass, K. H., Petronis, J. D., Folstein, M. F., Toung, J. K. T., Burns, H. D., and Kuhar, M. J.,** Effects of age on dopamine and serotonin receptors measured by positron tomography in the living brain, *Science,* 226, 1393, 1984.

153. **Perlmutter, J. S., Larson, K. B., Raichle, M. E., Markham, J., Mintun, M. A., Kilbourn, M. R. and Welch, J. J.,** Strategies for in vivo measurement of receptor binding using positron emission tomography, *J. Cereb. Blood Flow Metab.,* 6, 154, 1986.

154. **Fox, P. T. and Raichle, M. E.,** Stimulus rate dependence of regional cerebral blood flow in human striate cortex, demonstrated by positron emission tomography, *J. Neurophysiol.* 51, 1109, 1984.

155. **Perlmutter, J. S. and Raichle, M. E.,** Regional blood flow in hemi-parkinsonism, *Neurology,* 35, 1127, 1985.

156. **Perlmutter, J. S., Herscovitch, P., Powers, W. J., Fox, P. T., and Raichle, M. E.,** Standardized mean regional method for calculating global positron emission tomography measurements, *J. Cereb. Blood Flow Metab.,* 5, 476, 1985.

157. **Mazziotta, J. C.,** Physiologic neuroanatomy: new brain imaging methods present a challenge to an old discipline, *J. Cereb. Blood Flow Metab.,* 4, 481, 1984.

158. **Mazziotta, J. C. and Koslow, S. H.,** Assessment of goals and obstacles in data acquisition and analysis from emission tomography: report of a series of international workshops, *J. Cereb. Blood Flow Metab.,* 7, S1, 1987.

159. **Strother, S. and Perlmutter, J. S.,** Headholders for functional brain imaging, *J. Cereb. Blood Flow Metab.,* 7, S16, 1987.

160. **Fox, P. T., Perlmutter, J. S., and Raichle, M. E.,** A stereotactic method of anatomical localization for positron emission tomography, *J. Comput. Assist. Tomogr.,* 9, 141, 1985.

161. **Kearfott, K. J., Rottenberg, D. A., and Knowles, R. J. R.,** A new headholder for PET, CT, and NMR, *J. Comput. Assist. Tomogr.,* 8, 1217, 1984.

162. **Mazziotta, J. C., Phelps, M.E., Meadors, A. K., Ricci, A., Winter, J., and Bentson, J. R.,** Anatomical localization schemes for use in positron computed tomography using a specially designed headholder, *J. Comput. Assist. Tomogr.,* 6, 848, 1982.

163. **Bergstrom, M., Boethius, J., Eriksson, L., Grietz, T., Ribbe, T., and Widen, L.,** Head fixation device for reproducible position alignment in transmission CT and positron emission tomography, *J. Comput. Assist. Tomogr.,* 5, 136, 1981.

164. **Kempner, K., Stein, S. and Green, M.,** An image independent method of evaluating the efficacy of head restraint devices used in brain imaging, *J. Nucl. Med. Technol.,* 15, Ab 10, 1987.

165. **Conti, J., Deck, M. D. F., and Rottenberg, D. A.,** An inexpensive video patient repositioning system for use with transmission and emission computed tomographs, *J. Comput. Assist. Tomogr.,* 6, 417, 1982.

166. **Duara, R., Grady, C., Haxby, J., Ingvar, D., Sokoloff, L., Margolin, R. A., Manning, R. G., Cutler, N. R., and Rapoport, S. I.,** Human brain glucose utilization and cognitive function in relation to age, *Ann. Neurol.,* 16, 702, 1984.

167. **Kuhl, D. E., Phelps, M. E., Markham, C. H., Metter, E. J., Reige, W. H. and Winter, J.,** Cerebral metabolism and atrophy in Huntington's disease determined by ^{18}FDG and computed tomographic scan, *Ann. Neurol.,* 12, 425, 1982.

168. **Evans, A. C., Beil, C., Marrett, S., Thompson, C. J., and Hakim, A.,** Anatomical-functional correlation using an adjustable MRI-based region of interest atlas with positron emission tomography, *J. Cereb. Flow Metab.* 8, 513, 1988.

169. **Pelizzari, C. A., Chen, G. T. Y., Spelbring, D. R., Weichselbaum, R. R., Chen, C.-T.,** Accurate three-dimensional registration of CT, PET, and/or MR images of the brain, *J. Comput. Assist. Tomogr.,* 13, 20, 1989.

170. **Bohm, C., Greitz, T., Kingsley, D., Berggren, B. M., and Olsson, L.,** Adjustable computerized stereotaxic brain atlas for transmission and emission tomography, *AJNR,* 4, 731, 1983.

171. **Herholz, K., Pawlik, G., Wienhard, K., and Heiss, W.-D.,** Computer assisted mapping in quantitative analysis of cerebral positron emission tomograms, *J. Comput. Assist. Tomogr.,* 9, 154, 1985.

172. **Metter, E. J., Riege, W. H., Kuhl, D. E., and Phelps, M. E.,** Cerebral metabolic relationships for selected brain regions in healthy adults, *J. Cereb. Blood Flow Metab.,* 4, 1, 1984.

173. Tyler, J. L., Strother, S. C., Zatorre, R. J., Alivisatos, B., Worsley, K. J., Diksic, M., and Yamamoto, Y. L., Stability of regional cerebral glucose metabolism in the normal brain measured by positron emission tomography, *J. Nucl. Med.*, 29, 631, 1985.

174. Perlmutter, J. S., Powers, W. J., Herscovitch, P., Fox, P. T., and Raichle, M. E., Regional asymmetries of cerebral blood flow, blood volume, oxygen utilization and extraction in normal subjects, *J. Cereb. Blood Flow Metab.*, 7, 64, 1987.

175. Mazziotta, J. C., Phelps, M. E., Pahl, J. J., Huang, S.-C., Baxter, L. R., Riege, W. H., Hoffman, J. M., Kuhl, D. E., Lanto, A. B., Wapenski, J. A., and Markham, C. H., Reduced cerebral glucose metabolism in asymptomatic subjects at risk for Huntington's disease, *N. Engl. J. Med.*, 316, 357, 1987.

176. Berent, S., Giordani, B., Lehtinen, S., Markel, D., Penney, J. B., Buchtel, H. A., Starosta-Rubenstein, S., Hichwa, R., and Young, A. B., Positron emission tomographic scan investigations in Huntington's disease: cerebral metabolic correlates of cognitive function, *Ann. Neurol.*, 23, 541, 1988.

177. Cutler, N. R., Haxby, J. V., Duara, R., Grady, C. L., Kay, A. D., Kessler, R. M., Sundaram, M., and Rapoport, S. I., Clinical history, brain metabolism, and neuropsychological function in Alzheimer's disease, *Ann. Neurol.*, 18, 298, 1985.

178. Clark, C. M., Kessler, R., Buchsbaum, M. S., Margolin, R. A., and Holcomb, H. H., Correlational methods for determining regional coupling of cerebral glucose metabolism: a pilot study, *Biol. Psychiatry*, 19, 663, 1984.

179. Horwitz, B., Duara, R., and Rapoport, S. I., Intercorrelations of glucose metabolic rates between brain regions: application to healthy males in a state of reduced sensory input, *J. Cereb. Blood Flow Metab.*, 4, 484, 1984.

180. Ford, I., Confounded correlations: statistical limitations in the analysis of interregional relationships of cerebral metabolic activity, *J. Cereb. Blood Flow Metab.*, 6, 385, 1986.

181. Clark, C., Carson, R., Kessler, R., Margolin, R., Buchsbaum, M., DeLisi, L., King, C., and Cohen, R., Alternative statistical models for the examination of clinical positron emission tomography/fluorodeoxyglucose data, *J. Cereb. Blood Flow Metab.*, 5, 142, 1985.

182. Moeller, J. R., Strother, S. C., Sidtis, J. J., and Rottenberg, D. A., Scaled subprofile model: a statistical approach to the analysis of functional patterns in positron emission tomographic data, *J. Cereb. Blood Flow Metab.*, 7, 649, 1987.

183. Fox, P. T., Mintun, M. A., Reiman, E. M., and Raichle, M. E. Enhanced detection of focal brain responses using intersubject averaging and change-distribution analysis of subtracted PET images. *J. Cereb. Blood Flow Metab.*, 8, 642, 1988

184. Mintun, M. A., Fox, P. T., and Raichle, M. E., A highly accurate method of localizing regions of neuronal activation in the human brain with positron emission tomography, *J. Cereb. Flow Metab.*, 9, 96, 1989.

185. Petersen, S. E., Fox, P. T., Posner, M. I., Mintun, M., and Raichle, M. E., Positron emission tomographic studies of the cortical anatomy of single-word processing, *Nature*, 331, 585, 1988.

186. Reiman, E. M., Fusselman, J. J., Fox, P. T., and Raichle, M. E., Neuroanatomical correlates of anticipatory anxiety, *Science*, 243, 1071, 1989.

187. Creasy, H. and Rapoport, S. I., The aging human brain, *Ann. Neurol.*, 17, 2, 1985.

188. Gur, R. C., Gur, R. E., Obrist, W. D., Hungerbuhler, J. P., Younkin, D., Rosen, A. D., Skolnick, B. E., and Reivich, M., Sex and handedness differences in cerebral blood flow during rest and cognitive activity, *Science*, 217, 659, 1982.

189. Baxter, L. R., Jr., Mazziotta, J. C. Phelps, M. E., Selin, C. E., Guze, B. H., and Fairbanks, L., Cerebral glucose metabolic rates in normal human females versus normal males, *Psychiatr. Res.*, 21, 237, 1987.

190. Yoshii, F., Barker, W. W., Chang, J. Y., Loewenstein, D., Apicella, A., Smith, D., Boothe, T., Ginsberg, M. D., Pascal, S., and Duara, R., Sensitivity of cerebral glucose metabolism to age, gender, brain volume, brain atrophy, and cerebrovascular risk factors, *J. Cereb. Blood Flow Metab.*, 8, 654, 1988.

191. Geschwind, N. and Galaburda, A. M., Cerebral lateralization. Biological mechanisms, associations, and pathology. I. A hypothesis and a program for research, *Arch. Neurol.*, 42, 428, 1985.

192. Mazziotta, J. C. and Phelps, M. E., Results and strategies in studies of human sensory stimulation and deprivation with positron emission tomography, in *The Metabolism of the Human Brain Studied with Positron Emission Tomography*, Greitz, T., Ingvar, D. H., and Widen, L., Eds., Raven Press, New York, 1985, 315.

193. Yarowsky, P. J. and Ingvar, D. H., Neuronal activity and energy metabolism, *Fed. Proc.*, 40, 2353, 1981.

194. Fox, P. T. and Raichle, M. E., Focal physiological uncoupling of cerebral blood flow and oxidative metabolism during somatosensory stimulation in human subjects, *Proc. Natl. Acad. Sci. U.S.A.*, 83, 1140, 1986.

195. Lou, H. C., Edvinsson, L., and MacKenzie, E. T., The concept of coupling blood flow to brain function: revision required?, *Ann. Neurol.*, 22, 289, 1987.

196. **Fox, P. T., Raichle, M. E., Mintun, M. A. and Dence, C.,** Nonoxidative glucose consumption during focal physiologic neural activity, *Science,* 241, 462, 1988.
197. **Albers, R. W., Siegel, G. J., and Stahl, W. L.,** Membrane transport, in *Basic Neurochemistry,* Siegel, G., Agranoff, B., Albers, R. W., and Moulinoff, P., Eds., Raven Press, New York, 1989, chap. 3.
198. **Schwartz, W. J., Smith, C. B., Davidsen, L., Savaki, H., Sokoloff, L., Mata, M., Fink, D. J., and Gainer, H.** Metabolic mapping of functional activity in the hypothalamo-neurohypophysial system of the rat, *Science,* 205, 723, 1979.
199. **Kadekaro, M., Vance, W. H., Terrell, M. L., Gary, H., Jr., Elsenberg, H. M., and Sokoloff, L.** Effects of antidromic stimulation of the ventral root on glucose utilization system of the rat, *Proc. Natl. Acad. Sci. U.S.A.,* 84, 5492, 1987.
200. **Ackerman, R. F., Finch, D. M., Babb, T. L., and Engel, J., Jr.,** Increased glucose metabolism during long-duration recurrent inhibition of hippocampal pyramidal cells, *J. Neurosci.,* 4, 251, 1984.
201. **Yarowsky, P., Kadekaro, M., and Sokoloff, L.,** Frequency-dependent activation of glucose utilization in the superior cervical ganglion by electrical stimulation of the cervical sympathetic trunk, *Proc. Natl. Acad. Sci. U.S.A.,* 80, 4179, 1983.
202. **Lebrun-Grandie, P., Baron, J.-C., Soussaline, F., Loch'h, C., Sastre, J., and Bousser, M.-G.,** Coupling between regional blood flow and oxygen utilization in the normal brain, *Arch. Neurol.,* 40, 230, 1983.
203. **Wooten, G. F. and Collins, R. C.,** Metabolic effects on unilateral lesions of the substantia nigra, *J. Neurosci.,* 1, 285, 1981.
204. **Videen, T. O., Perlmutter, J. S., Mintun, M. A., and Raichle, M. E.,** Regional correction of positron emission tomography data for the effects of cerebral atrophy, *J. Cereb. Blood Flow Metab.,* 8, 662, 1988.
205. **Martin, W. R. W., Bechman, J. H., Caine, D. B., Adam, M. J., Harrop, R., Rogers, J. G., Ruth, T. J., Sayre, C. I., and Pate, B. D.,** Cerebral glucose metabolism in Parkinson's disease, *Can. J. Neurol. Sci.,* 11 (Suppl.), 169, 1984.

Chapter 2

NEUROTRANSMITTERS AND RECEPTORS IN THE BASAL GANGLIA

Anne B. Young and John B. Penney

TABLE OF CONTENTS

I. INTRODUCTION

The basal ganglia consist of a group of gray matter structures beneath the cerebral cortex and surrounding the thalamus and hypothalamus. They appear to be responsible for modulating and facilitating various motor and cognitive programs. Since the anatomy and physiology of the basal ganglia are extremely complex, the exact mechanisms by which the basal ganglia subserve these functions are unknown.

Considerable new information, however, has become available recently about the neurochemical anatomy of the internal organization of the striatum and its projections. The basal ganglia structures important to the control of movement include the caudate nucleus, the putamen, the globus pallidus (both internal and external segments), the subthalamic nucleus and the substantia nigra (pars compacta and pars reticulata) (Figure 1). Over the last three to four decades, the connections among these structures and between them and other regions of the brain have been worked out in some detail. Despite this extensive knowledge, questions about the function of these brain regions remain unanswered. In particular, diseases of the basal ganglia result in a variety of abnormal movements. These abnormal movements range from extreme hypokinesia to hyperkinesia. Parkinson's disease is the prototypic hypokinetic syndrome characterized by bradykinesia, rigidity, tremor, and loss of postural reflexes.[1] In contrast, Huntington's disease, the classic hyperkinetic syndrome, is characterized by chorea, abnormal saccadic eye movements, slowed and irregular fine motor coordination, and in advanced cases dystonia, rigidity and loss of postural reflexes.[2] Other presumed basal ganglia disorders which result in abnormal movements ranging from severe akinesia to severe hyperkinesia include progressive supranuclear palsy, Wilson's disease, Hallervorden-Spatz disease, dystonia musculorum deformans, other focal dystonias (blepharospasm, torticollis, cranial dystonia), hemiballismus, and striatonigral degeneration. These disorders also manifest superimposed abnormal movements such as dystonia, athetosis, and tremor. Although strength is preserved in most basal ganglia disorders, the speed, sequencing, and fluidity of individual movements or series of movements are greatly impaired.

Post-mortem biochemical studies have yielded important insights into basal ganglia pathophysiology but much information is still needed to complete our understanding of basal ganglia function. *In vivo* studies of basal ganglia function and biochemistry should provide important data on changes that occur early in various disease states. In this chapter, we will describe normal basal ganglia anatomy and neurochemical connections.

II. ANATOMY OF THE BASAL GANGLIA

Details of basal ganglia anatomy and physiology have been reviewed elsewhere.[3-9] Three decades ago the existence of the biogenic amine, dopamine, in brain was first demonstrated.[10] Shortly after this demonstration, investigators discovered a deficiency of dopamine in the brains of patients with Parkinson's disease.[11] Histofluoresence techniques were then developed which showed a major pathway from neuronal cell bodies in the substantia nigra pars compacta projecting to the caudate nucleus and putamen.[12-13] The subsequent development of specific therapies for Parkinson's disease was based on the biochemical observation that this pathway was defective in Parkinson's disease.[14] The nigrostriatal dopamine pathway is now known to influence basal ganglia function in a modulatory fashion controlling the activity of cortical inputs to the caudate/putamen and the activity of striatal interneurons and projection neurons.[15]

The primary afferent pathways to the caudate/putamen come not from the substantia nigra, but rather from the cerebral cortex. All areas of the cerebral cortex send somatotopically organized excitatory projections to some parts of the neostriatum (the olfactory tubercle, the nucleus accumbens, the caudate nucleus, and the putamen).[3,16] This corticostriatal pathway

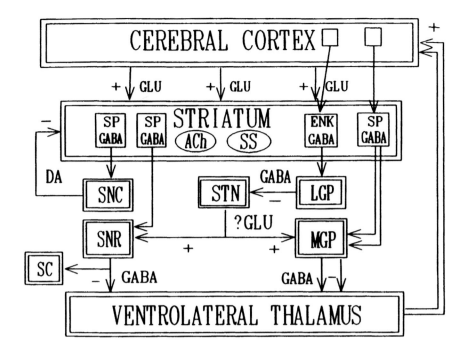

FIGURE 1. A simplified model of basal ganglia circuitry was constructed based on our current understanding of striatal functional anatomy. Abbreviations: LGP = lateral globus pallidus, MGP = medial globus pallidus, SNR = substantia nigra pars reticulata, SNC = substantia nigra pars compacta, STN = subthalamic nucleus, SC = superior colliculus, GLU = glutamic acid, ACh = acetylcholine, SS = somatostatin, ENK = enkephalin, DA = dopamine. (Modified from Young, A. B., Albin, R. L., and Penney, J. B., in *Neural Mechanisms in Disorders of Movement*, Crossman, A. R. and Sambrook, M. A., Eds., John Libbey, London, 1989, 17.)

apparently uses an excitatory amino acid as its neurotransmitter.[17,20] The neostriatum also receives input from a variety of other structures including the intralaminar nuclei of the thalamus (neurotransmitter unknown),[3,21] the substantia nigra pars compacta and ventral tegmental area (dopamine)[22] and the raphe nuclei (serotonin).[5,6]

The caudate/putamen itself contains several different neuronal types. The most abundant neuron is the medium spiny neuron which is thought to use gamma-aminobutyric acid (GABA) as its neurotransmitter.[23] These neurons comprise from 70 to 90% of the neurons within the caudate/putamen and often contain one or more of a number of neuropeptides in addition to GABA.[5,6,8] The medium spiny neurons project to the major output regions of the basal ganglia, which are discussed below. They also have a large number of recurrent axon collaterals that are distributed primarily within the dendritic field of the neuron.[25,26] In addition to the medium spiny neurons, there are also small numbers of large cholinergic interneurons (large aspiny neurons)[27] and small somatostatin/neuropeptide Y interneurons (small aspiny neurons).[28,29]

The neostriatal projection areas include the lateral globus pallidus (LGP), the medial globus pallidus (MGP), and the substantia nigra pars reticulata (SNr).[3,5-7,9] The majority of LGP, MGP, and SNr neurons are large projection neurons with extremely large dendritic fields. Interneurons within these areas are infrequent.[3] All pallidal neurons appear to use GABA as an inhibitory neurotransmitter.[30-32]

The LGP sends projections to the subthalamic nucleus[3,5,6] which also receives a direct excitatory (presumably glutamatergic) projection from the motor cortex. The subthalamic nucleus sends a reciprocal projection back to the striatum, LGP, MGP, and SNr.[3,5,6,33] The neurotransmitter and physiologic actions of the subthalamic nucleus neurons are excitatory and may be glutamatergic.[33-35]

The MGP and SNr send inhibitory GABAergic projections to the ventral tier nuclei of the thalamus.[3,5,6] They also send minor projections to the intralaminar thalamic nuclei and to various brainstem nuclei.[3,5,6] The ventral medial thalamus to which the SNr projects sends excitatory projections to the entire frontal lobe in the rat[36] and, in primates, to the prefrontal cortex with only minor projections to the premotor and supplementary motor cortices.[37,38] The MGP sends its major projection to the ventral lateral thalamic nucleus pars oralis, which in turn projects solely to the supplementary motor cortex.[39] The neurotransmitter of the excitatory thalamocortical pathway is unknown. Within the cerebral cortex itself, there are interconnections between supplementary motor cortex and other motor cortical regions.

A. STRIATAL INHOMOGENEITIES
Recently, additional complexities within the striatum have been described. Initial studies in rodent described heterogeneity of cell density, dopamine innervation, and cholinesterase staining within the caudate/putamen.[40-42] Subsequent studies using histological stains for acetylcholinesterase (AChE) demonstrated irregularities within the striatum in both fetal and adult brain.[43] During fetal development, regions of intense AChE staining have been termed "patches" or "striosomes" and lighter surrounding areas were termed "matrix".[5] In the adult, this pattern is reversed and the striosome stains less intensely for AChE than the matrix. Dense islands of dopamine terminals, "dopamine islands", were in the fetal and early postnatal developing striatum.[44,45] The dopamine islands become less distinct after birth as other dopamine terminals innervate the remaining areas of the striatum. In the fetus, the areas staining densely for AChE coincide with the dopamine islands. The birth dates of neurons in the striosomes are different from those of the matrix as are their inputs and outputs.[46]

Striosomal neurons receive inputs from dopamine cells in the medial substantia nigra pars compacta (SNc).[47,48] These striosomal cells project back primarily to the SNc, but not to the SNr.[49,50] Although the cortical inputs to striosomal neurons in the primate have not been well characterized, in the rat they originate primarily from medial frontal cortex, but not from other areas of prefrontal, motor or sensory cortex, or from the thalamus.[36,51] The medial frontal cortex in the rat receives projections from dopamine neurons in the ventral tegmental area.[22]

Striosomal neurons stain positively for glutamic acid decarboxylase (GAD)-like immunoreactivity; they also stain intensively for substance P, dynorphin, and possibly neurotensin.[5,6,52] The dendrites of the striosomal neurons appear to obey the boundaries of the striosomes and do not cross into the matrix.

In contrast, the matrix neurons receive inputs from motor, sensory, supplementary motor, and association cortices as well as from the intralaminar nuclei of thalamus.[53-55] The cells of the matrix also receive dopaminergic input from the dopamine cells in the SNc and the ventral tegmental area (VTA).[47,48] The level of dopaminergic input appears lower in the matrix than in the striosomes and the turnover of dopamine in the two regions is different.[56] The medium spiny neurons of the matrix are GABAergic and have projections to the SNr, MGP and LGP.[23,24,57] In the primate, each of these projections appears to be mediated by unique groups of neurons and there are only a limited number of striatal matrix neurons which project to all three areas.[6,58-60] The cells which project to the LGP contain high concentrations of enkephalin, and therefore, there are high concentrations of enkephalin-like immunoreactivity seen in the LGP as compared to the MGP or SNr.[61-63] In contrast, matrix projections to the MGP and the SNr contain high concentrations of substance P and dynorphin.[63-67]

B. FUNCTIONAL CONNECTIONS
Although an in-depth discussion of the functional anatomy of the basal ganglia is beyond the scope of this chapter, a number of lesion and metabolic studies in primate have impli-

cations for understanding basal ganglia physiology and positron emission tomography (PET). Specific lesions in basal ganglia afferents and efferents in primate have been made and animals then assessed with [^{14}C]-2-deoxy-D-glucose uptake. Similar studies have been carried out in rats and in some cases have been combined with receptor studies.

After lesions of the sensorimotor cerebral cortex, deoxyglucose uptake decreases prominently in both caudate/putamen and globus pallidus with less change in substantia nigra.[68,69] The striatal changes are presumably due primarily to loss of metabolism in corticostriatal terminals which normally excite striatal neurons. Loss of pallidal metabolism is presumably secondary to transneuronal effects through striatum since there are no known corticopallidal inputs. That the pallidum but not the nigra is affected suggests that cortical inputs may preferentially affect specific striatal projections to pallidum.

MPTP lesions of the substantia nigra pars compacta lead to distinct changes in striatal projection areas. Little change occurs in striatal glucose metabolism but deoxyglucose uptake is increased in lateral pallidum and unchanged in medial pallidum and pars reticulata of substantia nigra.[70,71] Deoxyglucose uptake is actually decreased in subthalamic nucleus. These results suggest that loss of nigrostriatal dopaminergic inputs preferentially disinhibit (or increase) striatal-lateral pallidal activity and thereby inhibit lateral pallidal (inhibitory) input to subthalamic nucleus. When primates, however, are treated with levodopa after MPTP lesions or made choreic with striatal injections of bicuculline, striatal-pallidal output is reduced and pallidal-subthalamic activity is increased resulting in inhibition of the subthalamic neurons. Lesions of the subthalamic nucleus and hypofunction of subthalamic neurons lead to chorea.

In Huntington's disease (HD), glucose metabolism in subthalamic nucleus cannot be measured, but one would predict that it would be increased because of disinhibition of the lateral pallidum. In symptomatic HD, striatal glucose metabolism decreases in concert with the progression of the disease[72] but in presymptomatic individuals glucose metabolism is normal.[73] In fact, in some persons with very early symptomatic HD, the glucose metabolism is within the 95% confidence levels of the mean of controls.[73] One possible explanation for this finding is that only a subgroup of striatal neurons is affected early in the disease and thus the loss of glucose metabolism is minor. Neuropathological data support this notion. Immunocytochemical data suggest that GABA/enkephalin neurons projecting to lateral globus pallidus and GABA/substance P neurons projecting to substantia nigra pars reticulata are affected early in HD whereas somatostatin and acetylcholine interneurons and GABA/substance P neurons projecting to medial pallidum and substantia nigra pars compacta are relatively spared early in the disease.[74-79] Loss of GABA/enkephalin neurons to lateral pallidum would disinhibit the pallidum which would in turn inhibit the subthalamic nucleus excessively leading to chorea. Later in the disorder, dystonia and parkinsonian features would become more prominent as other striatal projections became involved.

Although much remains to be explained in terms of complex circuitry, it appears that striatal afferents differentially affect the activity in striatal subcompartments. It is likely that certain diseases such as Huntington's disease, Parkinson's disease, and dystonia will also impact these compartments selectively.

III. NEUROTRANSMITTER RECEPTORS IN BASAL GANGLIA

Receptor-ligand interactions can be measured two different ways. The biological response to a receptor agonist or antagonist ligand can be measured directly by electrical, behavioral, or biochemical methods. Alternatively, the binding of the ligand to a biological preparation can be determined. By either method, a ligand-receptor interaction should be defined by its saturability, pharmacological and physiological specificity and its reversibility.[80] Since receptor molecules mediate the effects of neurohormones or neurotransmitters, changes in these receptor molecules in various disease states might explain certain aspects of the pathophysiology of neurological disorders.

Traditional biochemical measures of neurotransmitter receptors have examined the binding of high specific activity radiolabeled drugs or ligands to membrane homogenates from brain or other tissues.[80] Recently, autoradiographic techniques have been developed to look at both the biochemistry and pharmacology of receptor binding as well as the anatomy and localization of the binding sites.[81-83] These methods have allowed measurements of receptors in very small regions of the brain that could not be measured accurately using homogenate techniques (Figure 2).

A. DOPAMINE RECEPTORS
1. Properties and Subtypes
The interaction of dopamine with its receptors has been measured using behavioral, electrophysiological and biochemical techniques. Behavioral studies have assessed the effect of drugs on locomotor and stereotypic behavior or on rotation after unilateral nigrostriatal lesions.[84-88] These behavioral models allow the screening of large numbers of agonists and antagonists with relative ease.

The first biochemical measures of the dopamine receptor examined the effects of dopaminergic drugs on cyclic AMP formation in striatal slices.[89] Dopamine was found to increase cyclic AMP by stimulating adenylate cyclase. Although this stimulation was blocked by dopamine antagonists, the pharmacology of dopamine's effects in this assay differed substantially from the pharmacology of the dopaminergic drugs in rotational studies. Furthermore, the clinical potency of various antischizophrenic drugs was found to correlate well with their potency in the rotation assay and their affinity in membrane binding assays, but not as well with their potency in blocking activation of adenylate cyclase.[90-93]

Subsequently, membrane binding studies using radioactively labeled dopamine agonists and antagonists have demonstrated two types of binding sites in striatal membranes.[94-96] One site has a pharmacology very similar to that of the dopamine-stimulated adenylate cyclase, and is called the D-1 receptor.[97] The pharmacology of the other binding site resembles that of neuroleptic potency in the treatment of schizophrenia and in modifying rotational behavior in animals. This latter site is called the D_2 receptor.[94-96] Agonist stimulation of the D_2 receptor actually results in the inhibition of adenylate cyclase in striatal and pituitary membranes.[94-96] The possibility that D_1 and D_2 receptors occur together in the same membrane has been postulated, one to stimulate and the other to inhibit adenylate cyclase. Lesion studies, however, have suggested that at least some D_1 receptors are located on presynapic terminals whereas D_2 receptors appear to exist postsynaptically in striatum but also on the somata and dendrites of substantia nigra dopamine neurons.[99-103] For several years, investigators believed there were two additional binding sites, which were termed the D_3 and D_4 binding sites. However, it is currently believed that these two binding sites merely represented high affinity states of the D_1 and D_2 receptors.[94,95]

The behavioral consequences of D_1 receptor-induced activation of adenylate cyclase are poorly defined but they have many similarities to those of D_2 activation (although important differences also appear).[104,105] With the recent development of selective D_1 agonists and antagonists, specific D_1 induced behaviors can now be examined. The low affinity state of the D_1 receptor has micromolar affinity for dopamine and the high affinity state has nanomolar affinity for dopamine.[94,95] Thioxanthenes (such as *cis*-flupentixol) have nanomolar affinity for blocking the D_1 receptor, butyrophenones (such as haloperidol and spiroperidol) have micromolar affinity for blocking the D_1 receptor, and benzamides (such as sulpiride) are nearly inactive.[94-96] Specific antagonists at the D_1 site include SCH-22390 and SKF-83566.[96,106] Selective D_1 agonists include dihydroxynomifensine and SKF-38393. Labeled SCH-23390 appears to be the most specific D_1 receptor ligand available at the current time.[96,106]

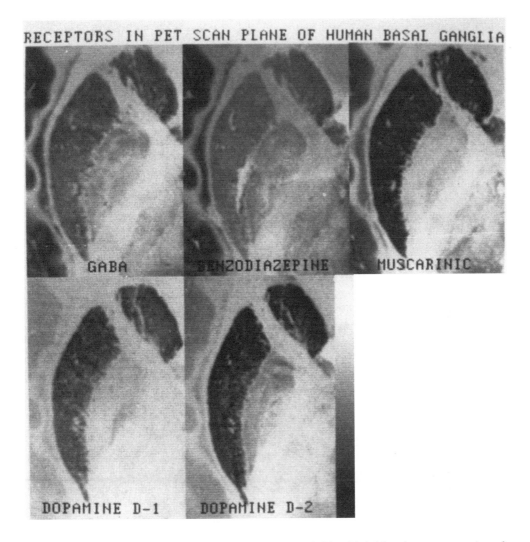

RECEPTORS IN PET SCAN PLANE OF HUMAN BASAL GANGLIA

GABA   BENZODIAZEPINE   MUSCARINIC

DOPAMINE D-1   DOPAMINE D-2

FIGURE 2. Receptor autoradiograms demonstrating the binding of tritium-labeled ligands to cryostat sections of a frozen, post-mortem human brain. The sections were cut in the horizontal plane through the most dorsal part of the medial globus pallidus. In each section the caudate nucleus is at the upper right, the thalamus is at the lower right, the insular cortex is at the extreme left, the claustrum is at mid left and the putamen is in the middle with the lateral globus pallidus to its right and the medial globus pallidus at the farther right. Top left: [³H]Muscimol binding (140 nM) to GABA$_A$ receptors. Binding is densest in layer 4 of cortex. Binding is high in the rest of cortex and in claustrum, moderate in caudate and putamen, and low to moderate in globus pallidus and thalamus. Top center: [³H]Flunitrazepam binding (23 nM) to benzodiazepine receptors. While the density of the binding is greater, the distribution of binding is identical to that of [³H]muscimol. Top right: [³H]Quinuclidinylbenzilate binding (1 nM) to muscarinic cholinergic receptors. Binding is densest in caudate and putamen, high in layer 1 of cortex, moderate in the rest of cortex, claustrum, and thalamus and low in the globus pallidus with medial globus pallidus having slightly more binding than lateral globus pallidus. Bottom left: [³H]SCH 23390 binding (500 pM) to dopamine D$_1$ receptors. Binding is high in caudate and putamen, low in cortex, claustrum, and medial globus pallidus, and very low in lateral globus pallidus and thalamus. Bottom center: [³H]Spiperone binding (275 pM) to dopamine D$_2$ receptors. Binding is high in caudate and putamen, low in cortex, caudate, and lateral globus pallidus, and very low in medial globus pallidus and thalamus.

D$_2$ receptors have very high affinity (nanomolar range) for all neuroleptics (butyrophenones, benzamides and phenothiazines).[94,95] The high affinity state of the D$_2$ receptor has nanomolar affinity for dopamine and the low affinity state, micromolar affinity.[94] The D$_2$ receptor inhibits adenylate cyclase in pituitary and striatum.[94,95] Drugs that act at the D$_2$ site result in marked behavioral effects in animals (rotation, locomotion, anti-Parkinsonian action, psychotomimetic action, emesis, and stereotypy).[95] In man, antagonists at the D_2 site are potent antipsychotic and antiemetic agents and produce signs of Parkinsonism. The most potent D_2 antagonists included the butyrophenones (haloperidol and spiroperidol) and the benzamides (sulpiride, tiapride).[96] The most potent agonists at the D_2 site are the ergot derivatives, pergolide, lisuride, and LY-171555.[96,107] In binding studies, [^{3}H]spiroperidol is commonly used to measure D_2 receptors.

At the current time, animal studies suggest that the maximal stimulation of a dopaminergic effect requires simultaneous activation of the D_1 and D_2 receptors. The two receptors appear to interact synergistically.[108-110] Thus a nonselective drug such as levodopa may significantly enhance the behavioral response to either a D_1 and D_2 agonist alone. If these findings can be confirmed in man, they will have important implications for the treatment of movement disorders.

2. Distribution

In rodents, D_1 receptors are most dense in the striatum and the nucleus accumbens.[111-114] Receptors are also relatively dense in entopeduncular nucleus (the murine equivalent of the medial segment of globus pallidus), ventral pallidum, and substantia nigra (particularly in pars reticulata). In cerebral cortex, particularly frontal regions, D_1 receptors are quite rich in the inner layers (V,VI). Moderate densities of D_1 receptors are seen in the amygdala and the hypothalamus.

There are three times as many D_1 and D_2 receptors in most neostriatal regions (caudate/putamen, nucleus accumbens, olfactory tubercle).[113,114] Nevertheless, they are denser in neostriatum than other areas. In the substantia nigra, D_2 receptors are more dense in the pars compacta than in the reticulata. Very few D_2 receptors are present in pallidal regions (most of them in lateral globus pallidus) or in the cerebral cortex.

In humans and primates, D_1 receptors are distributed in a fashion similar to that in rodents.[114,114a] D_1 receptors are very high in the caudate, putamen, nucleus accumbens, and olfactory tubercle. They are also high in the substantia nigra pars reticulata and the medial globus pallidus. The lateral globus pallidus and substantia nigra pars compacta have very few D_1 receptors. In cerebral cortex, they predominate in both the outer and inner layers of various regions, particularly the prefrontal areas.

D_2 receptors in humans and primates are present in levels about one-third that of D_1 receptors in neostriatum (caudate, putamen, nucleus accumbens, and olfactory tubercle).[114,114a] The D_2 receptors are present in moderate density in the substantia nigra pars compacta where D_1 receptors are very low. In primates and humans, D_2 receptors are observed in mild to moderate amounts in lateral globus pallidus, but not in the medial globus pallidus. Depending on the ligand used, there have been variable numbers of D_2 receptors observed in cerebal cortex.

Inhomogeneities in the striatal distribution of both D_1 and D_2 receptors have been observed in cat, primate and human brains.[113,114] There is some controversy, however, about whether the areas of densest D_2 receptor binding correspond one for one with the areas of densest D_1 receptor binding.[113-117] In adults, neither D_1 nor D_2 receptor inhomogeneities appear to correspond to striosomes as defined by acetylcholinesterase staining.

B. GABA RECEPTORS

GABA is the neurotransmitter used by the majority of neurons in the striatum, lateral and medial pallidum, and the substantia nigra pars reticulata.[23,24] Two classes of GABA receptors have been defined, $GABA_A$ and $GABA_B$ receptors. The $GABA_A$ receptors are postsynaptic receptors mediating chloride flux. These receptors are bicuculline-sensitive and are the classic GABA receptors mediating GABAergic inhibition. $GABA_B$ receptors also appear to mediate inhibition but through bicuculline-insensitive receptors. The $GABA_B$ receptor is located both presynaptically on the terminals of neurons which use transmitters other than GABA and postsynaptically. There are no selective antagonists at the $GABA_B$ receptor and the only selective agonist is baclofen.

$GABA_A$ receptors are complex structures which bind benzodiazepines, barbiturates and cage convulsants.[118] Benzodiazepine receptors are part of the complex, but GABAergic drugs and benzodiazepines interact with separate sites which interact in an allosteric fashion. The cage convulsants, of which picrotoxin is an example, bind to the chloride channel portion of the $GABA_A$ receptor. $GABA_A$ receptors are relatively dense in striatum, i.e., caudate/putamen, nucleus accumbens, and olfactory tubercle. A significant, but lesser number of these receptors is present in the lateral and medial globus pallidus and in the substantia nigra, both pars reticulata and pars compacta.[119-122a] Similar distributions are seen with tritiated ligands that bind to benzodiazepine receptors.

In animal models of Parkinson's disease, the numbers of GABA and benzodiazepine receptors in the lateral globus pallidus decrease whereas those in the medial globus pallidus and substantia nigra pars reticulata increase.[123] Haloperidol which blocks dopamine receptors leads to an increase in substantia nigra pars reticulata $GABA_A$ receptors. These studies suggest that dopamine has differential effects on striatal projections to lateral pallidum, medial pallidum and substantia nigra. Similar measurements have not been made from post-mortem Parkinson's brains. The few measurements that have been made indicate little change in striatum and a decrease in the number of pars compacta receptors, consistent with the loss of the intrinsic dopamine neurons.[124] However, most of these studies were carried out on patients who had received treatment. Untreated cases might show differences.

In animal models of Huntington's disease, $GABA_A$ and benzodiazepine receptors decrease in striatum and ventral thalamus and increase in lateral pallidum, entopeduncular nucleus and substantia nigra pars reticulata.[125,126] In Huntington's disease post-mortem studies, $GABA_A$ and benzodiazepine receptors decrease in striatum and ventral thalamus and increase in lateral pallidum and substantia nigra but change little in medial pallidum.[120] It is likely that there is differential damage to subsets of striatal neurons in Huntington's disease which could provide an explanation for these findings.[9]

C. ACETYLCHOLINE RECEPTORS

Muscarinic receptors measured with the nonselective antagonist quinuclidinylbenzilate are very dense in the caudate, the putamen, the nucleus accumbens, and the olfactory tubercle.[8] In contrast, the receptors in lateral and medial globus pallidus and substantia nigra are very low. Since the cholinergic neurons in the neostriatum are large aspiny interneurons, this localized high density of receptors in striatum is not surprising. There are no known cholinergic afferents to or efferents from the neostriatum.

More selective assays using ligands that labeled M1 receptors with [³H]pirenzepine and M2 receptors with [³H]-N-methylscopolamine in the presence of sufficient pirenzepine to block M1 receptors have been used to study M1 and M2 receptors in cat, monkey, and human striatum.[127,127a] M2 binding sites were homogeneously distributed except in ventral striatum where areas of dense and sparse binding were observed. M1 sites were denser than M2 sites and demonstrated regions of heterogeneity. These heterogeneities displayed areas of dense binding which often corresponded to acetylcholinesterase poor striosomes. The findings suggest that cholinergic systems may be compartmentalized in striatum based on receptor characteristics.

D. OPIATE RECEPTORS

The striatum and its projection areas contain very high concentrations of leucine-enkephalin and dynorphin.[8,66] Both peptides are colocalized with GABA in medium-spiny neurons.[128-130] Dynorphin/GABA containing cells project primarily to medial globus pallidus and substantia nigra pars reticulata, whereas enkephalin/GABA neurons have their major projection to the lateral globus pallidus.[63]

Opiate receptors are differentially located in the basal ganglia. In rats, mu opiate receptors are present in dense patches in striatum and are localized both on presynaptic dopamine terminals and postsynaptically on striatal neurons.[8] Delta and kappa opiate receptors appear predominantly on striatal somata and terminals. After striatal kainic acid lesions in rats, delta and mu opiate receptors decrease in globus pallidus and substantia nigra pars reticulata suggesting that the pallidal and nigral receptors are on striatal afferent terminals.[131]

A striking property of rodent and primate opiate receptors is that they are present in very low concentrations in the globus pallidus despite the very high levels of peptides in the same area. There is, thus, a striking mismatch in peptide levels vs. receptors. The functional significance of this mismatch is unclear.

IV. SUMMARY

Although other receptors could be discussed, those covered here are most likely to be measured using PET techniques. Methods for looking at presynaptic neuronal function using transmitter precursors or high affinity uptake inhibitors would complement the receptor ligands. It should be possible to use PET techniques to study the clinical aspects of basal ganglia circuitry in man. Studies of early or presymptomatic Parkinson's and Huntington's cases should provide information about which striatal markers are first affected by the disease. Most important in this regard would be to develop methods for looking at specific subgroups of striatal neurons, i.e., GABA/enkephalin neurons, GABA/substance P neurons, somatostatin interneurons, etc. Such information would further our understanding of the pathophysiology of basal ganglia disorders as well as suggest new therapies for the treatment of these diseases.

ACKNOWLEDGMENTS

Work on this chapter was supported by USPHS grants NS 15655 and 19613.

REFERENCES

1. **Marsden, C. D.**, The pathophysiology of movement disorders, *Neurol. Clin.*, 2, 435, 1984.
2. **Young, A. B., Shoulson, I., Penney, J. B., Starosta-Rubinstein, S., Gomez, F., Travers, H., Ramos-Arroyo, M. A., Snodgrass, S. R., Bonilla, E., Moreno, H., and Wexler, N. S.,** Huntington's disease in Venezuela: neurological features and functional decline, *Neurology*, 36, 244, 1986.
3. **Carpenter, M. B.,** Anatomy of the corpus striatum and brainstem integrating systems, in *Handbook of Physiology: The Nervous System II*, Vol. 1, Brooks, V. B., Ed., American Physiology Society, Washington, D.C., 1981.
4. **DeLong, M. R. and Georgopoulos, A. B.,** Motor functions of the basal ganglia, in *Handbook of Physiology: The Nervous System II*, Vol. 1, Brooks, V. B., Ed., American Physiology Society, Washington, D.C., 1981.
5. **Graybiel, A. M.,** Neurochemically specified subsystems in the basal ganglia, in *Functions of the Basal Ganglia. CIBA Foundation Symposium 107*, Evered, D. and O'Connor, M., Eds., Pitman, London, 1984, 114.
6. **Graybiel, A. M. and Ragsdale, C. W.,** Biochemical anatomy of the striatum, in *Chemical Neuroanatomy*, Emson, P. C., Ed., Raven Press, New York, 1983, 427.
7. **Penney, J. B. and Young, A. B.,** Speculations on the functional anatomy of basal ganglia disorders, *Annu. Rev. Neurosci.*, 6, 73, 1983.

8. **Young, A. B. and Penney, J. B.,** Neurochemical anatomy of movement disorders, *Neurol. Clin.*, 2, 417, 1984.

9. **Penney, J. B. and Young, A. B.,** Striatal inhomogenities and basal ganglia function, *Movement Disorders*, 1, 3, 1986.

10. **Carlsson, A.,** Occurence, distribution and physiological role of catecholamines in the nervous system, *Pharmacol. Rev.*, 11, 300, 1959.

11. **Birkmayer, W. and Hornykiewicz, O.,** The effect of 3,4-dihydroxyphenyl-L-alanine (DOPA) on the akinesia in Parkinson's disease, *Wien. Klin. Wschr.*, 73, 787, 1961.

12. **Dahlstrom, A. and Fuxe, K.,** Evidence for the existence of monoamine-containing neurons in the central nervous system, *Acta Physiol. Scand.*, 62 (Suppl. 232), 1, 1964.

13. **Ungerstedt, U.,** Stereotaxic mapping of the monamine pathways in the rat brain, *Acta Physiol. Scand.*, 82 (Suppl. 367), 1048, 1971.

14. **Cotzias, G. C., Papavasiliou, P. S., and Gellen, R.,** Modification of parkinsonism-chronic treatment with L-dopa, *N. Engl. J. Med.*, 280, 337, 1969.

15. **Kitai, S. T.,** Electrophysiology of the corpus striatum and brain stem integrating systems, in *Handbook of Physiology: The Nervous System II*, Vol. 1, Brooks, V. B., Ed., American Physiology Society, Washington, D.C., 1981, 997.

16. **Heimer, L, Zaborszky, L., Sahm, D. S., and Alheid, G. F.,** The ventral striatopallidothalamic projection. I. The striatopallidal link originating in the striatal parts of the olfactory tubercle, *J. Comp. Neurol.*, 255, 571, 1987.

17. **McGeer, P. L., McGeer, E. G., and Scherer, U., et al.,** A glutamatergic corticostriatal path?, *Brain Res.*, 128, 369, 1977.

18. **Kim, J. S., Hassler, R., Haug, P., and Paik, K. S,** Effect of frontal cortex ablation on striatal glutamic acid level in rat, *Brain Res.*, 132, 370, 1977.

19. **Fonnum, F., Storm-Mathisen, J., and Divac, I.,** Biochemical evidence for glutamate as a neurotransmitter in corticostriatal and corticothalamic fibers in rat brain, *Neuroscience*, 6, 863, 1978.

20. **Young, A. B., Bromberg, M. B., and Penney, J. B.,** Decreased glutamate uptake in subcortical areas deafferented by sensorimotor cortical ablation in the rat, *J. Neurosci.*, 1, 241, 1981.

21. **Herkenham, M. and Pert, C. B.,** Mosiac distribution of opiate receptors, parafascicular projections and acetylcholinesterase in rat striatum, *Nature*, 291, 415, 1981.

22. **Beckstead, R. M., Domesick, V. B., and Nauta, W. J. H.,** Efferent connections of the substantia nigra and ventral tegmental area in the rat, *Brain Res.*, 175, 191, 1979.

23. **Fonnum, F. Gottesfeld, A., and Grofova, I.,** Distribution of glutamate decarboxylase, choline acetyl-transferase and aromatic amino acid decarboxylase in the basal ganglia of normal and operated rats. Evidence for striatopallidal, striatoentopeduncular and striatonigral GABAergic fibres. *Brain Res.*, 158, 15, 1978.

24. **Nagy, J. I., Carter, D. A., and Fibiger, H. C.,** Anterior striatal projections to the globus pallidus, entopenduncular nucleus and substantia nigra in the rat: the GABA connection, *Brain Res.*, 158, 15, 1978.

25. **Park, M. R., Lighthall, J. W., and Kitai, S. T.,** Recurrent inhibition in the rat neostriatum, *Brain Res.*, 194, 359, 1980.

26. **Bishop, G. A., Chang, H. T., and Kitai, S. T.,** Morphological and physiological properties of neostriatal neurons: an intracellular horseradish peroxidase study in the rat, *Neuroscience*, 7, 179, 1982.

27. **Phelps, P. A. Houser, C. R., and Vaughn, J. E.,** Immunocytochemical localization of choline acetyl-transferase within the rat neostriatum: a correlated light and electron microscope study of cholinergic neurons and synapses, *J. Comp. Neurol.*, 238, 286, 1985.

28. **DiFiglia, M. and Aronin, N.,** Ultrastructural features of immunoreactive somatostatin neurons in the rat caudate nucleus, *J. Neurosci,*, 2, 1267, 1982.

29. **Vincent, S. R. and Johansson, O.,** Striatal neurons containing both somatostatin and avian pancreatic polypeptide (APP) like immunoreactivity and NADPH-diaphorase activity: a light and electron microscopic study, *J. Comp. Neurol.*, 217, 264, 1983.

30. **Di Chiara, G., Porceddu, M. L., Morelli, M., Mulas, M., and Gessa, G. L,** Evidence for a GABA-ergic projection from the substantia nigra to the ventromedial thalamus and to the superior colliculus of the rat, *Brain Res.*, 176, 273, 1979.

31. **Kilpatrick, I. C., Starr, M. S., Fletcher, A., James, T. A., and MacLeod, N. K.,** Evidence for a GABA-ergic nigrothalamic pathway in the rat. I. Behavioural and biochemical studies, *Exp. Brain Res.*, 40, 45, 1980.

32. **Penney, J. B. and Young, A. B.** GABA as the pallidothalamic neurotransmitter: implications for basal ganglia function, *Brain Res.*, 207, 195, 1981.

33. **Parent A., Hazrati, L. N., and Smith, Y.,** The organization of the subthalamic nucleus in primates: a neuroanatomical and immunohistochemical study, in *Neural Mechanisms in Disorders of Movement*, Crossman, A. R., Sambrook, M. A., Eds., John Libbey, London, 1989, 29.

34. **Nakanishi, H., Kita, H., and Kitai, S. T.,** Intracellular study of rat substantia nigra pars reticulata neurons in an in vitro slice preparation: electrical membrane properties and response characteristics to subthalamic stimulation, *Brain Res.*, 437, 45, 1987.

35. **Beitz, A. J.** personal communication, 1985.

36. **Herkenham, M.,** The afferent and efferent connections of the ventromedial thalamic nucleus in the rat, *J. Comp. Neurol.*, 153, 487, 1989.

37. **Ilinsky, I. A., Jouandet, M. L., and Goldman-Rakic, P. S.** Organization of the nigrothalamocortical system in the rhesus monkey, *J. Comp. Neurol.*, 236, 315, 1985.

38. **Yoshida, M., Yajima, K., and Uno, M.,** Differential activation of the two types of pyramidal tract neurons through the cerebellothalamocortical pathway, *Experientia*, 22, 331, 1966.

39. **Schell, G. R. and Strick, P. L.,** The origin of thalamic inputs to the arcuate premotor and supplementary motor areas, *J. Neurosci,*. 4, 539, 1984.

40. **Butcher, L. L. and Hodge, G. K.,** Postnatal development of acetylcholinesterase in the caudate-putamen nucleus and substantia nigra of rats, *Brain Res.*, 106, 223, 1976.

41. **Mensah, P. L.,** The internal organization of the mouse caudate nucleus: evidence for cell clustering and regional variations, *Brain Res.*, 137, 53, 1977.

42. **Olson, L. A., Seiger, A., and Fuxe, K.,** Heterogeneity of striatal and limbic dopamine innervation: highly fluorescent islands in developing and adult rats, *Brain Res.*, 44, 283, 1972.

43. **Graybiel, A. M. and Ragsdale, C. W., Jr.,** Histochemically distinct compartments in the striatum of human, monkey and cat demonstrated by acetylcholinesterase staining, *Proc. Natl. Acad. Sci. U.S.A.*, 75, 7523, 1978.

44. **Fuxe, K., Anderson, K. and Schwarcz, R., et al.,** Studies on different types of dopamine nerve terminals in the forebrain and their possible interactions with hormones and with neurons containing GABA, glutamate, and opioid peptides, *Adv. Neurol.*, 25, 199, 1979.

45. **Graybiel, A. M., Chesselet, M.-F., Wu, J.-Y., Eckenstein, F., and Joh, T. E.,** The relation of striosomes in the caudate nucleus of the cat to the organization of early-developing dopaminergic fibres, GAD-positive neuropil, and CAT-positive neurons, *Soc. Neurosci. Abstr.*, 9, 14, 1983.

46. **Graybiel, A. M. and Hickey, T. L.,** Chemospecficity of ontogenic units in the striatum: demonstration of combining [³H]thymidine neuronography and histochemical staining, *Proc. Natl. Acad. Sci. U.S.A.*, 79, 198, 1982.

47. **Gerfen, C. R., Baimbridge, K. G., and Miller, J. J.,** The neostrial mosaic: localization of compartmental distribution of calcium binding protein and parvalbumin in the basal ganglia of the rat and monkey, *Proc. Natl. Acad. Sci. U.S.A.*, 82, 8780, 1985.

48. **Jimenez-Castellanos, J. and Graybiel, A. M.,** Subdivisions of the dopamine containing A8-A9-A10 complex identified by their differential mesostriatal innervation of striosomes and extrastriosomal matrix, *Neuroscience*, 23, 223, 1987.

49. **Gerfen, C. R.,** The neostriatal mosaic: compartmentalization of corticostriatal input and striatonigral output systems, *Nature*, 311, 461, 1984.

50. **Gerfen, C. R.,** The neostriatal mosaic. I. Compartmental organization of projections from the striatum to the substantia nigra in the rat, *J. Comp. Neurol.*, 236, 454, 1985.

51. **Donoghue, J. P. and Herkenham, M.,** Neostriatal projections from individual cortical fields conform to histochemically distinct striatal compartments in the rat, *Brain Res.*, 365, 397, 1986.

52. **Goedert, M., Manthyth, P. W., Hunt, S. P., and Emson, P. C.** Mosaic distribution of neurotensin-like immunoreactivity in the cat striatum, *Brain Res.*, 274, 176, 1983.

53. **Selemon, L. D. and Goldman-Rakic, P. S.** Longitudinal topography and interdigitation of corticostriatal projections in the rhesus monkey, *J. Neurosci*, 5, 776, 1985.

54. **Ragsdale, C. W. and Graybiel, A. M.,** The fronto-striatal projection in the cat and monkey and its relationship to inhomogenities established by acetylcholinesterase histochemistry, *Brain Res.*, 208, 259, 1981.

55. **Goldman-Rakic, P. S.,** Cytoarchitectonic heterogenity of the primate neostriatum: subdivision into island and matrix cellular compartments. *J. Comp. Neurol.*, 205, 398, 1982.

56. **Doucet, G., Garcia, S., and Descarries, L.,** Radioautographic quantification of the dopamine innervation in adult rat neostriatum, *Soc. Neurosci. Abstr.*, 11, 1017, 1985.

57. **Ribak, C. E., Vaughn, J. E., and Roberts, E.,** The GABA neurons and their axon terminals in rat corpus striatum as demonstrated by GAD immunohistochemistry, *J. Comp. Neurol.*, 187, 261, 1979.

58. **Preston, R. J., Bishop, G. A., and Kitai, S. T.,** Medium spiny neuron projection from the rat striatum: an intracellular horseradish peroxidase study, *Brain Res.*, 183, 253, 1980.

59. **Parent, A., Bouchard, C., and Smith, Y.,** The striatopallidal and striatonigral projections: two distinct fiber systems in primate, *Brain Res.*, 303, 385, 1984.

60. **Beckstead, R. M. and Cruz, C. J.,** Striatal axons to the globus pallidus entopeduncular nucleus and substantia nigra come mainly from separate cell populations in the cat, *Neuroscience*, 19, 147, 1986.

61. **Cuello, A. C. and Paxinos, G.,** Evidence for a long leu-enkephalin striopallidal pathway in rat brain, *Nature*, 271, 178, 1978.
62. **Haber, S. N. and Elde, R. P.,** Correlation between met-enkephalin and substance P immunoreactivity in the primate globus pallidus, *Neuroscience*, 6, 1291, 1981.
63. **Haber, S. N. and Watson, S. J.,** The comparative distribution of enkephalin, dynorphin and substance P in the human globus pallidus and basal forebrain, *Neuroscience*, 14, 1011, 1985.
64. **Jessell, T. M., Emson, P. C., and Paxinos, G., et al.,** Topographical projections of substance P and GABA pathways in the striatal pallidonigral system: a biochemical and immunohistochemical study, *Brain Res.*, 152, 487, 1978.
65. **Christensson-Nylander, I., Herrera-Marschitz, M., Staines, W., Hokfelt, T., Terenius, L., Ungerstedt, U., Cuello, C., Oertel, W. H., and Goldstein, M.,** Striatonigral dynorphin and substance P pathways in the rat. I. Biochemical and immunohistochemical studies, *Exp. Brain Res.*, 64, 169, 1986.
66. **Watson, S. J., Khachaturian, H., Akil, H., et al.,** Comparison of the distribution of dynorphin systems and enkephalin systems in the brain, *Science*, 218, 1134, 1982.
67. **Reiner, A.,** The co-occurence of substance P-like immunoreactivity and dynorphin-like immunoreactivity in striatopallidal and striatonigral projection neurons in birds and reptiles, *Brain Res.*, 371, 155, 1986.
68. **Dauth, G. W., Gilman, S., Frey, K. A., and Penney, J. B., Jr.,** Basal ganglia glucose utilization after recent precentral ablation in the monkey, *Ann. Neurol.*, 17, 431, 1985.
69. **Gilman, S., Dauth, G. W., Frey, K. A., and Penney, J. B., Jr.,** Experimental hemiplegia in the monkey: basal ganglia glucose activity during recovery, *Ann. Neurol.*, 22, 370, 1987.
70. **Mitchell, I. J., Cross, A. J., Sambrook, M. A., and Crossman, A. R.,** Neural mechanisms mediating 1-methyl-4-phenyl-1,2,3,6-tetrahydropyridine-induced parkinsonism in the monkey: relative contributions of the striatopallidal and striatonigral pathways as suggested by 2-deoxyglucose uptake, *Neurosci. Lett.*, 63, 61, 1986.
71. **Porrino, L. J., Burns, R. S., Crane, A., Palombo, E., Kopin, I. J., and Sokoloff, L.,** Changes in local cerebral glucose utilization associated with Parkinson's syndrome induced by 1-methyl-4-phenyl-1,2,3,6-tetrahydropyridine (MPTP) in the primate, *Life Sci.*, 40, 1657, 1987.
72. **Young, A. B., Penney, J. B., Starosta-Rubinstein, S., Markel, D. S., Berent, S., Giordani, B., Ehrenkaufer, R., Jewett, D., and Hichwa R.,** PET scan investigations of Huntington's disease: cerebral metabolic correlates of neurologic features and functional decline, *Ann. Neurol.*, 20, 296, 1986.
73. **Young, A. B., Penney, J. B., Starosta-Rubinstein, S., Markel, D., Berent, S., Rothley, J., Betley, A., and Hichwa, R.,** Normal caudate glucose metabolism in persons at high-risk for Huntington's disease, *Arch. Neurol.*, 44, 254, 1987.
74. **Reiner, A., Albin, R. L., Anderson, K. D., D'Amato, C. J., Penney, J. B., and Young, A. B.,** Differential loss of striatal projection neurons in Huntington's disease, *Proc. Natl. Acad. Sci.*, U.S.A., 85, 5733, 1988.
75. **Ferrante, R. J., Kowall, N. W., Beal, M. F., Richardson, E. P., Bird, E. D., and Martin, J. B.,** Selective sparing of a class of striatal neurons in Huntington's disease, *Science*, 230, 561, 1985.
76. **Dawbarn, D., Dequidt, M. E., and Emson, P. C.,** Survival of basal ganglia neuropeptide Y — somatostatin neurons in Huntington's disease, *Brain Res.*, 340, 251, 1985.
77. **Feigenbaum, L. A., Graybiel, A. M., Vonsattel, J. P., Richardson, E. P., and Bird, E. D.,** Striosomal markers in the striatum in Huntington's disease, *Soc. Neurosci. Abstr.*, 12, 1328, 1986.
78. **Ferrante, R. J., Beal, M. F., Kowall, N. W., Richardson, E. P., and Martin, J. B.,** Sparing of acetylcholinesterase-containing neurons in Huntington's disease, *Brain Res.*, 411, 162, 1987.
79. **Beal, M. F., Mazurek, M. F., Ellison, D. W., Swartz, K. J., McGarvey, U., Bird, E. D., and Martin, J. B.,** Somatostatin and neuropeptide Y concentrations in pathologically graded cases of Huntington's disease, *Ann. Neurol.*, 23, 562, 1988.
80. **Young, A. B., Frey, K. A., and Agranoff, B. W.,** Receptor assays: in vivo and in vitro, in *Tracer Kinetic Studies of Cerebral and Myocardial Function: Positron Emission Tomography and Autoradiography*, Phelps, M., Mazziotta, J. C., and Schelbert, H., Eds., Raven Press, New York, 1985, 73.
81. **Young, W. S., III and Kuhar, M. J.,** A new method for receptor autoradiography [³H]opioid receptor labeling in mounted tissue sections, *Brain Res.*, 179, 255, 1979.
82. **Herkenham, M. and Pert, C. B.,** In vitro autoradiography of opiate receptors in rat brain suggest loci of "opiatergic" pathways, *Proc. Natl. Acad. Sci. U.S.A.*, 77, 5532, 1981.
83. **Penney, J. B., Pan, H. S., Young, A. B., Frey, K. A., and Dauth, G. W.,** Quantitative autoradiography of [3H]muscimol binding in rat brain, *Science*, 214, 1036, 1981.
84. **Ungerstedt, U.,** Postsynaptic supersensitivity after 6-hydroxydopamine induced degeneration of the nigrostriatal dopamine system, *Acta Physiol. Scand.*, Suppl. 367, 69, 1971.
85. **Ungerstedt, U.,** Central dopamine mechanisms and unconditioned behavior, in *The Neurobiology of Dopamine*, Horn, A. S., Kork, J., and Westerink, B. H. C., Eds., Academic Press, London, 1979, 577.

86. **Pijnenberg, A. J. J., Honig, W. M. M., and Von Rossum, J. M.**, Inhibition of d-amphetamine-induced locomotor activity by injection of haloperidol into the nucleus accumbens of the rat, *Psychopharmacology*, 41, 87, 1975.

87. **Quinton, R. M. and Halliwell, G. E.**, Effects of methylDOPA on the amphetamine excitatory response in reserpenized rats, *Nature*, 200, 178, 1963.

88. **Randup, A., Munkvad, I., and Udsen, P.**, Adrenergic mechanisms and amphetamine induced abnormal behavior, *Acta Pharmacol. Toxicol,.* 20, 145, 1963.

89. **Kebabian, J. W., Petzold, G. L., and Greengard, P.**, Dopamine sensitive adenylcyclase in caudate nucleus of rat brain and its similarity to the "dopamine receptor", *Proc. Nat. Acad. Sci. U.S.A.*, 69, 2145, 1972.

90. **Creese, I., Burt, D. R., and Snyder, S. H.**, Dopamine receptor binding predicts clinical and pharmacological potencies of anti-schizophrenic drugs, *Science*, 192, 481, 1976.

91. **Creese, I., Burt, D., and Snyder, S. H.**, Dopamine receptor binding enhancement accompanies lesion-induced behavioral supersensitivity, *Science*, 197, 596, 1977.

92. **Seeman, P., Chau-Wong, M., Tedesco, J., and Wong, K.**, Brain receptors for antipsychotic-drugs and dopamine direct binding assays, *Proc. Natl. Acad. Sci. U.S.A.*, 72, 4376, 1975.

93. **Seeman, P., Lee, T., Chau-Wong, M., and Wong, K.**, Antipsychotic drug doses and neuroleptic-dopamine receptors, *Nature*, 26, 717, 1976.

94. **Grigoriadis, D. and Seeman, P.**, The dopamine/neuroleptic receptor, *Can. J. Neurol. Sci.*, 11, 108, 1984.

95. **Leff, S. E. and Creese, I.**, Dopamine receptors re-explained, *TIPS*, 463, 1983.

96. **Stoof, J. C. and Kebabian, J. W.**, Two dopamine receptors: biochemistry, physiology, and pharmacology, *Life Sci.*, 35, 2281, 1984.

97. **Kebabian, J. W., and Calne, D. B.**, Multiple receptors for dopamine, *Nature (London)*, 277, 93, 1979.

98. **Onali, P., Olianas, M. C., and Gessa, G. L.**, Characterization of dopamine receptors mediating inhibition of adenylate cyclase activity in rat striatum, *Mol. Phamacol.*, 28, 138, 1985.

99. **Dubois, A., Savasta, M., Curet, O., and Scatton, B.**, Autoradiographic distribution of the D-1 agonist [3H]SKF 38393, in the rat brain and spinal cord. Comparison with the distribution of D-2 dopamine receptors, *Neuroscience*, 19, 125, 1986.

100. **Dawson, T. M., Gehlert, D. R., Filloux, F. M., and Wamsley, J. K.**, A quantitative autoradiographic comparison of density and localization of dopamine D-1 and D-2 receptors in rat brain: effects of neurotoxins, *Soc. Neurosci. Abstr.*, 12, 481, 1986.

101. **Filloux, F. M., Dawson, T. M., Gehlert, D. R., and Wamsley, J. K.**, A quantitative comparison of the effects of unilateral striatal and nigral neurotoxin lesion in the rat brain on [3H]-SCH 23390 and [3H]-Forskolin binding sites, *Soc. Neurosci. Abstr.*, 12, 481 1986.

102. **Herrera-Marschitz, M. and Ungerstedt, U.**, Evidence that striatal efferents relate to different dopamine receptors, *Brain Res.*, 323, 269, 1984.

103. **Spano, P. F., Trabucchi, M., and DiChiara, G.**, Localization of nigral dopamine-sensitive adenylate cyclase on neurons originating in the corpus striatum, *Science*, 196, 1343, 1977.

104. **Barone, P., Davis, T. A., Braun, A. R., and Chase, T. N.**, Dopaminergic mechanisms and motor function: characterizations of D-1 and D-2 dopamine receptor interactions, *Eur. J. Pharmacol.*, 123, 109, 1986.

105. **Christensen, A. V., Arnt, J., Hyttel, J., Larsen, J. J., and Svendsen, O.**, Pharmacological effects of a specific dopomaine D-1 agonist SCH 23390 in comparison with neuroleptics, *Life Sci.*, 34, 1529, 1984.

106. **Hyttel, J.**, SCH 23390 — The first selective dopamine D-1 antagonist, *Eur. J. Pharmcol.*, 91, 153, 1983.

107. **Titus, R. D., Kornfeld, E. C., Jones, N. D., Clemens, J. A. Smalstig, E. B., Fuller, R. W., Hahn, R. A., Hynes, M. D., Mason, N. R., Wong, D. T., and Foreman, M. M.**, Resolution and absolute configuration of an ergoline-related dopamine agonist trans-4,4a,5,6,7,8,8a,9-octohydro-5-propyl-1H(or 2H)-pyrazolo [3,4-g]quinilone. *J. Med. Chem.*, 26, 1112, 1983.

108. **Carlson, J. J., Bergstrom, D. A., and Walters, J. R.**, Stimulation of both D-1 and D-2 dopamine receptors appears necessary for full expression of postsynaptic effects of dopamine agonists: a neurophysiological study, *Brain Res.*, 400, 205, 1987.

109. **Walters, J. R., Bergstrom, S. A., Carlson, J. H., Chase, T. N., Braun, A. R.**, D1 dopamine receptor activation required for postsynaptic expression of D2 agonist effects, *Science*, 236, 719, 1987.

110. **Robertson, G. S. and Robertson, H. A.**, Synergistic effects of D_1 and D_2 dopamine agonists on turning behavior in rat, *Brain Res.*, 384, 387, 1986.

111. **Dawson, J. T., Gehlert, D. R., Yamamura, H. I., Barnett, A., and Wamsley, J. K.**, D-1 dopamine receptors in rat brain: autoradiographic localization using [3H]SCH 23390, *Eur. J. Pharmacol.*, 108, 323, 1985.

112. **Schultz, D. W., Stanford, E. J., Wyrick, S. W., and Mailman, R. B.**, Binding of [^{3}H]SCH 23390 in rat brain: regional distribution of effects of assay conditions and GTP suggest interactions at a D1-like dopamine receptor, *J. Neurochem.*, 45, 1601, 1985.

113. **Richfield, E. K., Debowey, D. L., Penney, J. B., and Young, A. B.**, Basal ganglia and cerebral cortical distribution of dopamine D-1 and D-2 receptors in neonatal and adult cat brain, *Neurosci. Lett.*, 73, 203, 1986.

114. **Richfield, E. K., Young, A. B., and Penney, J. B.** Comparative distribution of dopamine D-1 and D-2 receptors in the basal ganglia of turtle, pigeon, rat, cat and monkey, *J. Comp. Neurol.*, 262, 446, 1987.

114a. **Cortes, R., Camps, M., Gueye, B., Probst, A., and Palacious, J. M.**, Dopamine receptors in human brain: autoradiographic distribution of D_1 and D_2 sites in Parkinson syndrome of different etiology, *Brain Res.*, 483, 30, 1989.

115. **Graybiel, A. M.**, Dopaminergic and cholinergic systems in the striatum, in *Neural Mechanisms in Disorders of Movement*, Crossman, A. R. and Sambrook, M. A., Eds., John Libbey, London, 1989, 3.

116. **Joyce, J. N. and Winokur, A.**, Loss of dopamine D1 and preservation of D2 receptors in Huntington's chorea striatum, relationship to the striosomal organization of the striatum, *Soc. Neurosci. Abstr.*, 13, 214, 1987.

117. **Beckstead, R. M.**, The distributions of dopamine D1 & D2 receptors are partially complementary in the cat basal ganglia, *Soc. Neurosci. Abstr.*, 13, 190, 1987.

118. **Olsen, R. W.**, GABA-benzodiazepine-barbiturate receptor interactions, *J. Neurochem.*, 37, 1, 1981.

119. **Penney, J. B. and Young, A. B.**, Quantitative autoradiography of neurotransmitter receptors in Huntington's disease, *Neurology*, 32, 1391, 1982.

120. **Walker, F. O., Young, A. B., Penney, J. B., Dorovini-Zis, K., and Shoulson, I.** Benzodiazepine receptors in early Huntington's disease, *Neurology*, 34, 1237, 1984.

121. **Penney, J. B. and Pan, H. S.**, Quantitative autoradiography of GABA and benzodiazepine binding in studies of mammalian and human basal ganglia function, in *Quantitative Receptor Autoradiography*, Boast, C., Snowhill, E. W., and Altar, C. A., Eds., Alan R. Liss, New York, 1986, 29.

122. **Uhl, G. R., Hackney, G. O., Torchia, M., Stranov, V., Tourtellotte, W. W., Whitehouse, P. J., Tran, V., and Strittmatter, S.**, Parkinson's disease: nigral receptor changes support peptidergic role in nigrostriatal modulation, *Ann. Neurol.*, 20, 194, 1985.

122a. **Zezula, J., Cortes, R., Probst, A., and Palacious, J. M.**, Benzodiazepine receptor sites in the human brain: autoradiographic mapping, *Neuroscience*, 25, 771, 1988.

123. **Pan, H. S., Penney, J. B., and Young, A. B.**, GABA and benzodiazepine receptor changes induced by unilateral 6-hydroxydopamine lesions of the medial forebrain bundle, *J. Neurochem.*, 45, 1396, 1985.

124. **Rinne, U. K.**, Brain neurotransmitter receptors in Parkinson's disease, in *Movement Disorders*, Marsden, C. D. and Fahn, S., Eds., Butterworth Scientific, London, 1982, 59.

125. **Pan, H. S., Frey, K. A., Young, A. B., and Penney, J. B.**, Changes in [^{3}H]muscimol binding in substantia nigra, entopeduncular nucleus, globus pallidus and thalamus after striatal lesions as demonstrated by quantitative autoradiography, *J. Neurosci*, 3, 1189, 1983.

126. **Pan, H. S., Penney, J. B. and Young, A. B.**, Characterization of benzodiazepine receptor changes in substantia nigra, globus pallidus and entopeduncular nucleus after striatal lesions, *J. Pharmacol. Exp. Ther.*, 230, 768, 1984.

127. **Nastu, M. A. and Graybiel, A. M.** Autoradiographic localization and biochemical characteristics of M1 and M2 muscarinic binding sites in the striatum of the cat, monkey and human, *J. Neurosci.*, 8, 1052, 1988.

127a. **Cortes, R., Probst, A., and Palacious, J. M.**, Quantitative light microscopic autoradiographic localization of cholinergic muscariniz receptors in the human brain: forebrain, *Neuroscience*, 20, 65, 1987.

128. **Oertel, W. H., Riethmuler, G., Mugnaini, E., et al.**, Opioid peptide-like immunoreactivity localized in GABAergic neurons of rat neostriatum and central amygdaloid nucleus, *Life Sci.*, 33 (Suppl. 1), 73, 1983.

129. **Penny, G. R., Afsharpour, S., and Kitai, S. T.**, The glutamate decarboxylase-, leucine enkephalin-, methionine enkephalin-, and substance-P immunoreactive neurons in the neostriatum of the rat and cat, *Neuroscience*, 17, 1011, 1986.

130. **Aronin, N. DiFiglia, M., Graveland, G. A., Schwartz, W. J., and Wu, J.-Y.**, Localization of immunoreactive enkephalins in GABA synthesizing neurons of the rat striatum, *Brain Res.*, 300, 376, 1984.

131. **Abou-Khalil, B., Young, A. B., and Penney, J. B.**, Evidence for the presynaptic localization of opiate binding sites on striatal efferent fibers, *Brain Res.*, 323, 21, 1984.

132. **Young, A. B., Albin, R. L., and Penney, J. B.**, Neuropharmacology of basal ganglia functions: relationship to pathophysiology of movement disorders, in *Neural Mechanisms in Disorders of Movement*, Crossman, A. R. and Sambrook, M. A., Eds., John Libbey, London, 1989, 17.

Chapter 3

TRACER STUDIES OF NEURORECEPTOR KINETICS *IN VIVO*

Albert Gjedde

TABLE OF CONTENTS

I. INTRODUCTION

The development of methodology for *in vivo* functional imaging made it possible to quantify the distribution of radioactivity in the brain following the administration of radioligands binding to neuroreceptors. The importance of mathematical tracer techniques to the interpretation of data obtained with positron emission tomography (PET) has been introduced in Chapter 1. This chapter describes the application of mathematical models to the analysis of radioligand uptake data obtained with PET to enable the measurement of ligand-receptor binding kinetics.

II. COMPARTMENTAL ANALYSIS

Drugs and chemicals that act in brain often do so specifically, i.e., by association with membrane proteins designed to receive endogenous neurotransmitters and neuromodulators, although the endogenous ligands may not always be known. The existence of chemical receptors was suspected before the turn of the century in the form of Langley's[1] concept of a 'receptive' substance and Ehrlich's[2] 'side-chain' theory but modeling did not begin until the discovery of the binding of oxygen to specialized proteins that made direct observation of receptor-ligand interaction possible. When the binding of oxygen to myoglobin was first observed to be a function of the oxygen tension in the solution,[3] the relationship between the quantities of bound and free oxygen corresponded exactly to the relationship between the invertase reaction velocity and substrate concentration later derived by Michaelis and Menten.[4] Bohr[5] published an equation for the interaction between hemoglobin and oxygen which antedated the equation suggested by Hill[6] for receptor sites that interact cooperatively.

In conventional kinetic models, an organ consists of a number of compartments corresponding to the different states of a tracer. The compartments reflect the fate of the tracer and represent a specific theory of the biochemistry of an organ. The concept of compartments can be ascribed to Sheppard[7] who defined compartments as volumes, real or kinetic, in which the concentration of a tracer or its derivatives everywhere remains the same. In kinetic terms, Rescigno and Beck[8] interpreted this definition to mean that a compartment must obey the expression

$$\frac{dM}{dt} = J(t) - k M \tag{1}$$

where M is the quantity of tracer in the compartment, k a constant, and $J(t)$ an arbitrary flux as a function of time. The concentration of the tracer is determined as the ratio between M and the volume in which it is dissolved. In this context, a tracer is any compound which can be labeled. All concentration gradients are placed at the interfaces between compartments. Normally, these interfaces are cell membranes or chemical reactions involving transporter, receptor, or enzyme proteins.

The purpose of the kinetic analysis of tracer uptake is to measure the size of the compartments and the velocity of exchanges between the compartments. The number and definition of compartments relevant to each tracer must be known before attempts can be made to quantify the tracer exchanges between compartments.

The transfer of a tracer, applied at time zero, from one compartment to another observes a simple mathematical expression of conservation of mass. The basis of the formalism is the use of transfer coefficients, k, that are less rigidly defined than in classical compartmental analysis. The transfer coefficients operate on concentrations, C, measured in volumes, V. In combination, the basic variables define clearances ($K = kV$), masses ($M = VC$), or fluxes ($J = kVC$). The variables are sometimes numbered consecutively, unlike the transfer constants of traditional compartmental analysis that are numbered on the basis of their destination and origin. In the present discussion, variables belonging to general cases will be numbered while variables belonging to specific cases will be lettered.

Although M symbolizes a mass, it can also conveniently be thought of as a *measured* quantity of tracer in a sample of brain. This usage is necessitated by the limitation that it is not possible, *in vivo*, to determine tracer concentrations per unit water volume.

According to Equation 1, the fundamental expression of exchange of tracer between the two compartments of a closed system must be

$$\frac{dM_2}{dt} = k_1 V_1 C_1 - k_2 V_2 C_2 \tag{2}$$

where M_2 is the net gain of tracer in compartment 2 as a function of the time t. V_1 and V_2 are the actual volumes of compartments 1 and 2, and k_1 and k_2 descriptive transfer coefficients.

The symbols C_1 and C_2 represent concentrations of the tracer or its metabolites that retain the label in the respective compartments. The symbols, therefore, need not refer to the same chemical species. The product of k_1 and V_1 defines a clearance, K_1, which reflects perfusion when there are no barriers to diffusion of the tracer between the circulation and the compartment. The product of V_2 and C_2 defines the mass M_2.

The general solution to Equation 2 is

$$M_2 = e^{-k_2 T} \left[M_2(0) + K_1 \int_0^T C_1 e^{k_2 t} \, dt \right] \tag{3}$$

which is an example of a convolution integral. In principle, Equation 3 is a transcendental equation which can be solved for K_1 or k_2 only by iteration and may have zero, one, or two solutions. Special cases include $C_1 = 0$ ("wash-out") and $M_2(0) = 0$ ("fill-in").

The purpose of autoradiography or positron tomography is normally the quantitation of one or more of the coefficients in Equation 2. In actual practice, one or more independent variables and one dependent variable are measured as function of time and the desired coefficients estimated by regression analysis, using a suitable computerized optimization program.

III. ANALYSIS OF K_1 AND k_2

In most organs, capillaries are no barrier to the entry of small polar solutes. In brain, however, they do constitute such a barrier, as noted above. In brain, the concentration difference of many tracers between the two sides of the endothelium is initially so great that the endothelium often is the only significant barrier that these tracers meet in brain. For these tracers, the brain is an organ of only two compartments, the vascular compartment and the tissue space, separated by the blood-brain barrier.

Although easy to define, endothelial permeability is measurable only as an indirect index of 'clearance' (K_1). The quantity of tracer transported from blood to brain in a given period of time is a function of P (often given in units of cm s^{-1} or nm s^{-1} and thus akin to a velocity of transfer through the barrier), S, the area of endothelial surface available for transport (measured in cm^2 g^{-1} or ml^{-1}), and the integral of the concentration difference across the endothelium or barrier.

Unfortunately, the magnitudes of K_1 and k_2 do not reflect the permeability-surface area product in a simple manner because the tracer concentration is dropping in the capillary as the tracer travels from the arterial to the venous end. The definitive derivation of the relationship between transendothelial clearance, perfusion (F), and the permeability-surface area product (*PS*) of the endothelium was made by Bohr[9] during his examination of the oxygen diffusion capacity of the pulmonary endothelium

$$\frac{PS}{F} = -\alpha \ln \frac{\Delta C_v}{\Delta C_a} \tag{4}$$

where α is the solubility of the tracer in the sample of blood relative to that in tissue and plasma water (serves as a correction for protein binding or other sequestration in blood), ΔC_v the concentration difference between tissue and blood at the venous exit from the endothelium, and ΔC_a the concentration difference at the arterial entry to the endothelium. If α is not unity, and tracer clearance is determined initially when tissue concentrations can be assumed to be negligible, Crone[10] showed that the equation modifies to

$$PS = -\alpha F \ln (1 - E_o) \tag{5}$$

where E_o, the so-called 'first pass' extraction fraction, is the K_1/F ratio. In theory, therefore, this equation is only valid for extraction fractions measured in the presence of negligible tissue concentrations. When the colloquial 'first pass' extraction expression is used, negligible tissue concentration is actually referred to. The reason is that the capillary concentration of the tracer must fall exponentially if the transport remains unidirectional. Only when extravascular concentrations remain negligible, do Equations 3 and 5 together yield

$$K_1 = F\left(1 - e^{-PS/[\alpha F]}\right) = \frac{M - M_a}{\int_0^T C_a \, dt} \tag{6}$$

It follows from the definition of the steady-state distribution volume V_e that the definition of k_2 must be [11]

$$k_2 = \frac{K_1}{V_e} = \frac{F}{V_e}\left(1 - e^{-PS/[\alpha F]}\right) \tag{7}$$

It is the purpose of the two-compartment analysis to estimate the coefficients of transfer (K_1 and k_2) between compartment 1 and compartment 2 in brain, i.e., a process that occurs *inside* brain where the residues of compartments 1 and 2 cannot be detected separately. The exact interpretation of the physiological or pathophysiological meaning of K_1 depends on the known properties of the tracer in relation to the permeability of the endothelium, blood flow to the regions of brain, and binding of the tracer to proteins or other agents in blood plasma.

Equation 2 can be integrated to yield M, the sum of M_1 and M_2, when $M_2(0) = 0$

$$M = V_a C_a + (K_1 + k_2 V_a)\int_0^T C_a \, dt - k_2 \int_0^T M \, dt \tag{8}$$

where C_a is the arterial concentration, measured in whole-blood or a subcompartment of blood; and where V_a is the vascular volume of distribution of the tracer in brain, equal to the plasma water volume in brain when the tracer concentration C_a is actually distributed and measured only in plasma water. The coefficients of Equation 8 can be obtained by 'four-dimensional' linear regression in which the dimensions include three independent variables (i.e., C_a and the two integrals) and one dependent variable (i.e., M)

$$Y = p_1 X_1 + p_2 X_2 + p_3 X_3 \tag{9}$$

where $p_{(i)}$ denotes the coefficient of the independent variable $X_{(i)}$.

The coefficient K_1 can be isolated in Equation 8,

$$K_1 = \frac{M + k_2 \int_0^T M_e \, dt - V_a C_a}{\int_0^T C_a \, dt} \tag{10}$$

where M_e is the total mass of tracer in the extravascular water pool, equal to $V_2 C_2$. If only a single value of M is known, the value of M_e must be calculated on the basis of Equation 3 and known values of the transfer coefficients. If k_2 is not known, the calculation of K_1 on the basis of a single measurement of M requires both negligible backflux and a known or negligible product of V_a and C_a. The product of V_a and C_a can be measured with a second tracer which remains in compartment 1 but backflux cannot easily be ruled out on the basis of single measurement, as discussed above.

Alternatively, with the same number of experiments and a single tracer, both K_1 and V_a can be estimated by terminating the experiments at different times after administration of the tracer. In experimental animals, results of a series of experiments can be compared only after normalization of the individual observations. Normalization is the division of the radioactivity in brain by the arterial radioactivity concentrations of tracer obtained in individual experiments

$$V = \frac{M}{C_a} = V_a + K_1 \left(\frac{\int_0^T C_a \, dt - \left[\dfrac{\int_0^T M_e \, dt}{V_e} \right]}{C_a} \right) \tag{11}$$

where there M/C_a ratio represents the measured volume of distribution and V_e is the measured volume of the extravascular pool, equal to the K_1/k_2 ratio. The equation can be further simplified to

$$V = V_a + K_1 \Theta - k_2 \left(\frac{\int_0^T M_e \, dt}{C_{a2}} \right) \tag{12}$$

in which Θ indicates the $\int_0^T C_a \, dt / C_a$ ratio. Θ has unit of time and represents a modified time variable. It is apparent that V remains a linear function of Θ for as long as the $\int_0^T M_e \, dt / V_e$ ratio is negligible compared to $\int_0^T C_a \, dt$. The requirement for absent backflux is a very large value of V_e, i.e., very low tissue/blood concentration ratios. Equation 12 underlies the so-called 'slope-intercept' or 'Patlak' plot.[12,13]

When T and Θ approach infinity

$$V(\infty) \to \frac{K_1}{k_2} + V_a = V_e + V_a \tag{13}$$

which confirms that V_e is the steady-state extravascular volume of distribution of the tracer, relative to the arterial concentration.

The measured permeabilities of the blood-brain barrier to hydrophilic substances are low, of the order of 1 to 10 nm s^{-1}. Most substrates of brain metabolism are hydrophilic and few lipophilic substances exist in solution in plasma water (for obvious reasons). However, facilitated diffusion allows hydrophilic nutrients to cross much more readily than do inert polar nonelectrolytes.

IV. ANALYSIS OF k_3 AND k_4

Certain tracers interact in some manner with the brain to escape the build-up in the interstitial fluid that leads to backflux and eventually to steady-state. The kinetic equivalent of this interaction is 'trapping' of the tracer.

Trapping can be described as a process imposed by a hypothetical additional compartment reflecting transport (e.g., into the intracellular space), binding (e.g., to receptor sites), or metabolism (e.g., by chemical reactions that sequester the label for a shorter or longer time). In the compartmental analysis, the process is represented by a transfer coefficient (k_3) leading to the additional compartment, and a transfer coefficient (k_4) leading from the compartment. Entry into compartment 3 competes with the likelihood of transfer back into compartment 1. This competition is described by two diffferential equations

$$\frac{dM_2}{dt} = K_1 C_1 - (k_2 + k_3) M_2 + k_4 M_3 \tag{14}$$

and

$$\frac{dM_3}{dt} = k_3 M_2 - k_4 M_3 \tag{15}$$

where M_2 and M_3 represent the exchangeable (compartment 2) and trapped (compartment 3) quantities of tracer.

The integration of Equations 14 and 15 for M, the total content of labeled material in the tissue, including the original tracer and its derived forms, has been extended to three compartments by Blomqvist[14] and further extended to include k_4 by Evans[15]

$$M = V_a C_a + (K_1 + [k_2 + k_3 + k_4] V_a) \int_0^T C_a \, dt$$

$$+ K_1 [k_3 + k_4] + k_2 k_4 V_a) \int_0^T \left[\int_0^t C_a \, du \right] dt$$

$$- (k_2 + k_3 + k_4) \int_0^T M \, dt - k_2 k_4 \int_0^T \left[\int_0^t M \, du \right] dt \tag{16}$$

where M is the sum of M_1, M_2, and M_3 in brain, and V_a and C_a represent V_1 and C_1, respectively. The equation is soluble for the coefficients by 'six-dimensional' linear regression in which the six dimensions include the five independent variables (i.e., C_a, the integrals, and the integrals of integrals) and the one dependent variable (i.e., M).

$$Y = p_1 X_1 + p_2 X_2 + p_3 X_3 + p_4 X_4 + p_5 X_5 \tag{17}$$

where $p_{(i)}$ denotes the coefficient of independent variable $X_{(i)}$.

Equations 14 and 15 can also be solved for K, the net clearance of tracer into the third compartment, equal to the product of k_3 and V_f where V_f is the distribution volume $K_1/K_1/(K_2 + K_3)k_2 + k_3)$

$$K = \frac{M - \dfrac{k_2}{k_2 + k_3}\left(M_e - k_4 \displaystyle\int_0^T M_m\, dt\right) - V_a C_a}{\displaystyle\int_0^T C_a\, dt} \tag{18}$$

where M_e is the quantity of tracer in the extravascular, exchangeable pool representing M_2, M_m the quantity of tracer in the pool of metabolic or other trapping represented by M_3. The ratio $k_2/(k_2 + k_3)$ defines an 'escape potential', r_e. From the definitions of V_e, V_f, and r_e, it follows that $V_f = r_e V_e$.

The following variations of the solution are of special interest: first, the magnitude of k_3 may be negligible compared to the magnitude of k_2. This is the two-compartment situation discussed above. Second, k_3 may be of the same order of magnitude as k_2. The probabilities of backflux and binding are then equally great. On the average, half of the tracer molecules enter the third compartment and the remaining half return to compartment 1 (e.g., the vascular compartment). The rate of net transfer to the third compartment is only 50% percent of the rate of initial uptake. The fraction ('entrapment') that net uptake represents of the rate of initial uptake is $1 - r_e$ where r_e is the 'escape potential' referred to above. Third, it is possible that the magnitude of the coefficient k_3 is much greater than the magnitude of the coefficient k_2. The last case requires two-compartment analysis because the value of k_3 is so high that it retains very little influence over the accumulation of tracer in the brain.

When k_4 is negligible, Equations 14 and 15 yield

$$K = \frac{M - r_e M_e - M_a}{\displaystyle\int_0^T C_a\, dt} \tag{19}$$

where M_a is the radioactivity in the vascular space in brain, equal to the product of C_a and V_a. This is the solution first introduced by Sokoloff et al.[16] for deoxyglucose and discussed in detail by Gjedde.[17,18]

The complete solution of Equations 14 and 15 for the volume of distribution of the tracer in brain is

$$V = V_a + r_e \frac{M_e}{C_a} + K\left(\frac{\displaystyle\int_0^T C_a\, dt - \left[\displaystyle\int_0^T \frac{M_m\, dt}{V_m}\right]}{C_a}\right) \tag{20}$$

where V_m is a 'metabolic' or 'trapping' pool equal to the ratio $(K_1 k_3/(k_2 k_4))$. Note the similarity with Equation 11.

The higher the value of the $K_1 k_3$ product relative to the value of the $k_2 k_4$ product, i.e., the larger V_m, the lower the probability of escape of the tracer from brain. When Θ is sufficiently small and V_m sufficiently large (i.e., when k_4 is sufficiently small), the equation reduces to

$$V = K(\Theta - \Theta_m) + r_e V'_f + V_a \cong K\Theta + r_e V'_f + V_a \tag{21}$$

where V'_f is the measured (steady- or nonsteady-state) M_e/C_a ratio; Θ the normalized integral introduced in Equation 12; and Θ_m the time spent by the label in the metabolite pool, calculated as $\int_0^T M_m \, dt/(C_a V_m)$.

When the ratio between the compound free in brain and the compound free in blood no longer changes rapidly, the ratio M_e/C_a eventually approaches V_f. The graphical representation of this case is a straight line. K is the slope of the line and $r_e V_f + V_a$ the ordinate intercept (see 'slope-intercept' or 'Patlak' plot above).

If the volume of distribution observed in a region of binding is divided by the volume of distribution in a region of no binding, the ratio between the volumes of distribution observed in the two regions eventually reaches the linear relationship

$$\frac{V^{(1)} - V_a}{V^{(2)} - V_a} \cong r_e k_3 \Theta + r_e^2 \qquad (22)$$

which is the basis for the so-called 'ratio' method which derives the value k_3 from the slope and the intercept of the relationship between the ratio of the measured volumes of distribution in region of binding ($V^{(1)}$) and a region of no binding ($V^{(2)}$).

However, if k_4 is not negligible, the three-compartment tracers must eventually approach an equilibrium defined by the four coefficients of Equations 14 and 15. At steady-state, the 'equilibrium volume' of distribution is

$$V(\infty) \rightarrow \frac{K_1}{k_2} \left(1 + \frac{k_3}{k_4} \right) + V_a = V_e + V_m + V_a \qquad (23)$$

where the K_1/k_2 ratio is the volume V_e, and the k_3/k_4 ratio the V_m/V_e ratio. The k_3/k_4 ratio is a convenient measure of the tissue's 'binding potential' (r_B), imposed by the presence of binding sites.

A. RECEPTOR BINDING

The definitions of k_3 and k_4 follow from the Michaelis-Menten equation that describes the association and dissociation of the ligand-receptor complex as functions of the concentrations of ligand and inhibitor(s). However, true ligand *concentration* is unknown *in vivo*. Instead, only the *content* of ligand in the exchangeable pool, M_e, can be estimated. Therefore, the binding equation must be modified accordingly[19]

$$\frac{dB}{dt} = k_{on} \left[\frac{B_{max} - (B + B_I)}{V_d} \right] M_e - k_{off} B \qquad (24)$$

where k_{on} is the bimolecular association rate constant, k_{off} the dissociation rate, B_{max} the maximal tracer binding capacity and V_d the volume of tissue in which the ligand is dissolved. This volume is defined as the ratio between the content of free ligand and the concentration of free ligand in tissue water. B is the quantity of bound ligand, and B_I the total quantity of bound inhibitors, assumed constant in the present analysis. This constancy is not strictly true, however, if the ligand concentration C changes significantly.

The difference between B_{max} and B_I has been designated B'_{max} to indicate the number of receptor sites available for binding of the ligand in question. Note that B'_{max} is defined only when C and C_I are constants or negligible. By simple comparison of Equation 24 with Equations 14 and 15, the transfer coefficients k_3 and k_4 can be identified as follows

$$k_3 = k_{on} B'_{max}/V_d \qquad (25)$$

and

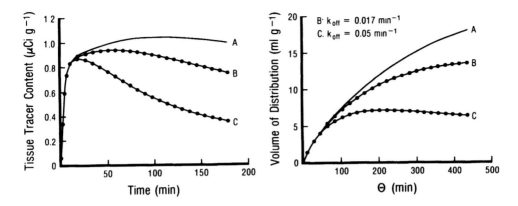

FIGURE 1. Simulated approach to steady-state volume of distribution of three labeled tracers with different values of k_{off} corresponding to 'binding potentials' of 5 (standard, A), 3 (B), and 1 (C). B_{max} is the same, 25 pmol g^{-1}, in the three cases. Other values as listed in Table 3. Left panel shows simulated uptake in measured units of radioactivity vs. real time. Abscissa: Time (minutes). Ordinate: Radioactivity in sample of brain *in vivo* (μCi g^{-1}). Right panel shows simulated uptake in converted units of volume of distribution vs. normalized arterial time-activity integral. Abscissa: Normalized integral (minutes). Ordinate: Volume of distribution (ml g^{-1}). Each line represents a different value of k_{off}: A is the standard value of 0.01 min^{-1} representing 'spiperone', B-0.017 min^{-1}, C-0.05 min^{-1}.

$$k_4 = k_{off} + k_{on} \frac{M_e}{V_d} = k_{off} \left(1 + \frac{C}{K_D} \right) \tag{26}$$

where M_e is the quantity (mass) of tracer available for binding.

Since k_3 and k_4 are arbitrary assignations of the different components of the differential equations, it appears that k_3 is independent of the injected dose of tracer while k_4 is a function of the free tracer concentration and therefore not a constant when M_e is not constant or negligible. This definition of k_4 is not new to receptor kineticists; it is known as the 'observed k' used to calculate k_{on} when k_{off} has been determined.

According to Equation 23, the k_3/k_4 ratio represents the ratio between B'_{max}/V_d and $K_D + C$ at steady-state, e.g., when C attains a constant level. This ratio is the unitless 'binding potential' r_B. Note that the magnitude of r_B depends on the volume of distribution and concentration of the ligand. The higher the concentration of the ligand, the lower the magnitude of r_B. Thus, during the approach to equilibrium, the measured distribution space V, equal to the ratio $[M_a + M_e + M_b]/C_a$, rises to the steady-state value $V(\infty)$

$$V(\infty) \rightarrow V_e \left(1 + \frac{B'_{max}/V_d}{K_D + C(\infty)} \right) + V_a \tag{27}$$

Simulated examples of the approach to equilibrium are given in Figures 1 and 2, illustrating the effect of different values of k_{off} in Figure 1, and the effect of different values of B_{max} in Figure 2.

In positron emission tomography, it is often possible to do several studies in the same subject, and these studies may therefore be repeated with different total doses of radioligand. The highest ligand concentrations reduce the binding potential to zero and the equilibrium volume to its minimum value, equal to the partition coefficient $V_e + V_a$ of the ligand. By nonlinear regression, Equation 27 allows estimates to be made of $V_e + V_a$, B'_{max}, and the k_{off}/k_{on} ratio, or K_D.

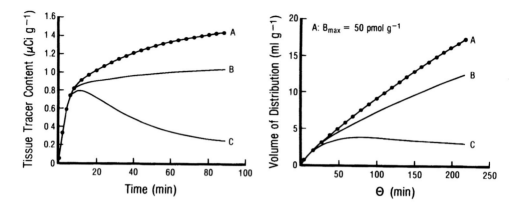

FIGURE 2.   Simulated uptake of the 'standard' radioligand by a radioligand-binding region in brain in the absence and presence of an elevated number of binding sites in brain. Left panel and right panel axes as in Figure 1. Each of the three graphs represents a different number of binding sites. A is the case of binding sites with a twofold elevated B_{max} of 50 pmol g^{-1}. B is the 'standard' case of B_{max} 25 pmol g^{-1} and k_{off} = 0.01 min^{-1}. C is the case of no specific binding (nonbinding region).

B. RECEPTOR BLOCKADE

The quantity B'_{max} represents the number of receptors available for occupation by the labeled ligand. If the receptor is blocked by a competitor, the total quantity of receptor sites in the tissue (B_{max}) is reduced by a factor that depends on the receptor's affinity for the competitor

$$B'_{max} = B_{max} \frac{K'_I}{K'_I + C_I} \tag{28}$$

where B_{max} is the maximal quantity of bound ligand, K'_I the competitor's apparent inhibition constant ('IC$_{50}$') and C_I its concentration in brain water. In the simplest cases, the apparent inhibition constant is the affinity of the competitor in the presence of the ligand[20]

$$K'_I = K_I\left(1 + \frac{C}{K_D}\right) \tag{29}$$

where C is the free ligand concentration and K_D the dissociation constant of the ligand. Both of these equations follow from simple inhibition kinetics when an inhibitor competes with the ligand for binding. Thus, the quantity of bound inhibitor is also a function of the ligand concentration

$$B_I = \frac{B_{max}C_I}{C_I + K_I\left(1 + \frac{C}{K_D}\right)} \tag{30}$$

and K'_I can be a constant only when C is negligible or invariant. This condition also applies to B'_{max} and k_3. Like K_D, K_I is the ratio between the magnitudes of k_{Ioff} and for k_{Ion} for the inhibitor.

Blockade involves prior occupancy of the receptor by the blocking agent, unlike saturation which involves significant occupation of the receptor by the labeled ligand during the course of study, or displacement which involves clearance of the labeled ligand from the receptor by an unlabeled competitor or by the unlabeled ligand itself.

TABLE 1
Distribution and Binding Constants For N-[^{11}C]Methylspiperone Binding in Human Caudate in The Absence and Presence of Unlabeled Haloperidol *In Vivo*

Variable		Before haloperidol	After haloperidol
K_1	(ml g^{-1} min^{-1})	0.15	0.21
k_2	(min^{-1})	0.051	0.077
k_3	(min^{-1})	0.087	0.010[a]
V_e	(cerebellum; ml g^{-1})	3.0	2.7
V_f	(ml g^{-1})	1.1	2.4[a]
ρ	(relative to cerebellum; ratio)	4.1	0.0[a]

[a] Significantly different from pre-haloperidol value (paired *t*-test) at $P < 0.05$.

Adapted from Wong, D. F., Gjedde, A., Wagner, H. N., Jr., et al., *J. Cereb. Blood Flow Metab.*, 6, 137, 1986.

The measure of blockade is saturation, defined as the ratio between bound inhibitor and the maximal binding capacity at equilibrium. In a receptor-controlled brain function, occupancy of the receptor by an agonist is the factor responsible for the magnitude of the response. Occupancy is a function of the affinity and concentrations of the ligands that compete for occupation. When a single competitor contributes to the occupancy, the degree of saturation by the inhibitor can be calculated from the ratio

$$s = \frac{C_I}{K'_I + C_I} = 1 - \frac{k_3^{(I)}}{k_3} \qquad (31)$$

where $k_3^{(I)}$ is the value of k_3 measured in the presence of inhibition. The degree of saturation is also an index of the degree of occupancy established by any pharmacological agent bound to the receptor.

The apparent volume of distribution of the ligand (V_f) increases when binding is blocked because k_3 declines as less tracer is removed from the free ligand pool.

V. SOLUBILITY AND NONSPECIFIC BINDING

Nonspecific binding refers to the sequestration of some fraction of the tracer by attachment to 'sites' that cannot be saturated in the range of concentrations available for study. Depending on the mechanism involved, nonspecific binding can also be manifested as a change of solubility. In this sense, nonspecific binding is all binding to sites of sufficiently low affinity and high capacity to escape saturation at the chosen ligand concentrations. Some nonspecific sites may also be saturable but nonspecific binding will be defined here as binding to sites that cannot be saturated and are of such low affinity that equilibrium is 'instantaneous' for all practical purposes.

The nonspecific binding simulates an expansion of distribution space for free ligand such as to render the concentration of free ligand in tissue water lower than suspected from the sample content. At equilibrium, nonspecific binding can be simulated by an expansion of the equilibrium distribution volume of the type expressed in Equation 23,

$$V_d = V_w(1 + \rho) \qquad (32)$$

where ρ is the 'binding potential' of nonspecific or low-affinity binding (see Table 1), corresponding to the k_3/k_4 ratio for specific binding, and V_w is the volume of water measured

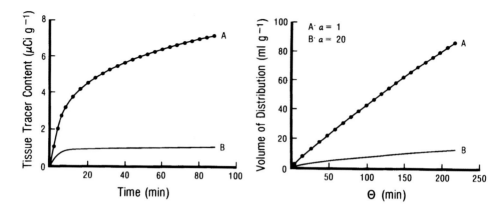

FIGURE 3.   Simulated uptake of the 'standard' radioligand by a radioligand-binding region in brain as a function of the degree of protein binding in blood. Left panel and right panel axes as in Figure 1. The two graphs represent different degrees of protein binding. A is the case of no protein binding in blood (α = 1, f_1 = 1). B is the 'standard' case of 5% free radioligand in blood (α = 20, f_1 = 0.05).

in the absence of nonspecific binding. Although the legality of estimating the degree of nonspecific binding at nonsteady-state is questionable, Mintun et al.[21] used Equations 14 and 15 to estimate the degree of nonspecific binding of radiolabeled ligand in brain on the basis of measurements of free fraction in plasma *in vitro*. The reciprocal of the volume of distribution in brain was defined as f_2

$$f_2 = \frac{1}{V_d} \tag{33}$$

The free fraction in arterial samples was defined by Mintun et al.[21] as

$$f_1 = \frac{1}{\alpha} \tag{34}$$

where α is the solubility of the ligand in the sample relative to water (Equation 4). Thus

$$f_2 = \frac{f_1}{V_e} \tag{35}$$

according to which f_2 can be calculated when f_1 and V_e are known. If the ligand distributes only in a fraction of the total tissue water, e.g., only in extracellular fluid, V_w refers only to the volume of water in the extracellular space. Note that f_1 is a proper fraction while f_2 strictly, is the reciprocal of a volume with units of g ml^{-1} or ml ml^{-1}. The influence of protein (or other) binding in plasma on the brain uptake of the radioligand is simulated in Figure 3.

Values of f_1 and f_2 of [^{18}F]fluorospiperone were measured in monkey and man by Perlmutter et al. The values were 4 to 6% for f_1 and 1 to 2% for f_2 in monkey[22] and 5% for f_1 and 0.7% for f_2 in man.[23] Values for f_1 for other ligands have been reported also to be close to 5%. The consequences of protein binding in plasma for the measurement of blood-brain barrier permeability-surface area product are exemplified in Table 2 in which protein binding was corrected for in one study only.

Additional sites to which the radioligand may attach can only be distinguished from the sites under investigation if they differ significantly with respect to affinity to the ligand. In

TABLE 2

Influence of Plasma Protein Binding on Apparent Permeability of Radioligands

Tracer	PS (ml g^{-1} min^{-1})	Correction for protein binding	Ref.
Fluorospiperone	2.80	Yes	Perlmutter et al.[23,a]
Methylspiperone	0.22	No	Wong et al.[26,a]
Fluorospiperone	0.20	No	Logan et al.[34,b]
Fluoroethylspiperone	0.09	No	Huang et al.[27,b]

[a] Humans.
[b] Baboons.

these cases, they act as binding sites of such low-affinity that they can be simulated by nonspecific binding. The presence of additional sites, e.g., the low-affinity HT$_2$ sites for *NMSP* in neostriatum, may affect the analysis by causing the degree of nonspecific binding to vary between regions. The analysis of Wong et al.[24] allowed for this possibility, as shown in Table 1 in which the term ρ indicates the 'binding' potential (k_5/k_6) of the 'additional' sites assumed to be HT$_2$ sites.

VI. SIMULATION OF RADIOLIGAND UPTAKE

In the present discussion, the kinetic behavior of radioligands interacting with neuroreceptor sites in the brain has been illustrated by simulated uptake curves created by a simple numerical integration included in the FORTRAN routine listed below. The routine can also form the core of a least-squares nonlinear regression analysis available from the author:

```
SUBROUTINE SIMUL(P,NP,CA,CAI,TIM,ACT,NT,N,SA)
REAL P(NP),CA(NT),CAI(NT),TIM(NT),ACT(NT),INTERV(NT)
REAL K1,K1I,K2,K2I,K3,K3I,K5,KMET,
REAL ME,MI,MM,KON,KONI,KONS,KOFF,KOFFI,KOFFS
CALL FRACTNS(P,NP,F1,F2,F1I,F2I)
CALL PSPRODS(P,NP,PS1,PS2,PS1I,PS2I,CBF,VA)
CALL BMAXVAL(P,NP,BMAX,BMAXS)
CALL AFFINIT(P,NP,KON,KOFF,KONS,KOFFS,KONI,KOFFI,KMET)
CALL INITIAL(P,NP,CA,CAI,NT,ME,MI,MM,B,BI,BS)
KON=KON*F2
KONS=KONS*F2
KONI=KONI*F2I
K1=CBF-CBF*EXP(-PS1*F1/CBF)
K1I=CBF-CBF*EXP(-PS1I*F1I/CBF)
K2=K1*PS2*F2/(PS1*F1)
K2I=K1I*PS2I*F2I/(PS1I*F1I)
K3=KON*BMAX
K3I=KONI*BMAX
K5=KONS*BMAXS
DO 100 J=1,NT
DO 100 I=1,N
CALL INTRAPO(STEP,CA,CAI,C,CI,TIM,J,I,NT,N)
C=C/SA
DB=K3*ME-KON*ME*(B+BI)-KOFF*B
```

```
    DBS=K5•ME – KONS•ME•BS – KOFFS•BS
    DBI=K3I•MI – KONI•MI•(B + BI) – KOFFI•BI
    DMM=KMET•ME
    DIN=K1•C – K2•ME
    DII=K1I•CI – K2I•MI
    DME=DIN – DB – DBS – DMM
    DMI=DII – DBI
    ME=STEP•DME + ME
    MM=STEP•DMM + MM
    MI=STEP•DMI + MI
    B=STEP•DB + B
    BS=STEP•DBS + BS
    BI=STEP•DBI + BI
100 ACT(J)=(ME + MM + B + BS + VA•C)•SA
    RETURN
    END
```

in which CA(NT) is the arterial tracer input function, NT the number of measurements of the arterial tracer concentration, i.e., the number of points on the arterial input curve, and TIM are the times of the arterial concentrations measurements. The concentrations of the inhibitor are CAI(NT). Thus, two separate compounds are considered, the radioligand, represented by CA, TIM, ME, B, BS, and MM, and an inhibitor, represented by CAI, TIM, MI, and BI. STEP is the step size employed during the numerical integration. Each interval between two arterial concentration measurements is divided into N steps chosen by the user. The concentration change for each step is determined by intrapolation performed by the subroutine INTRAPO. PS1 and PS2 are the *PS*-products of transport in the two directions through the blood-brain barrier. In the absence of facilitated diffusion of the radioligand, PS1 = PS2. ACT(NT) are the measured radioactivities in brain.

The differentials are represented by DME, DB, DBI, DBS, DMM, and DMI. The significance of the coefficients K1, K2, K3, K1I, K3I, KON, KOFF, KONI, KOFFI, KONS, KOFFS, and K5 has been discussed in detail above. KMET is the coefficient of metabolism of the tracer in arterial blood. Labeled metabolites of the tracer may be generated in the circulation and then either (1) pass or (2) not pass into the brain. Labeled metabolites may also be generated in brain tissue, (3) pass back or (4) not pass back into the circulation and/or (5) bind to the specific sites in question. If the labeled ligand is present at concentrations above tracer concentrations, (6) metabolites may further block the specific sites to a significant extent. In the routine listed above, only possibility (4) has been considered.

P(NP) are the 19 parameter values needed for the constants in the routine. Most of these values are listed in Table 3 for simulations illustrated in Figures 1-4. The values of the constants are set by the subroutines FRACTNS, PSPRODS, BMAXVAL, and AFFINIT. The initial conditions of the numerical integration are fixed by the subroutine INITIAL. In the simulation, it is assumed that CA are in units of radioactivity but CAI in units of concentration. Hence, the specific activity SA is supplied to convert radioactivity units to concentration units, and hence also to enable the routine to simulate the effects of different specific activities on binding of the radioligand. When the routine is used for nonlinear regression, the number of parameters must be reduced to four or less, on the basis of reasonable assumptions.

VII. *IN VIVO* ANALYSIS OF BINDING

A. IRREVERSIBLE BINDING: DETERMINATION OF k_3

The main distinction observed below is the distinction between 'reversible' and 'irre-

TABLE 3

'Standard' *In Vivo* Receptor Kinetic Values Used in Simulations. Values Were Chosen to Represent Averages of Values Reported for 'Spiperone' and Spiperone Analog Binding in Human Caudate

Variable	Value	Unit
$PS = -\alpha F \ln(1 - K_1/F)$	3	ml g^{-1} min^{-1}
F	0.5	ml g^{-1} min^{-1}
$\alpha = 1/f_1$	20	Ratio
$V_d = 1/f_2$	50	ml g^{-1}
K_1	0.15	ml g^{-1} min^{-1}
k_2	0.06	min^{-1}
k_3	0.05	min^{-1}
k_4	0.01	min^{-1}
$V_e = f_1/f_2 = K_1/k_2$	2.5	ml g^{-1}
$r_B = k_3/k_4$	5	Ratio
$k'_{on} = k_{on}/V_d$	0.002	g pmol^{-1} min^{-1}
k_{off}	0.01	min^{-1}
k_{on}	0.1	min^{-1} nM^{-1}
K_D	0.1	nM
$B_{max} = k_3/k'_{on}$	25	pmol g^{-1}
SA	1	μCi pmol^{-1}

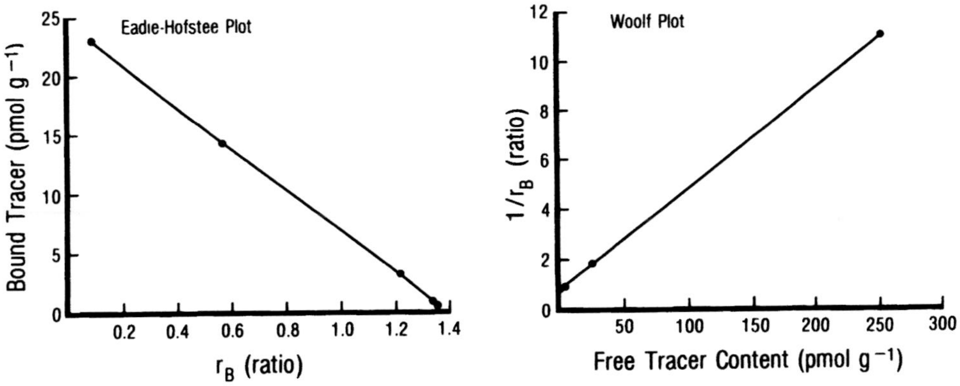

FIGURE 4. Simulated use of Eadie-Hofstee (left panel) and Woolf (right panel) plots to illustrate relationships between bound ligand, free ligand, and binding potential, at assumed equilibrium ($\Theta = 250$ min), determined as a function of the specific activity of the tracer in the injected bolus. The five points on each line represent diferent specific activities. The points nearest the bottom of the graphs represent the 'standard' specific activity of 1 μCi pmol^{-1} used in Figures 1—3. In declining order, the additional specific activities are 0.1 μCi pmol^{-1}, 0.01 μCi pmol^{-1}, 0.001 μCi pmol^{-1}, 0.0005 μCi mol^{-1}, and no specific binding (nonbinding region). In both plots, B_{max} is 25 pmol g^{-1}, and K_D is 0.1 nM as listed in Table 3.

versible' binding, referring to the presence or absence of noticeable loss of tracer from the brain during the study. It must be known in advance whether bound ligand dissociates from binding and hence escapes from brain, or whether the ligand remains trapped. As explained above, irreversibility is a feature of high values of the product of V_e and the k_3/k_4 ratio (binding potential) and can be predicted on the basis of the expected volume of distribution at equilibrium: the higher the equilibrium M/C_a ratio, the lower the chance of reversibility in a given period of study.

Steady-state M/C_a ratios of the order of 10 or more are likely to be associated with irreversible binding during the first hour. Irreversible trapping is characteristic of the high-affinity binding of certain receptor ligands, e.g., the substituted butyrophenones spiroperidol and methylspiperone, to receptors in the basal ganglia.

The purpose of the analysis of irreversible binding is the estimation of k_3. Regression analysis of the irreversible binding yields estimates of K_1, k_2, k_3, K, and V_f. Since the irreversible case, by definition, fails to reach equilibrium in the period of study, it is not logically possible to determine the equilibrium constants B'_{max} and K_D directly by this procedure. When k_{on} is a constant, the value of k_3 is an observed index of the receptor density that varies with B'_{max} and V_d. The value of B'_{max} may vary because the actual receptor number varies or because some receptors are blocked by endogenous or exogenous competitors. V_d may vary with variations of protein or other low-affinity binding in the tissue.

Equation 31 predicts an inverse proportionality between the concentration of a blocking agent (inhibitor) and the value of k_3. Equation 31 can be rearranged to yield the formula for a modified 'Woolf' plot[25]

$$\frac{1}{k_3^{(1)}} = \frac{1}{k_3} + \left[\frac{V_{le}}{k_{on}K_I\left(1 + \frac{C}{K_D}\right)}\right]\frac{C_{l_a}(\infty)}{B_{max}} \tag{36}$$

where V_{le} is the steady-state partition of haloperidol between brain and plasma and C_{l_a} the steady-state arterial concentration of the inhibitor.

Wong et al.[24,26] determined the values of K_1, k_2, and k_3 for tracer N-methylspiperone (*NMSP*) in neostriatum and cerebellum ($k_3 = 0$) in the human brain. The *NMSP* binding was blocked with a therapeutic dose of haloperidol. Unblocked, the net binding rate of *NMSP (K)* was 0.094 ml g^{-1} min^{-1}, and blocked it was 0.023 ml g^{-1} min^{-1}. As listed in Table 1, the distribution of *NMSP* (V_f) increased from 1.1 to 2.4 ml g^{-1} and hence approached the value of V_e expected of a region with no binding (e.g., cerebellum) and the corresponding value of k_3 declined from 0.09 to 0.01 min^{-1} after the blockade. Thus, at plasma concentrations of 2 to 3 n*M*, haloperidol blocked 90% of the *NMSP* binding sites.

Assuming a constant value for the $V_{le}/[k_{on} K_I]$ term ('D_w' = 186 min ml g^{-1}) and negligible C (tracer dose), Wong et al.[24] calculated the values of the B_{max} and K'_I for the D_2 dopamine receptors and haloperidol, respectively, in the human brain from the slope and abscissa intercept of Equation 36. The weakness of this indirect approach is the need to assume values for constants that cannot be verified in each experiment.

B. REVERSIBLE BINDING: DETERMINATION OF r_B

Completely irreversible trapping or binding is rare. In most cases, sooner or later, an equilibrium (i.e., $dC/dt = 0$) is approached between the quantities of tracer in the circulation, free tracer in brain, and tracer bound to receptors or converted to metabolites.

The purpose of the kinetic analysis of reversible binding is the estimation of the maximal value of the 'binding potential' r_B which equals the k_3/k_4 ratio only in the presence of truly negligible levels of the tracer, i.e., when $C(\infty)$ is negligible compared to K_D in Equations 27 and 37. The values of k_3 and k_4 are estimated by linear regression to Equation 16. The analysis must therefore be extended to include a significant portion of the approach to equilibrium, although the equilibrium need not be reached completely to estimate the binding potential. From measurements of the transfer coefficients, or from measurements of volumes of distribution at steady-state (see below), it is possible to calculate binding potentials for a variety of radioligands. Experimental results of such calculations are exemplified in Table 4.

The transfer coefficients cannot be determined by Equations 14 and 15 when k_4 is not

TABLE 4
Binding Potentials at Tracer Doses of Selected Radioligands

Ligand	Receptor	$r_B = k_3/k_4$	Ref.
Methylspiperone	Dopamine D_2	> 10	Arnett et al.[35,a]
Bromospiperone	Dopamine D_2	6.7	Crawley et al.[36,a]
Fluorospiperone	Dopamine D_2	6.4	Logan et al.[34,b]
Raclopride	Dopamine D_2	3.0	Farde et al.[33,a]
SCH-23 390	Dopamine D_1	2.0	Farde et al.[33,a]
Methylspiperone	Serotonin HT_2	1.5	Wong et al.[37,a]
Haloperidol	Dopamine D_2	1.1	Logan et al.[34,b]

[a] Humans.
[b] Baboons.

a constant. This transfer coefficient ceases to be a constant when the ligand concentration C changes significantly relative to K_D (Equation 37). Therefore, under ordinary circumstances, it is not possible to determine the transfer coefficients and hence the k_3/k_4 ratio under nonsteady-state conditions when the ligand concentration is significant, i.e., when the radioligand is not really a tracer. However, if the unlabeled ligand can be given so far in advance that its concentration in the circulation and brain tissue is approximately constant, as required by Equation 26, and if the plasma concentration of the ligand can be determined, it becomes possible to determine the k_3/k_4 ratio at different degrees of saturation of the receptor sites and hence to calculate the binding constants. This type of experiment is essentially a blockade with the ligand as its own inhibitor.

There is one additional possibility. Huang et al.[27] have proposed to solve Equations 14 and 24 directly by a two-step numerical procedure (e.g., Runge-Kutta) in which the six coefficients V_a, K_1, k_2, B_{max}, k_{off}, and k_{on}/V_d are estimated simultaneously. The procedure is very close to the method of simulation used in the present text. The first step, during which ligand concentrations are negligible, yields estimates of V_a, K_1, k_2, $k_{on} B_{max}/V_d$, and k_{off} (4 + 1 parameters). This step is basically a standard determination of K_1-k_4 according to Equation 16. The second step, during which the previously estimated coefficients are kept constant, yields k_{on}/V_d and B_{max} separately (2 parameters). The procedure does not require complete equilibrium. In theory, a single low-specific activity injection would suffice but the number of parameters is then too great (6) to yield accurate estimates.

C. EQUILIBRIUM BINDING: DETERMINATION OF B_{max} AND K_D

Equation 23 defines an equilibrium volume of distribution. According to Equation 27, the equilibrium volume declines when the receptors are saturated. Thus, when the ligand concentration rises in the distribution space, the equilibrium volume falls, as shown by equation 27. The actual amounts of ligand held in the compartment can be determined by multiplying the volume of distribution with the arterial concentration of the ligand, $C_a(\infty)$. Multiplication with the arterial concentration yields the total quantity of tracer in the region at equilibrium.

$$M(\infty) = M_e + \frac{B_{max} C}{K_D + C} + M_a \tag{37}$$

Equation 37 can be rearranged to yield the equation underlying the linearized plot attributed to Eadie,[28] Scatchard,[29] Hofstee,[30] and Rosenthal[31]

$$B = -[V_d K_D] r_B + B_{max} \tag{38}$$

where r_B is the binding potential equal to the B/M_e ratio. The ordinate intercept is B_{max} and the slope is $-V_d K_D$. By definition, at equilibrium, and when binding is negligible

$$M_e(\infty) = V_d\, C(\infty) = V_e C_a(\infty) \qquad (39)$$

and

$$B = V_m\, C_a(\infty) \qquad (40)$$

where $V_e = K_1/k_2$ and $V_m = r_B V_e$. Since k_3 and k_4 cannot be estimated under nonsteady-state circumstances when the ligand concentration is significantly above tracer level, it is usually not possible to calculate B and M_e by regression. Fortunately, M_e and B can be determined in several other ways. Thus, if a particular region of the brain is known not to contain any receptor sites for the ligand under investigation, then, at *steady-state*, $M_e + M_a$ is by definition the tracer content in that region. If no such region exist, then Equation 27 must be used to determine the volume of distribution of the free ligand (V_e) as the volume of distribution of the ligand at very high values of $C(\infty)$. This can be performed by nonlinear regression of Equation 27 to simultaneously determined values of $V(\infty)$ and $C_a(\infty)$. The third method of estimating M_e measures the volume of distribution of an enantiomer of the tracer which does not bind to the receptor sites under study but to all other sites in exactly the same manner and with the same physical properties as the tracer itself.

The bound quantity B can similarly be determined as the difference between the quantity of tracer in a binding region and the quantity of tracer in a nonbinding region. If a nonbinding region does not exist, then the bound quantity must be determined from the volumes $V_e + V_a$, recorded at complete saturation

$$B = M(\infty) - (M_a + M_e) = M(\infty) - (V_e + V_a)\, C_a(\infty) \qquad (41)$$

according to which, at equilibrium

$$V_m = \frac{M}{C_a} - (V_e + V_a) \qquad (42)$$

The 'Woolf' plot of Equation 37 is

$$\frac{1}{r_B} = \frac{M_e}{B_{max}} + \frac{V_d K_d}{B_{max}} \qquad (43)$$

which basically is identical to Equation 36. Examples of the Eadie-Hofstee-Scatchard-Rosenthal and Woolf plots of the same receptor kinetic data obtained *in vivo* are given in Figure 4.

Calculation of the 'binding potential' r_B at (at least) two different ligand concentrations allowed Farde et al.[32,33] to determine the neostriatal B_{max} value and K_D of the dopamine D_2 receptor ligand raclopride in this manner. The concentration of free ligand was estimated as the quantity of tracer in cerebellum at each dose of tracer raclopride injected. The same procedure allowed Logan et al.[34] to calculate the neostriatal B_{max} in baboons.

REFERENCES

1. **Langley, J. N.**, On the physiology of the salivary secretion. II. On the mutual antagonism of atropin and pilocarpin, having special reference to their relation in the submaxillary gland of the cat, *J. Physiol.*, 1, 339, 1878.
2. **Ehrlich, P.**, Uber den jetzigen Stand der Chemotherapie, *Ber. Dtsch. Chem. Ges.*, 42, 17, 1909.
3. **Bohr, C.**, *Experimentelle Untersuchungen uber die Sauerstoffaufnahme des Blutfarbstoffes*, Copenhagen, 1885.
4. **Michaelis, L. and Menten, M. L.**, Die Kinetik der Invertinwirkung, *Biochem. Z.* 49, 333, 1913.
5. **Bohr, C.**, Theoretische Behandlung der quantitativen Verhaltuisse bei der Sauerstoffaufnahme des Haemoglobins, *Zentralbl. Physiol.*, 23, 1, 1904.
6. **Hill, A. V.**, The possible effects to aggregation of the molecules of haemoglobin on its dissociation curves, *J. Physiol.*, 40, 4, 1910.
7. **Sheppard, C. W.**, The theory of the study of transfers within a multi-compartmental system using isotopic tracers, *J. Appl. Phys.*, 19, 70, 1948.
8. **Rescigno, A. and Beck, J. S.**, Compartments, in *Foundations of Mathematical Biology 2*, Rosen, R., Ed., Academic Press, New York, 1972, 255.
9. **Bohr, C.**, Uber die spezifische Tatigkeit der Lungen bei der respiratorischen Gasaufnahme und ihr Verhalten zu der durch die Alveolarwand stattfindenden Gasdiffusion, *Skand. Arch. Physiol.*, 22, 221, 1909.
10. **Crone, C.**, The permeability of capillaries in various organs as determined by use of the 'indicator diffusion' method, *Acta Physiol. Scand.* 58, 292, 1963.
11. **Lassen, N. A. and Gjedde, A.**, Kinetic analysis of the uptake of glucose and some of its analogs in the brain, using the single capillary model: comments on some points of controversy, in *Lecture Notes in Biomathematics 48: Tracer Kinetics and Physiologic Modeling*, Lambrecht, R. M. and Rescigno, A., Eds., Springer Verlag, New York, 1983, 387.
12. **Gjedde, A.**, High- and low-affinity transport of D-glucose from blood to brain, *J. Neurochem.*, 36, 1463, 1981.
13. **Patlak, C., Blasberg, R. G., and Fenstermacher, J. D.**, Graphical evaluation of blood-to-brain transfer constants from multiple-time uptake data, *J. Cereb. Blood Flow Metab.* 3, 1, 1983.
14. **Blomqvist, G.**, On the construction of functional maps in positron emission tomography, *J. Cereb. Blood Flow Metab.*, 4, 629, 1984.
15. **Evans, A. C.**, A double integral form of the three-compartmental, four-rate-constant model for faster generation of parameter maps, *J. Cereb. Blood Flow Metab.*, 7 (Suppl. 1), S453, 1987.
16. **Sokoloff, L., Reivich, M., Kennedy, C., des Rosiers, M. H., Patlak, C. S., Pettigrew, K. D., Sakurada, O., and Shinohara, M.**, The [^{14}C]deoxyglucose method for the measurement of local cerebral glucose utilization: theory, procedure, and normal values in the conscious and anesthetized albino rat, *J. Neurochem.*, 28, 897, 1977.
17. **Gjedde, A.**, Calculation of glucose phosphorylation from brain uptake of glucose analogs in vivo: a re-examination, *Brain Res. Rev.*, 4, 237, 1982.
18. **Gjedde, A.**, Does deoxyglucose uptake in the brain reflect energy metabolism?, *Biochem. Pharmacol.*, 36, 1853, 1987.
19. **Gjedde, A. and Wong, D. F.**, Positron tomographic quantitation of neuroreceptors in human brain in vivo with special reference to the D2 dopamine receptors in caudate nucleus, *Neurosurg. Rev.*, 10, 9, 1987.
20. **Dixon, M.**, The determination of enzyme inhibitor constants, *Biochem. J.*, 55, 170, 1953.
21. **Mintun, M. A., Raichle, M. E., Kilbourn, M. R., Wooten, G. F., and Welch, M. J.**, A quantitative model for the in vivo assessment of drug binding sites with positron emission tomography, *Ann. Neurol.* 15, 217, 1984.
22. **Perlmutter, J. S., Larson, K. B., Raichle, M. E., Markham, J., Mintun, M. A., Kilbourn, M. R., and Welch, M. J.**, Strategies for in vivo measurement of receptor binding using positron emission tomography, *J. Cereb Blood Flow Metab.*, 66, 154, 1986.
23. **Perlmutter, J. S., Kilbourn, M. R., Raichle, M. E., and Welch, M. J.**, MPTP-induced up-regulation of in vivo dopaminergic radioligand-receptor binding in humans, *Neurology*, 37, 1575, 1987.
24. **Wong, D. F., Gjedde, A., Wagner, H. N., Jr., Dannals, R. F., Douglass, K. H., Links, J. M., and Kuhar, M. J.**, Quantification of neuroreceptors in the living human brain. II. Inhibition studies of receptor density and affinity, *J. Cereb. Blood Flow Metab.*, 6, 147, 1986.
25. **Haldane, J. B. S.**, Graphical methods in enzyme chemistry, *Nature*, 179, 832, 1957.
26. **Wong, D. F., Gjedde, A., and Wagner, H. N., Jr.**, Quantification of neuroreceptors in the living human brain. I. Irreversible binding of ligands, *J. Cereb. Blood Flow Metab.*, 6, 137, 1986.
27. **Huang, S. C., Bahn, M. M., Barrio, J. R., Hawkins, R. A., Hoffmann, J. M., Satyamurthy, N., Bida, G. T., Mazziotta, J. C., and Phelps, M. E.**, A double-injection procedure for measurement of dopamine-D2 receptor density (B_{max}) and ligand-receptor association constant (k_a) using 3-2'-[^{18}F]fluoroethylspiperone (FESP) and PET, *J. Cereb. Blood Flow Metab.*, 7 (Suppl. 1), S359, 1987.

28. **Eadie, G. S.,** The inhibition of cholinesterase by physostigmine and prostigmine, *J. Biol. Chem.,* 146, 85, 1942.

29. **Scatchard, G.,** The attractions of proteins for small molecules and ions, *Ann. N.Y. Acad. Sci.,* 51, 600, 1949.

30. **Hofstee, B. H. J.,** Graphical analysis of single enzyme systems, *Enzymologia,* 17, 273, 1954—1956.

31. **Rosenthal, H.** A graphic method for the determination and presentation of binding parameters in a complex system, *Anal. Biochem.* 20, 525, 1967.

32. **Farde, L., Hall, H., Ehrin, E., and Sedvall, G.,** Quantitative analysis of D2 dopamine receptor binding in the living human brain by PET, *Science,* 231, 258, 1986.

33. **Farde, L., Halldin, C., Stone-Elander, S., and Sedvall, G.,** PET analysis of human dopamine receptor subtypes, using ¹¹C-SCH 23390 and ¹¹C-raclopride, *Psychopharmacology,* 92, 278, 1987.

34. **Logan, J., Wolf, A. P., Shiue, C. Y., and Fowler, J. S.,** Kinetic modeling of receptor-ligand binding applied to positron emission tomographic studies with neuroleptic tracers, *J. Neurochem.,* 48, 73, 1987.

35. **Arnett, C. D., Wolf, A. P., Shiue, C. Y., Fowler, J. S., MacGregor, R. R., Chistman, D. R., and Smith, M. R.,** Improved delineation of human dopamine receptors using [¹⁸F]-N-methylspiroperidol and PET, *J. Nucl. Med.* 27, 1878, 1986.

36. **Crawley, J. C. W., Crow, T. J., Johnstone, E. C., Oldland, S. R. D., Owen, F., Owens, D. G. C., Poulter, M., Pufter, O., Smith, T., Veall, N., and Zanelli, G. D.,** Dopamine D2 receptors in schizophrenia studied in vivo, *Lancet,* II, 224, 1986.

37. **Wong, D. F., Gjedde, A., Dannals, R. F., Lever, J. R., Hartig, P., Ravert, H., Wilson, A., Links, J., Villemagne, V., Braestrup, C., Harris, J., and Wagner, H. N., Jr.,** Quantification of neuroreceptors in living human brain: equilibrium binding kinetic studies with dopamine and serotonin receptors, *J. Cereb. Blood Flow Metab.,* 7 (Suppl. 1), S356, 1987.

Chapter 4

DOPAMINE RECEPTOR STUDIES WITH POSITRON EMISSION TOMOGRAPHY

Joel S. Perlmutter

TABLE OF CONTENTS

I. INTRODUCTION

This chapter will review the different approaches that have been proposed to measure dopaminergic radioligand-receptor binding *in vivo* using positron emission tomography (PET). I will highlight the relevant observations suggesting PET could be a useful tool to measure *in vivo* binding, discuss the development and charactristics of appropriate dopaminergic radioligands, summarize different methods of data analysis, and review the clinical applications involving patients with involuntary movement disorders.

II. BACKGROUND

Involuntary movement disorders such as parkinsonism, various forms of dystonia, Huntington's disease, Tourette's syndrome, and tardive dyskinesias are thought to involve abnormalities of central dopaminergic pathways. Analysis of dopaminergic receptors in the brain should enhance our understanding of alterations of dopaminergic pathways that either contribute to the pathophysiology of these conditions or play a major role in pharmacotherapy. Until recently, however, receptor-binding measurements utilized *in vitro* binding techniques and were limited to post-mortem studies.

The basic principles underlying *in vitro* methodology should be understood as they form the bases for the development of *in vivo* studies. *In vitro* techniques expose homogenized tissue or tissue slices to solutions containing various concentrations of radioligand.[1] After equilibrium has occurred (at which point no additional radioligand will bind even with more prolonged incubation), tissue radioactivity is quantified. Total radioactivity includes radioligand bound to nonspecific as well as to specific binding sites. The amount of nonspecific binding is exquisitely dependent on assay conditions as well as investigator technique. Nonspecific binding is usually quantified by performing identical experiments without and with an excess of unlabeled high affinity ligand to block specific binding. With excess unlabeled ligand, tissue radioactivity represents radioligand bound only to nonsaturable, nonspecific binding sites. Without excess unlabeled ligand, tissue activity reflects both nonspecific and specific binding. Specific binding then is calculated by subtracting nonspecific binding, identified with excess unlabeled ligand, from total tissue activity, measured in the absence of unlabeled ligand. By varying the concentration of radioligand in a series of such paired assays, specific binding is measured as a function of free radioligand in the *in vitro* system. Subsequent data analysis permits estimation of the number of available specific binding sites (B_{max}) as well as the equilibrium dissociation constant, K_d, the reciprocal of which is the equilibrium affinity constant. K_d is the concentration of ligand that results in 50% binding of available receptor sites. This is equivalent to the ratio of the two individual rate constants that describe the interaction between ligand and receptor, the dissociation rate constant of ligand-receptor complex and the asociation rate constant of ligand for receptor. These individual rate constants cannot be measured with equilibrium techniques.

In vitro equilibrium analyses have produced exciting, but at times, conflicting findings. For example, some investigators have reported increased dopaminergic receptor binding and others have found no change in patients with Parkinson's disease.[2-11] Discrepancies arise, not only because of differences in ante-mortem drug therapy, but also from technical factors involved in *in vitro* binding assays.[11-13] Furthermore, *in vitro* studies using autopsy material permit measurements at only one point in time for each subject. Noninvasive techniques to measure *in vivo* radioligand-receptor binding in living subjects would be of great value to clarify the role of rceptors in the pathogenesis of disease, and to determine whether pharmacotherapy affects receptor function and whether such alterations produce changes in clinical response to treatment.

Positron emission tomography (PET) is a nuclear medicine imaging technique that

TABLE 1
Radioligands That Have Been Synthesized for
Positron Emission Tomographic Studies of
Dopamine Receptors

Radioligands	Ref.
^{18}F-haloperidol	Tewson et al.[17]
^{11}C-pimozide	Crouzel et al.[18]
^{18}F-spiperone	Maeda et al.[19]
^{11}C-spiperone	Fowler et al.[20]
^{75}Br-SCH23390	DeJesus et al.[21]
^{11}C-N-methylspiperone	Wagner et al.[22], Burns et al.[23]
^{76}Br-bromospiperone	Maziere et al.[24]
^{18}F-N-methylspiperone	Arnett et al.[25]
^{18}F-benperidol	Arnett et al.[26]
^{18}F-pipamperone	Shiue et al.[27]
^{11}C-raclopride	Ehrin et al.[28]
^{75}Br-bromospiperone,	Moerlein et al.[29]
^{75}Br-brombenperidol,	
^{75}Br-bromperidol	
^{11}C-SCH 23390	Halldin et al.[30]
^{18}F-fluoroethylspiperone	Coenen et al.[31]
^{18}F-fluoropropylspiperone	Welch et al.[32]
^{11}C-eticlopride	Halldin et al.[33]

measures the regional distribution of a previously administered radionuclide (see Chapter 1).[14] In effect, it produces an *in vivo* autoradiograph from a living subject. Previous studies in animals suggested that such autoradiographs could be useful in delineating dopaminergic receptors. After intravenous (IV) administration of radioligands with high affinity for dopaminergic receptors, such as radiolabeled spiperone, areas of brain rich in dopaminergic receptors (e.g., striatum) accumulate higher amounts of radioactivity than regions relatively devoid of specific binding sites (e.g., cerebellum).[15,16] Thus, these autoradiographs permit imaging of the distribution of specific binding sites and such studies provided the basis for *in vivo* PET investigations.

III. RADIOCHEMISTRY

Based upon these encouraging findings, radiochemists began to synthesize dopaminergic ligands labeled with positron-emitting radionuclides such as ^{11}C, ^{18}F, ^{75}Br, or ^{76}Br that would be suitable for PET studies.[17-33] Most of these labeled ligands have been either butyrophenones or substituted benzamides that preferentially bind to D_2 dopaminergic sites (see Table 1). *In vivo* binding of these radioligands is evaluated by IV administration to animals as described above. Wagner and collaborators first demonstrated that after IV administration of ^{11}C-N-methylspiperone (^{11}C-NMSP) to a living human, PET could identify preferential accumulation of radioactivity in striatum in an analogous fashion to animal studies.[22]

The development of dopaminergic radioligands for PET studies, however, is a complicated process and can take as long as 3 to 5 years. Thus, it is necessary to understand the intertwining factors that contribute to the selection of appropriate radioligands.[26,32] Some of these factors are extensions of important characteristics of radioligands for *in vitro* assays, whereas others have unique importance for *in vivo* PET studies in living subjects.

One factor that is equally important for *in vitro* and *in vivo* studies is the availability of radioligand. Radioligands for *in vitro* studies are labeled with long-lived isotopes and frequently are purchased and stored until used for each experiment. Less commonly, a newly developed or unusual radioligand must be custom synthesized. Radioligands for PET studies, on the other hand, are labeled with positron-emitting radionuclides with relatively short half lives (e.g., ^{11}C — 20 min, ^{18}F — 110 min, ^{75}Br — 98 min). This forces each team of investigators to synthesize their own radioligands or have access to a nearby facility willing to do so. The short half-lives of these radionuclides dictate that synthesis, subsequent separation from unwanted reaction products, and quality control procedures must be quick. In some cases, this requires the development of new analogs of existing ligands.[32] In addition, radiation exposure of chemists and technicians should be minimized by the use of relatively fast and simple procedures when possible. In the future, automated, robotic techniques hopefully will diminish the impact of this latter limitation.[34]

Another characteristic common to desirable radioligands for *in vitro* and *in vivo* studies is low nonspecific binding in brain tissue. Low nonspecific binding increases the contrast between receptor-rich and receptor-poor brain regions. Since nonspecific binding under *in vitro* conditions is sensitive to assay conditions and the *in vivo* environment of receptors in tissue is very diferent from *in vitro* conditions, one would not expect nonspecific binding to be comparable in these two conditions. For example, after IV injection of ^{18}F-haloperidol, the distribution of radioactivity reveals less contrast between striatum and cerebellum than after injection of ^{18}F-spiperone. Since *in vitro* nonspecific binding for these two ligands is similar, the difference could, in part, reflect relativeley lower nonspecific binding *in vivo* of spiperone.[35,36] High specific activity of a radioligand decreases nonspecific binding since it contains fewer unlabeled ligand molecules. Unlabeled ligand competes with labeled ligand for receptor sites. Thus, after a low specific activity injection, a relativeley lower fraction of the total labeled ligand binds to receptor sites producing an image with less contrast between receptor-rich and receptor-poor regions. Nonspecific binding of radioligand in blood also impacts *in vivo* studies. Radioligand must penetrate the blood-brain barrier (BBB) to reach brain receptors, and some investigators suggest that only free (i.e., not bound) radioligand in blood is available to cross the BBB. Thus, radioligands that have a high degree of binding in blood such as ^{18}F-spiperone (e.g., 90 to 95% bound)[37,38] accumulate relatively slowly in brain tissue.

Another important consideration common to *in vitro* and *in vivo* assays is radioligand specificity. Spiperone and its labeled derivatives specifically bind predominantly to D_2 dopaminergic sites and S_2 serotonergic sites.[39-41] Fortunately, these different receptor sites are, to a degree, anatomically separate. D_2 sites predominate in striatum, and S_2 sites predominate in frontal cortex.[39-43] The degree of anatomic separation may have important species variability. Furthermore, relative distribution of receptor types potentially could change under pathologic conditions. Thus, one must cautiously interpret alterations in receptor binding based upon normal distributions. Alternatively, radioligands with greater specificity would limit this potential source of error. For example, ^{11}C-raclopride has greater specificity for D_2 dopaminergic sites with much lower affinity for serotonergic receptors.[42] Recently, ^{11}C-labeled SCH 23390 has been synthesized for use in PET studies.[33] This radioligand has relatively high specificity for D_1 dopaminergic receptor sites and will permit its evaluation with the development of proper methodology.

There are several characteristics of radioligands that are important only for *in vivo* studies. For example, the radioligand must have a sufficiently long half-life to permit necessary PET and/or blood measurements. The required length of an experiment depends upon the rate of radioligand delivery to brain tissue, subsequent penetration of the BBB, affinity for receptor binding sites and the method of data analysis. An equilibrium-based method of analysis requires sufficient time for equilibrium or near-equilibrium to occur, whereas a nonsteady-state dynamic technique does not have this constraint (see below). Additionally, some methods not only require measurements of total radioactivity in blood, which can be accomplished relatively quickly, but also measurements of the accumulation of radiolabeled metabolites in blood. The latter is a more complicated process involving separation of radioligand from labeled metabolites, and the radionuclidic half-life must be sufficiently long to ensure that enough radioactivity remains in each sample for reasonable counting statistics.[26,32,37]

In vivo tissue assays also can be complicated by the accumulation of radiolabeled metabolites of the originally administered radioligand.[32,37] For example, 30 min after IV injection of ^{18}F-spiperone, approximately 50% of radioactivity in arterial blood is associated with labeled metabolites.[37] An ideal radioligand would not be metabolized in the brain or periphery during the course of the PET study. If peripheral metabolism occurs, as in the case of ^{18}F-spiperone, then labeled metabolites should not cross the BBB. Finally, if labeled metabolites cross the BBB or are produced within the brain itself then these labeled metabolites should not bind to receptor sites. The latter would be an extremely difficult problem to surmount in data analysis.

The chosen radioligand must also satisfy the receptor binding characteristics necessary for the method of analysis as well as for the objectives of the investigations. Initially, high affinity, irreversibly bound ligands, such as ^{11}C-NMSP,[23] were thought most desirable since these characteristics provided images with enhanced contrast between receptor-rich and receptor-poor brain regions. Others prefer to use a lower affinity ligand, such as ^{11}C-raclopride, which approaches equilibrium much faster.[42] The importance of this factor depends upon the method of data analysis as described below. Additionally, if an appreciable molar mass of ligand is injected with the radiolabeled ligand, a lower affinity ligand is less likely to cause a clinically apparent pharmacologic effect upon the subject. This is particularly important in parkinsonian patients who can have an exacerbation of symptoms in such a situation.[44] Thus, the objectives of an investigation also influence the choice of an appropriate radioligand.

Finally, the toxicity of the radioligand or its labeled metabolites must be evaluated. This includes not only pharmacologic effects but also radiation exposure to the subject. The latter constrains the amount of administered radioactivity. This limits the total radioactivity within the field of view of the PET which subsequently limits statistical counting accuracy. In general, short-lived radionuclides like [11]C (half-life = 20 min) permit larger amounts of radioactivity to be administered but the radioactivity decays quicker. This is an advantage if one wants to obtain frequent, early PET measurements of tissue radioactivity or perform repeated studies in the same subject, in the same study session. On the other hand, if one wants to monitor the brain activity for longer periods of time, then [18]F (half-life = 110 min) or [76]Br (half-life = 16.2 h) are more suitable.

In summary, the selection of an appropriate radioligand must be based on a number of factors including the objectives of the proposed investigation. Obviously, the choice must be carefully made since the development of radiochemical syntheses is often complicated and time-consuming.

IV. METHODS OF DATA ANALYSIS

After IV administration of a dopaminergic radioligand such as labeled spiperone, autoradiographic images show that areas of brain known to have high concentrations of dopaminergic receptors, like striatum, accumulate higher amounts of radioactivity than areas known to be relatively devoid of dopaminergic receptors, such as cerebellum. Although these images show evidence of specific binding, direct quantitative measurement of dopaminergic binding cannot be made from the regional radioactivity distribution alone. Other factors, such as regional radioligand delivery, intravascular content of radioactivity, volume of distribution, nonspecific binding, and the presence of labeled metabolites of the radioligand must be taken into account.[37] Even simple ratios comparing radioactivity from striatum and cerebellum can be misleading indicators of true changes in receptor binding.[12,37,45]

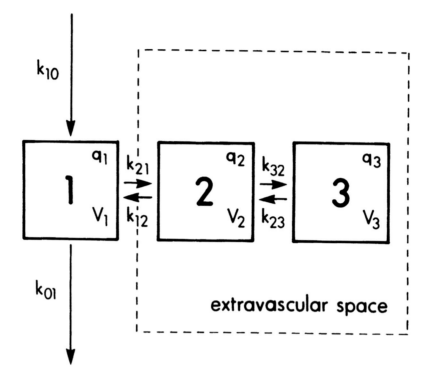

FIGURE 1.   The 3-compartment model employed to analyze positron emission tomographic (PET) data of radioligand-receptor binding is shown. Compartment 1 represents the intra-vascular space; compartment 2, the free and nonspecifically bound tracer within the cerebral extravascular space; and compartment 3, the specific binding sites within the extravascular space. Together these compartments contain all radiotracer within the field of view of the PET. Directions of passage of tracer into and out of the field of view as well as its movements between compartments are indicated by the arrows. Following conventional compartmental analysis notation, the turnover rate constants k_{ij} denote fractions of radiotracer in compart-ments j that move per unit time into compartments i. Zero subscript denotes the surroundings external to all compartments and to the PET region of interest. Tracer enters the field of view of the PET via flowing blood. q_i is the quantity of radiotracer in compartment i and V_i is the volume of that compartment. Different dynamic methods vary in the assumptions made to simplify the model or its implementation. (From Perlmutter, J. S., *Trends Neurosci.*, in press. With permission.)

Two general approaches for the study of dopaminergic radioligand-receptor binding with PET have been developed. These can be divided into dynamic and equilibrium methods.[46] Dynamic methods use sequential PET scans to measure time-dependent changes in the distribution of radioactivity after administration of radioligand.[47] The PET data are analyzed with a compartmental model that represents the *in vivo* behavior of the radioligand (Figure 1).[37,47] After IV injection, radioligand is distributed within the intravascular space as free tracer and as tracer bound to nonspecific sites in plasma. Specific sites might also exist, such as serotonergic sites on platelets for spiperone binding, but are usually ignored in these analyses. Unbound ligand is free to cross the BBB and enter the cerebral extravascular space. Within the extravascular space, ligand can be free, nonspecifically bound or specif-ically bound to saturable sites (i.e., receptors). This is the basis of the three-compartment model shown in Figure 1. More precisely, five compartments have been described. Since association-dissociation kinetic rate constants for nonspecific binding are assumed to be much larger than the compartmental rate constants, the free and the nonspecifically bound moieties on either side of the BBB can be viewed as a single compartment. In this manner the five compartments are collapsed to three.[37,47] Each compartment corresponds to a volume in which radioligand can distribute or, alternatively, to a biochemical state in which it can exist. In this three-compartment model, compartment 1 represents the intravascular space; compartment 2, the free and nonspecifically bound tracer within the cerebral extravascular space; and compartment 3, the specific binding sites within the brain tissue. Together these three compartments comprise all of the radioactivity within the field of view of the PET.

The directions of passage of radioactive moieties into and out of the field of view as well as movements between compartments are indicated by the arrows in Figure 1. Using standard compartmental modeling notation,[48,49] the turnover rate constants k_{ij} denote fractions of radioligand in compartments j that move into compartments i per unit time. The interpretation of these turnover rate constants in terms of relevant physiologic variables depends upon the particular assumptions and implementation of a given method.

After compartments and relevant parameters have been identified, mathematical equations are formulated that describe the time-dependent tracer conservation conditions. Tracer conservation conditions assume that the change in radioactivity content of a compartment is equivalent to the difference between the flux of radioactivity into and the flux out of the compartment. These equations can be found in several recent papers and will not be restated here.[36,37,46,47] Radioactive decay must be either explicitly included in the model or the PET and blood data must be corrected for decay before further processing. This formulation results in a set of differential equations which can be integrated analytically or numerically. The integrated equations express the time-dependent radioligand content within each compartment in terms of the modeling parameters. Parameter estimation schemes then can be employed to calculate the best estimates of the modeling parameters that yield the optimum fit to the observed data (Figures 2 and 3).

Different dynamic methods vary in the assumptions made to simplify the model or its implementation. Although several published approaches using dynamic methods appear to be dramatically different, almost all are based upon this same three-compartment model.[36,37,45-47,50,51] The complexity of the assumptions, mathematical equations, and subtleties of implementation often make it difficult to comprehend fully the differences among methods. Even mathematical notation for similar variables used by different groups varies and leads to frequent confusion.[37]

A. NONSTEADY-STATE METHOD

The dynamic method first introduced by Mintun et al.[47] and later modified[37] is a nonsteady-state approach based upon the three-compartment model described above and has been applied to PET data using ^{18}F-spiperone as the radioligand. This method makes a number of assumptions beyond the usual compartmental assumptions. These include:

1. Only unbound radioligand in the plasma can cross the BBB.
2. Transport of unbound radioligand across the BBB is bidirectional and occurs by passive diffusion.
3. Only free ligand within the extravascular space is available to bind to specific receptors (i.e., nonspecifically bound ligand is not available for specific binding).
4. Free and nonspecifically bound radioligand in vascular and extravascular spaces are essentially in equilibrium at all times. Thus, as free radioligand crosses the BBB or binds to specific sites, the relative proportions of free to the sum of nonspecifically bound plus free radioligand remain constant throughout the length of the study.
5. Nonspecific binding is constant throughout different regions of brain, and in particular, is the same in striatum and cerebellum.
6. The physical distribution space of ^{18}F-spiperone is equivalent to the tissue water space.
7. Association of ligand and receptor follows bimolecular association kinetics, and dissociation of radioligand-receptor complex follows unimolecular kinetics.

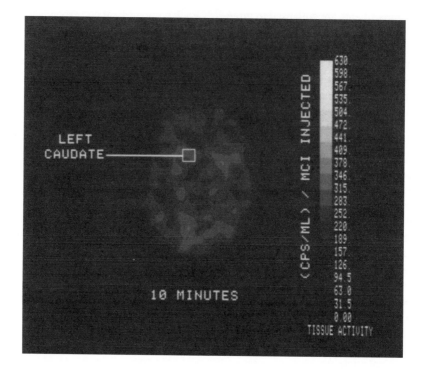

A

FIGURE 2.   After injection of ^{18}F-spiperone into a patient with untreated MPTP-induced parkinsonism, 39 sequential PET scans were obtained.[38] The first five scans were 2 min long and the rest were 5 min. Three of the 5-min-long scans are shown (A, B, and C). Each began at the time indicated below each image, and the counts per second (CPS) per milliliter were decay corrected to the time of injection of ^{18}F-spiperone. Furthermore, CPS/ML were normalized to millicuries (mCi) of ^{18}F-spiperone injected. The position of the caudate regions was determined by a stereotactic localization technique that is independent of the appearance of the images.[65] Radioactivity increases preferentially in the region of the caudate and putamen at increasing times after administration of ^{18}F-spiperone, as displayed in the three images. (From Perlmutter, J. S., *Trends Neurosci.*, in press. With permission.)

8.   Receptor sites are not saturated by radioligand during the course of the PET study.
9.   Labeled metabolites of the radioligand do not cross the BBB and are not produced within the brain tissue (i.e., all radioactivity in the extravascular space is associated with radioligand).

The validity and limitations of these assumptions have been addressed previously and will be discussed briefly below.[26,36,37,47]

This model is represented by a set of differential equations.[37] Several of the variables are either measured directly with PET (e.g., regional radioactivity in brain), obtained independently (e.g., free fraction of radioligand in arterial blood, regional blood flow and blood volume) or assumed. The accumulation of radiolabeled metabolites in arterial blood is measured throughout the course of the experiment. The volumes of compartments 2 and 3 are assumed to be equal to extravascular water space, which is known independently. It also is assumed that in the cerebellum, there are no specific receptors for ^{18}F-spiperone and the turnover rate constants between compartments 2 and 3 are zero (i.e., no third compartment containing receptors). In this region of brain, only two unknown parameters remain to be estimated: the nonspecific binding fraction in compartment 2 (f_2) and the local permeability-

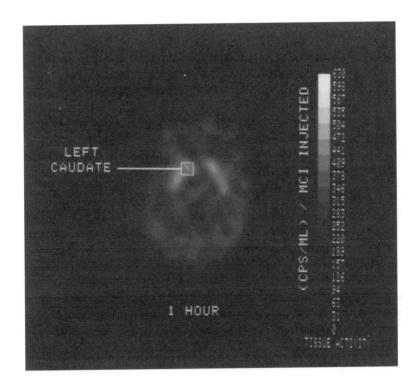

B

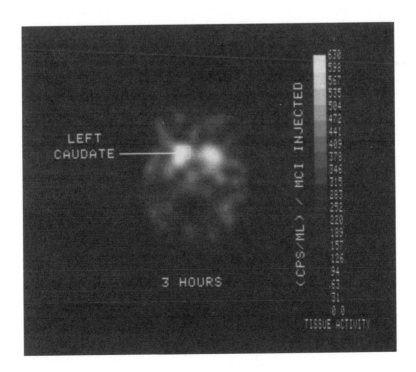

C

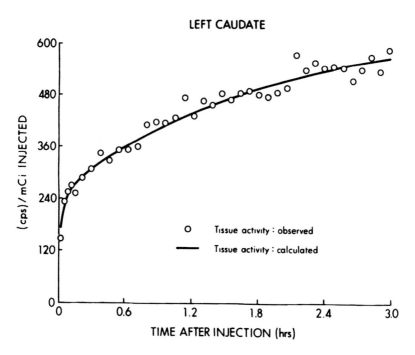

LEFT CAUDATE

○ Tissue activity : observed

— Tissue activity : calculated

FIGURE 3.   After injection of ^{18}F-spiperone into a patient with MPTP-induced parkinsonism, 39 sequential PET scans were obtained. A stereotactic localization technique was employed to obtain regional measurements of radioactivity from the scans.[65] Values for the left caudate are shown. The solid curve shows the calculated fit of a nonsteady-state, 3-compartment model that represents the *in vivo* behavior of ^{18}F-spiperone after injection (see Figure 1). The model takes into consideration the nonspecific binding of the radioligand, arterial-blood radioactivity and the production of ^{18}F-labeled metabolites within the blood[37,38] (From Perlmutter, J. S., *Trends Neurosci.*, in press. With permission.)

surface-area product PS. This value of f_2 then is assumed to be the same in striatum, reducing the number of unknown parameters there to four: (1) the local PS, (2) the dissociation rate constant, (3) the association rate constant k_a, and (4) the maximum number of available specific binding sites, B_{max}. If the specific activity of the radioligand is very high and the number of available specific binding sites occupied by radioligand during the course of the experiment is very low, then two parameters, the association rate constant k_a and B_{max}, always appear as a product and cannot be determined independently. This gives rise to a new term, the combined forward rate constant defined as the product of k_a and B_{max}. Although this may appear to be a significant compromise in our ability to study receptor pharmacology with PET, it has not proven to be so in practice (see below).[38]

This also raises an important area of divergence among different investigators. Some investigators propose to measure B_{max}. To understand how this is done it is necessary to define, in more commonly understood physiologic terms, one of the turnover rate constants from the three-compartment model.

$$k_{32} = f_2[B_{max} - c_3(t)]k_a \qquad (1)$$

k_{32} represents the fraction of radioligand in compartment 2 that enters compartment 3 per unit time; $c_3(t)$ represents the time-dependent concentration (note $c_3(t) = q_3(t)/V_3$) of radioligand-receptor complex; and the other variables are defined above. For radioligand preparations with high specific activity, $c_3(t)$ is small with respect to B_{max} (i.e., radioligand occupies only a small number of the available receptor sites) and the term $B_{max} - c_3(t)$ is approximately equal to B_{max}. Under these conditions

$$k_{32} = f_2 B_{max} k_a \qquad (2)$$

and B_{max} and k_a cannot be determined independently. On the other hand, if the specific activity is relatively low, $B_{max} - c_3(t)$ cannot be approximated by B_{max}, and Equation 1 cannot be simplified to Equation 2. Furthermore, the apparent number of available specific binding sites decreases since excess unlabeled ligand blocks or competes for available receptor sites. If k_a were assumed to remain constant for at least two separate injections of radioligand with different specific activities, k_a and the true B_{max} could be estimated.[36,46] Theoretically, one might be able to perform this entire estimation with one lower specific activity injection,[46] but this remains to be demonstrated.

There are several factors that should be kept in mind when considering the use of an unlabeled ligand (either as an unlabeled form of the administered radioligand or a different ligand) to alter the apparent number of available binding sites. A different unlabeled ligand that arrives at and/or binds to receptor sites faster than the radioligand might have an advantage if one wants to block a number of available binding sites prior to radioligand arrival.[52] This approach assumes that radioligand delivery to tissue is unaltered by the unlabeled ligand. Alterations in regional blood flow should be considered if this affects the results of the binding study. This depends on the choice of unlabeled ligand, radioligand and method of data analysis. Furthermore, radiation exposure to the subject increases if additional injections of radioligand are required. Lower amounts of radioactivity could be injected with each individual administration but the relative contrast between radioactivity in receptor-rich and receptor-poor brain regions diminishes (especially after lower specific activity injection or pretreatment with a different unlabeled ligand) and statistical counting accuracy decreases. More importantly, the additional amount of unlabeled ligand, which is most commonly a dopaminergic antagonist, could cause a pharmacologic effect in some patients. In particular, parkinsonian patients could suffer a temporary exacerbation of symptoms because of the dopaminergic blockade. In patients with diseases thought to result from relative excess of dopaminergic activity such as Tourette's syndrome or tardive dyskinesia, this might not be a limiting factor.

Implementation of the nonsteady-state method requires sequential PET scans and arterial-blood samples to be collected for 2.5 to 3 h after the administration of a radioligand such as ^{18}F-spiperone.[37,38] Independent measurements of regional blood flow and blood volume can be made for each subject using PET with ^{15}O-labeled radiotracers. This is not absolutely necessary for studies with ^{18}F-spiperone as errors in regional blood flow and blood volume make only modest errors in estimates of relevant binding variables.[47] Measurements of the free fraction of radioligand in arterial blood as well as sequential measurements of total radioactivity and radiolabeled metabolites of the radioligand are also performed. These data then are processed using one of the above nonsteady-state models and a parameter estimation scheme to obtain the best fit to the observed data (see Figures 2 and 3).

Several points regarding the nonsteady-state method need emphasis. First, it is assumed that nonspecific binding in the cerebellum is the same as in the striatum. Implicit in this assumption is that no specific binding occurs in cerebellum. Logan et al.[36] show that stereoselective blocking with (+) butaclamol (which blocks D_2 dopaminergic receptors) reduces the uptake of ^{18}F-spiperone in cerebellum and suggest that this indicates the presence of saturable binding sites. It is important to note that the difference was demonstrable only at relatively late times after injection. The impact of the resulting error in the estimate of nonspecific binding (actually the estimate of the free fraction in compartment 2, f_2), results in a modest error in the estimate of the combined forward rate constant (the product of k_a and B_{max}).[47] From a practical point of view, the greatest disadvantage of using the nonsteady-state method with ^{18}F-spiperone is the length of time required for the study, at least 2 to 3 h after radioligand injection.[36,37,47] Hopefully, a ligand with faster kinetics (i.e., rapid association and reversibility), such as raclopride, would permit a much shorter study.[42]

B. STEADY-STATE METHOD

Wong et al.[45] have proposed a different dynamic method for the estimation of dopaminergic receptor binding. Their method also requires sequential PET scans after the injection of the radioligand,[11]C-NMSP. The study only requires scanning to continue for as long as 60 to 90 min, shorter than required for the nonsteady-state method using ^{18}F-spiperone. Additionally, individual measurements of regional blood flow and blood volume are not required. The same three-compartment model is employed to represent the *in vivo* behavior of radioligand but a graphical evaluation appropriate for steady-state data is used for analysis.[53] Additional assumptions necessary for implementation of this technique include: (1) during the course of the PET study, steady state occurs for radioligand transfer between blood and receptor sites in brain tissue; (2) there is equal tracer delivery to cerebellum (i.e., the reference region) and striatum (i.e., region of interest); (3) arterial-blood radioactivity due to ^{11}C-NMSP can be represented by a simple power function (i.e., $C_a(T) = aT^{-b}$, where $C_a(T)$ represents the arterial-blood concentration of ^{11}C-NMSP at time T and "a" and "b" are arbitrary constants); (4) there is no entry into brain of labeled metabolites of ^{11}C-NMSP (the same assumption is made for radioligands used with the nonsteady-state methods discussed above); and (5) the dissociation rate constant of ^{11}C-NMSP is negligible. If the rate of specific binding of ^{11}C-NMSP is relatively small compared to the transport rate constant from brain to blood (i.e., $k_3 \ll k_2$; using notation of Wong and co-workers[45]) then the tissue-activity data from the cerebellum can be used as an internal filter to estimate the time-dependent arterial-blood concentration of ^{11}C-NMSP.[45,46] This eliminates the need for arterial-blood sampling for the measurement of ^{11}C-NMSP or labeled metabolites. This steady-state technique permits estimation of a variable (k_3 in the notation of Wong et al.[45]) that represents the product of k_a and the available number of specific binding sites B_{max}, similar to the combined forward rate constant noted above.

Wong et al.[52] also proposed an extension of this method to estimate B_{max} for ^{11}C-NMSP and the equilibrium inhibitory constant for an unlabeled competitive ligand with weaker affinity for D_2 dopaminergic receptors (e.g., haloperidol). The technique requires two separate PET studies, before and 4 h after administration of 5 to 7.5 mg of haloperidol. To analyze the data, the following additional assumptions are made: (1) the concentration of free radioligand in brain tissue is negligible compared to K_d or at least is time-invariant; (2) haloperidol does not alter ^{11}C-NMSP delivery to brain tissue; (3) the partition coefficient of haloperidol is the same as that for ^{11}C-NMSP (this is required to estimate the concentration of haloperidol in the brain using the estimate of the partition coefficient for ^{11}C-NMSP and the serum level of haloperidol); and (4) a value for the *in vivo* dissociation rate constant of haloperidol is independently available. Given these assumptions, this method permits the estimation of B_{max} as well as the apparent inhibitory constant of haloperidol. Application of this method yielded reasonable values of B_{max} (9.4 pmol/g) and the inhibition constant for haloperidol (1.4 n*M*) for the caudate of four normal volunteers.[52]

C. EQUILIBRIUM METHOD

Many of the complexities of dynamic methods are avoided in a seemingly simpler equilibrium approach using ^{11}C-raclopride as the radioligand.[54] This method assumes that equilibrium occurs between ^{11}C-raclopride and brain receptor sites *in vivo* during the course of the PET study. Each study requires only a single PET scan including striatum and cerebellum performed about 42 min after tracer injection. Data are analyzed in a fashion analogous to *in vitro* binding studies. This requires measurement of free and specifically bound fractions of radioligand in brain tissue. Based upon *in vitro* observations, Farde and co-workers[54] note that nonspecific binding of raclopride is very low. They assume that under *in vivo* conditions all (or at least a known large fraction) of the radioactivity in cerebellum is "free" and bound to neither receptor sites (same assumption as the dynamic methods) nor to nonspecific sites (a markedly different assumption from that used for analysis of labeled spiperone compounds). Furthermore, it is assumed that striatal radioactivity comprises only radioligand bound to specific receptors and "free" ^{11}C-raclopride. Thus, the difference between striatal and cerebellar radioactivities represents specifically bound ^{11}C-raclopride. Values for specifically bound and free radioligand must be calculated multiple times (in some cases, five different studies were performed on individual subjects), each time after an injection of ^{11}C-raclopride with a different specific activity. The maximum number of specific binding sites B_{max} and the equilibrium dissociation constant K_d are estimated with a nonlinear regression analysis of the rearranged Scatchard equation

$$\text{Bound} = \frac{B_{max} \times \text{free}}{K_d + \text{free}} \qquad (3)$$

using the five values for Bound (i.e., specifically bound) and free. The values calculated for B_{max} and K_d using this technique were similar to values that the group has measured in unpublished studies on post-mortem human brain.[54] If just a single study is done on an individual, then values of K_d and B_{max} from a normal sample must be used. The measured specifically bound (i.e., Bound) radioactivity then can be compared to the "expected" Bound calculated with the above equation using the normal values for K_d and B_{max}.

This method of analysis of *in vivo* binding assumes equilibrium conditions and therefore must be reviewed very cautiously. It is assumed that equilibrium is reached 42 min after radioligand injection. To support this assumption, Farde et al.[54] showed that values of K_d calculated from data obtained at 36 and 42 min after injection were similar and that the ratio of concentrations of ^{11}C-raclopride in plasma and cerebellum was constant beginning 2 min after radioligand injection. On the one hand, it is not clear if the decay-corrected concentrations of regional radioactivity in striatum and cerebellum reached a constant value at 42 min or if they continued to decline with time (measurements were made for only a total of about 50 min). The effect of not reaching equilibrium on the outcome of the data analysis must be evaluated. This could be increasingly important to know as the time to reach equilibrium could change in pathologic conditions. They also assumed that all ^{11}C in the brain is still bound to unmetabolized ^{11}C-raclopride and cited data showing that after 45 min less than 90% of radioactivity in the brain was still due to unchanged ^{11}C-raclopride.[55] Finally, the assumption of no nonspecific binding needs to be more thoroughly evaluated and effects of this potential source of error investigated.

The advantages of this method include the need to acquire only a single PET scan after the injection of radioligand to obtain regional measurements from striatum and cerebellum. ^{11}C-raclopride as the radioligand offers the advantages of relatively fast entry into the brain as well as increased specificity for central D_2 dopaminergic receptors with very low affinity for other receptor sites.[54] A disadvantage of their method is the need for several separate PET studies in each subject to calculate K_d and B_{max}. This requires return visits by the subject and the additional assumption that the physiologic state of receptor number and function remain constant until the entire set of studies has been completed. Overall, the studies with the equilibrium method and ^{11}C-raclopride have demonstrated close agreement between *in vitro* and *in vivo* binding and are very encouraging.

V. APPLICATIONS

Most of the peer-reviewed published PET studies of dopaminergic receptor binding in humans have investigated parkinsonian patients. Rutgers et al.[56] found no consistent abnormalities of striatal-to-cerebellar or left-right ratios of radioactivity 1 h after administration of ^{11}C-NMSP to hemiparkinsonian patients. They did find lower striatal-to-cerebellar ratios in patients not taking medication compared to those taking levodopa and/or bromocriptine.

Although the latter suggests that drug treatment alters radioligand uptake, changes in receptors are difficult to deduce from striatal-to-cerebellar ratios (as discussed above).[37,45]

Similarly, Baron et al.[57] measured striatal-cerebellar ratios of regional radioactivity after injection of [^{76}Br]bromospiperone in seven patients with progressive supranuclear palsy (PSP). The mean ratio for patients (1.32; range, 0.90 to 1.57) was significantly lower than seven selected, age-matched controls (1.74; range, 1.45 to 1.95). This demonstrates diminished striatal uptake of [^{76}Br]bromospiperone in PSP patients and suggests that there is a loss of dopaminergic receptor binding. Further quantification of the exact nature of the change would require application of a mathematical model.

Lindvall et al.[58] used ^{11}C-raclopride and an equilibrium PET method to investigate receptor binding in two parkinsonian patients taking levodopa before and after transplantation of adrenal medullary grafts to the right putamen. The surgery was performed in the hope that the grafted tissue would produce dopamine *in situ*. The striatal-to-cerebellar ratios before and after surgery were not different from controls. In one subject (the 63 year old), a small dose (about 10 μg) of unlabeled raclopride was injected with ^{11}C-raclopride followed by a study using a saturating dose of unlabeled raclopride (about 200 μg). No comment was made about the clinical effect from this dose of raclopride. In this patient, B_{max} was calculated using the equilibrium method discussed above and found to be reduced compared to values from younger, healthy controls. B_{max} was essentially unchanged after surgery. It would be interesting to know whether this difference existed in comparison to age-matched controls.

In a preliminary communication, Leenders et al.[59] used ^{11}C-NMSP and reported that the mean striatal-cerebellar ratio for four untreated parkinsonian patients (3.81) was not significantly different from seven normal elderly controls (4.00), whereas 5 PD patients treated with levodopa had a significantly lower mean ratio (3.19 +/− 0.32). The authors noted that these results suggest that levodopa causes down-regulation of dopamine receptors. Further study and analysis is necessary to confirm this.

Hagglund and co-workers,[60] using ^{11}C-NMSP, found no significant difference in receptor binding between six parkinsonian and two control subjects. These findings must be viewed cautiously as the data were analyzed with an early version of the steady-state method[37,50,61] that subsequently was modified.[45] They also reported that a single patient with Huntington's disease had lower striatal receptor binding than controls. Of course, caudate atrophy and volume averaging could result in spuriously lower regional measurements of radioactivity and contribute to this finding.[62]

We have measured dopaminergic receptor binding with ^{18}F-spiperone in one of the few untreated, symptomatic patients with parkinsonism induced by 1-methyl-4-phenyl-1,2,3,6-tetrahydropyridine (MPTP).[38] We used the nonsteady-state dynamic method to analyze the data (see Figures 2 and 3). Recall that this technique determines a combined forward rate constant equal to the product of the maximum number of available specific binding sites, B_{max}, and the association rate constant of ^{18}F-spiperone and receptor, k_a, as well as a binding-site dissociation rate constant. Both the combined forward rate constant and the dissociation rate constants were elevated in the patient compared to ten normals, whereas nonspecific binding in blood and brain were normal. Although generalizations based upon findings in a single patient must be considered tentative, these results fit well with clinical observations. Patients with MPTP-induced parkinsonism often show improvement in symptoms with relatively low doses of levodopa and early development of dose-dependent involuntary movements.[63] These signs of behavioral supersensitivity are consistent with the increase in the combined forward rate constant found in this study. However, the clinical importance of changes in the individual rate constants remains to be determined.

Further studies in parkinsonian patients as well as in patients with other involuntary movements disorders such as Huntington's disease, Tourette's syndrome, and idiopathic dystonia are in progress. In addition to studies of D_2 dopaminergic receptors, the role of D_1 receptors will soon be evaluated using newly developed specific ligands.[33]

VI. CONCLUDING REMARKS

There are a number of different radioligands and methods of data analysis applied to PET studies of dopaminergic receptor binding. Each has its own merits. All investigators, however, must pay meticulous attention to methodologic details to insure reliable and accurate studies. One must carefully choose the appropriate radioligand for a given investigation, and it is crucial to understand the assumptions, advantages, and limitations of the method of data analysis. With these caveats in mind, further studies promise to yield unique insights into the pathophysiology of involuntary movement disorders and the response to pharmacotherapy.

ACKNOWLEDGMENTS

I want to thank Steve Moerlein for useful discussions and the Division of Radiation Sciences for expert technical and intellectual support. This work was supported by NIH grants NS06833, HL13851, AGO3991, Teacher Investigator Development Award NS00929, the Greater St. Louis Chapter of the American Parkinson's Disease Association, and the generous contributions from Mrs. Donald Danforth and Mr. and Mrs. Jefferson Miller.

REFERENCES

1. **Hrdina, P. D.**, General principles of receptor binding, in *Neuromethods*, Part 4, *Receptor Binding*, Boulton, A. A., Baker, G. B., and Hrdina, P. D., Eds., Humana Press, Clifton, NJ, 1986.
2. **Reisine, T., Fields, J., and Yamamura, H.**, Neurotransmitter receptor alterations in Parkinson's disease, *Life Sci.*, 21, 335, 1977.
3. **Lee, T., Seeman, P., Rajput, A., Farley, I. J., and Hornykiewicz, O.**, Receptor basis for dopaminergic supersensitivity in Parkinson's disease, *Nature*, 273, 59, 1978.
4. **Rinne, U., Sonninen, V., and Laaksonen, H.**, Responses of brain neurochemistry to levodopa treatment in Parkinson's disease, *Adv. Neurol.*, 24, 259, 1979.
5. **Quik, M., Spokes, E., MacKay, A., and Bannister, R.**, Alterations in ^{3}H-spiperone binding in human caudate nucleus, substantia nigra and frontal cortex in the Shy-Drager syndrome and Parkinson's disease, *J. Neurol. Sci.*, 43, 429, 1979.
6. **Olsen, R., Reisine, T., and Yamamura, H.**, Neurotransmitter receptors—biochemistry and alterations in neuropsychiatric disorders, *Life Sci.*, 27, 801, 1980.
7. **Rinne, U., Lonnberg, P., and Koskinen, V.**, Dopamine receptors in parkinsonian brain, *J. Neural Transm.*, 51, 97, 1981.
8. **Rinne, U., Rinne, J. O., Rinne, J. K., et al.**, Brain receptor changes in Parkinson's disease in relation to the disease process and treatment, *J. Neural Transm.*, (Suppl.), 18, 279, 1983.
9. **Bakobza, B., Ruberg, M., Scatton, B., Javoy-Agid, F., and Agid, Y.**, [^{3}H]spiperone binding, dopamine and HVA concentration in Parkinson's disease and supranuclear palsy, *Eur. J. Pharmacol.*, 99, 167, 1984.
10. **Guttman, M. and Seeman, P.** L-dopa reverses the elevated density of D_2 dopamine receptors in Parkinson's diseased striatum, *J. Neural Transm.*, 64, 93, 1985.
11. **Guttman, M., Seeman, P., Reynolds, G. P., et al.**, Dopamine D_2 receptor density remains constant in treated Parkinson's disease, *Ann. Neurol.*, 19, 487, 1986.
12. **Bennett, J. P., Jr. and Wooten, G. F.**, Dopamine denervation does not alter in vivo ^{3}H-spiperone binding in rat striatum: implications for external imaging of dopamine receptors in Parkinson's disease, *Ann. Neurol.*, 19, 378, 1986.
13. **Perlmutter, J. S. and Raichle, M. E.**, In vitro or in vivo receptor binding: where does the truth lie?, *Ann. Neurol.*, 19, 384, 1986a.
14. **Raichle, M. E.**, Neuroimaging, *Trends Neurosci.*, 9, 525, 1986.
15. **Laduron, P. M., Janssen, P. F. M., and Leysen, J. E.**, Spiperone: a ligand of choice for neuroleptic receptors, *Biochem. Pharmacol.*, 27, 317, 1978.
16. **Kuhar, M. J., Murrin, L. C., Malouf, A. T., and Klemm, N.**, Dopamine receptor binding in vivo: the feasibility of autoradiographic studies *Life Sci.*, 22, 203, 1978.

17. **Tewson, T. J., Raichle, M. E., and Welch, M. J.,** Preliminary studies with [¹⁸F]haloperidol: a radioligand for in vivo studies of the dopamine receptors, *Brain Res.*, 192, 291, 1980.

18. **Crouzel, C., Mestelan, G., Kraus, E., Lecomte, J. M., and Comar, D.,** Synthesis of a ¹¹C-labelled neuroleptic drug: pimozide, *Int. J. Appl. Radiat. Isot.*, 31, 545, 1980.

19. **Maeda, M., Tewson, T. J., and Welch, M. J.,** Synthesis of high specific activity ¹⁸F-spiroperidol for dopamine receptor studies, *J. Labelled Compd. Radiopharmaceut.*, 18, 102, 1981.

20. **Fowler, J. S., Arnett, C. D., Wolf, A. P., MacGregor, R. R., Norton, E. F., and Findley, A. M.,** (¹¹C)spiroperidol: synthesis, specific activity determination, and biodistribution in mice, *J. Nucl. Med.*, 23, 437, 1982.

21. **DeJesus, O. T., Van Moffaert, G. J., Glock, D., Goldberg, L. I., and Friedman, A. M.,** Synthesis of a radiobrominated analog of SCH 23390, a selective dopamine D1/DA1 antagonist, *J. Labelled Compd. Radiopharmaceut.*, 23, 919, 1986.

22. **Wagner, H. N., Burns, H. D., Dannals, R. F., et al.,** Imaging dopamine receptors in the human brain by positron tomography, *Science*, 221, 1264, 1983.

23. **Burns, H. D., Dannals, R. F., Langstrom, B., et al.,** (3-N-[¹¹C]Methyl)spiperone, a ligand binding to dopamine receptors: radiochemical synthesis and biodistribution studies in mice, *J. Nucl. Med.*, 25, 1222, 1984.

24. **Maziere, B., Loc'h, C., Hantraye, P., et al.,** ⁷⁶Br-bromospiroperidol: a new tool for quantitative imaging of neuroleptic receptors, *Life Sci.*, 35, 1349, 1984.

25. **Arnett, C. D., Fowler, J. S., Wolf, A. P., Shiue, C.-Y., and McPherson, D. W.,** [¹⁸F]-N-methylspiroperidol: the radioligand of choice for PETT studies of the dopamine receptor in human brain, *Life Sci.*, 36, 1359, 1985a.

26. **Arnett, C. D., Shiue, C.-Y., Wolf, A. P., Fowler, J. S., Logan, J., and Watanabe, M.,** Comparison of three ¹⁸F-labeled butyrophenone neuroleptic drugs in the baboon using positron emission tomography, *J. Neurochem.*, 44, 835, 1985b.

27. **Shiue, C.-Y., Fowler, J. S., Wolf, A. P., Watanabe, M., and Arnett, C. D.,** Syntheses and specific activity determinations of no-carrier-added (NCA) ¹⁸F-labeled butyrophenone neuroleptics—benperidol, haloperidol, spiroperidol, and pipamperone, *J. Nucl. Med.*, 26, 181, 1985.

28. **Ehrin, E., Farde, L., De Paulis, T., et al.,** Preparation of ¹¹C-labelled raclopride, a new potent dopamine receptor antagonist: preliminary PET studies of cerebral dopamine receptors in the monkey, *Int. J. Appl. Radiat. Isot.*, 36, 269, 1985.

29. **Moerlein, S. M., Laufer, P., Stocklin, G., Pawlik, G., Wienhard, K., and Heiss, W. D.,** Evaluation of ⁷⁵Br-labelled butyrophenone neuroleptics for imaging cerebral dopaminergic receptor areas using positron emission tomography, *Eur. J. Nucl. Med.*, 12, 211, 1986.

30. **Halldin, C., Sone-Elander, S., Farde, L., Ehrin, E., Fasth, K. J., Lanstrom, B., and Sedvall, G.,** Preparation of ¹¹C-labelled SCH 23390 for the in vivo study of dopamine D-1 receptors using positron emission tomography, *Int. J. Radiat. Appl. Instrum.*, 37, 1039, 1986.

31. **Coenen, H. H., Lauger, P., Stocklin, G., Wienhard, K., Pawlik, G., Bocher-Schwarz, H. G., and Weiss, W. D.,** 3-N-(2-[¹⁸F]-fluoroethyl)-spiperone: a novel ligand for cerebral dopamine receptor studies with PET, *Life Sci.*, 40, 81, 1987.

32. **Welch, M. J., Katzenellenbogen, J. A., Mathias, C. J., et al.,** N-(3-[¹⁸F]Fluoropropyl)-spiperone: the preferred ¹⁸F labeled spiperone analog for positron emission tomographic studies of the dopamine receptor, *Nucl. Med. Biol.*, 15, 83, 1988.

33. **Halldin, C., Stone-Elander, S., Farde, L., and Sedvall, G.,** Synthesis of ¹¹C-eticlopride, a new selective D₂-receptor ligand, *J. Nucl. Med.*, 28, 625, 1987.

34. **Brodack, J. W., Kilbourn, M. R., Welch, M. J., and Katzenellenbogen, J. A.,** Application of robotics to radiopharmaceutical preparation: controlled synthesis of fluorine-18 16-alpha-fluoroestradiol-17-beta, *J. Nucl. Med.*, 27, 714, 1986.

35. **Welch, M. J., Kilbourn, M. R., Mathias, C. J., Mintun, M. A., and Raichle, M. E.,** Comparison in animal models of ¹⁸F-spiroperidol and ¹⁸F-haloperidol: potential agents for imaging the dopamine receptor, *Life Sci.*, 33, 1687, 1983.

36. **Logan, J., Wolf, A. P., Shiue, C.-Y., and Fowler, J. S.,** Kinetic modeling of receptor-ligand binding applied to positron emission tomographic studies with neuroleptic tracers, *J. Neurochem.*, 48, 73, 1987.

37. **Perlmutter, J. S., Larson, K. B., Raichle, M. E., Markham, J., Mintun, M. A., Kilbourn, M. R., and Welch, M. J.,** Strategies for in vivo measurement of receptor binding using positron emission tomography, *J. Cereb. Blood Flow Metab.*, 6, 154, 1986.

38. **Perlmutter, J. S., Kilbourn, M. R., Raichle, M. E., and Welch, M. J.,** MPTP-induced up-regulation of in vivo dopaminergic radioligand-receptor binding in humans, *Neurology*, 37, 1575, 1987.

39. **Palacios, J. M., Niehoff, D. L., and Kuhar, M. J.,** [³H]spiperone binding sites in brain: autoradiographic localization of multiple receptors, *Brain Res.*, 213, 177, 1981.

40. **Altar, C. A., Kim, H., and Marshall, J. F.**, Computer imaging and analysis of dopamine (D_2) and serotonin (S_2) binding sites in rat basal ganglia or neocortex labeled by [^{3}H]spiroperidol, *J. Pharmacol. Exp. Ther.*, 233, 527, 1985.

41. **List, S. J. and Seeman, P.**, Resolution of dopamine and serotonin receptor components of [^{3}H]spiperone binding to rat brain regions, *Proc. Natl. Acad. Sci. U.S.A.*, 78, 2620, 1981.

42. **Farde, L., Ehrin, E., Eriksson, L., et al.**, Substituted benzamides as ligands for visualization of dopamine receptor binding in the human brain by positron emission tomography, *Proc. Natl. Acad. Sci. U.S.A.*, 82, 3863, 1985.

43. **Lyon, R. A., Titeler, M., Frost, J. J., et al.**, ^{3}H-3-N-methylspiperone labels D_2 dopamine receptors in basal ganglia and S_2 serotonin receptors in cerebral cortex, *J. Neurosci.*, 6, 2941, 1986.

44. **Larson, S. M., Di Chiro, G., Burns, R. S., et al.**, PET imaging of dopamine receptors in MPTP-induced parkinsonism, *J. Nucl. Med.*, 25, P57, 1984.

45. **Wong, D. F., Gjedde, A., and Wagner, H. N., Jr.**, Quantification of neuroreceptors in the living human brain. I. Irreversible binding of ligands, *J. Cereb. Blood Flow Metab.*, 6, 137, 1986a.

46. **Huang, S. C., Barrio, J. R., and Phelps, M. E.**, Neuroreceptor assay with positron emission tompography: equilibrium versus dynamic approaches, *J. Cereb. Blood Flow Metab.*, 6, 515, 1986.

47. **Mintun, M. A., Raichle, M. E., Kilbourn, M. R., Wooten, G. F., and Welch, M. J.**, A quantitative model for the in vivo assessment of drug binding sites with positron emission tomography, *Ann. Neurol.*, 15, 217, 1984.

48. **Jacquez, J. A.**, *Compartmental Analysis in Biology and Medicine*, Elsevier, New York, 1972.

49. **Godfrey, K.**, *Compartmental Models and Their Application*, Academic Press, New York, 1983.

50. **Wong, D. F., Wagner, H. N., Jr., Dannals, R. F., et al.**, Effects of age on dopamine and serotonin receptors measured by positron tomography in the living human brain, *Science*, 226, 1393, 1984.

51. **Swart, J. A. A. and Korf, J.**, In vivo dopamine receptor assessment for clinical studies using positron emission tomography, *Biochem. Pharmacol.*, 36, 2241, 1987.

52. **Wong, D. F., Gjedde, A., Wagner, H. N., Jr., Dannals, R. F., Douglass, K. H., Links, J. M., and Kuhar, M. J.**, Quantification of neuroreceptors in the living human brain. II. Inhibition studies of receptor density and affinity, *J. Cereb. Blood Flow Metab.*, 6, 147, 1986b.

53. **Patlak, C., Blasberg, R. G., and Fenstermacher, J. D.**, Graphical evaluation of blood-to-brain transfer constants from multiple-time uptake data, *J. Cereb. Blood Flow Metab.*, 3, 1, 1983.

54. **Farde, L., Hall, H., Ehrin, E., and Sedvall, G.**, Quantitative analysis of D_2 dopamine receptor binding in the living human brain by PET, *Science*, 231, 258, 1986.

55. **Kohler, C., Hall, H., Ogren, S. O., and Gawell, L.**, Specific in vitro and in vivo binding of ^{3}H-raclopride. A potent substituted benzamide drug with high affinity for dopamine D_2 receptors in the rat brain, *Biochem Pharmacol.*, 34, 2251, 1985.

56. **Rutgers, A. W. F., Lakke, P. W. F., Paans, A. M. J., Vaalburg, W., and Korf, J.**, Tracing of dopamine receptors in hemiparkinsonism with positron emission tomography (PET)., *J. Neurol. Sci.*, 80, 237, 1987.

57. **Baron, J. C., Maziere, B., Loc'h, C., Cambon, H., Sgouropoulos, P., Bonnet, A. M., and Agid, Y.**, Loss of striatal [^{76}Br]bromospiperone binding sites demonstrated by positron emission tomography in progressive supranuclear palsy, *J. Cereb. Blood Flow Metab.*, 6, 131, 1986.

58. **Lindvall, O., Backlund, E.-O., Farde, L., et al.**, Transplantation in Parkinson's disease: two cases of adrenal medullary grafts to the putamen, *Ann. Neurol.*, 22, 457, 1987.

59. **Leenders, K. L., Herold, S., Palmer, A. J., et al.**, Human cerebral dopamine system measured in vivo using PET, *J. Cereb. Blood Flow Metab.*, 5, S1257, 1985.

60. **Hagglund, J., Aquilonius, S.-M., Eckernas, S.-A., Hartvig, P., Lundquist, H., Gullberg, P., Langstrom, B.**, Dopamine receptor properties in Parkinson's disease and Huntington's chorea evaluated by positron emission tomography using ^{11}C-N-methyl-spiperone, *Acta Neurol. Scand.*, 75, 87, 1987.

61. **Eckernas, S.-A., Aquilonius, S.-M., Hartvig, P., Hagglund, J., Lundqvist, H., Nagren, K., and Langstrom, B.**, Positron emission tomography (PET) in the study of dopamine receptors in the primate brain: evaluation of a kinetic mode using ^{11}C-N-methyl-spiperone, *Acta Neurol. Scand.*, 75, 168, 1987.

62. **Mazziotta, J. C., Phelps, M. E., Plummer, D., and Kuhl, D. E.**, Quantitation in positron emission computed tomography. V. Physical-anatomical effects, *J. Comput. Assist. Tomogr.*, 5, 734, 1981.

63. **Ballard, P. A., Tetrud, J. W., and Langston, J. W.**, Permanent human parkinsonism due to 1-methyl-4-phenyl-1,2,3,6-tetrahydropyridine (MPTP): seven cases, *Neurology*, 35, 949, 1985.

64. **Perlmutter, J. S.**, New insights into the pathophysiology of Parkinson's disease: the challenge of positron emission tomography, *Trends Neurosci.*, in press.

65. **Fox, P. T., Perlmutter, J. S., and Raichle, M. E.**, A stereotactic method of anatomical localization for positron emission tomography, *J. Comput. Assist. Tomogr.*, 9, 141, 1985.

Commentary to Chapter 4

G. Frederick Wooten

DIFFERENT METHODS OF MEASURING BINDING TO THE EFFECTOR LIGAND BINDING SITES OF NEUROTRANSMITTER RECEPTORS: A NOTE OF CAUTION

Discrepancies among various binding studies aimed at the characterization of the density or concentration of D_2 dopamine receptors in the striatum of patients with Parkinson's disease (PD) and in animal models of PD are apparent. As discussed by Perlmutter in the preceding chapter, several groups using *in vivo* PET techniques found neither differences in striatal D_2 dopamine receptor binding site density between patients with PD and age matched controls nor asymmetries in striatal D_2 dopamine receptors in patients with highly asymmetric parkinsonian symptoms.[1-3] In contrast, several *in vitro* studies of post-mortem parkinsonian striatum using crude membrane preparations have reported increases in the density of D_2 dopamine receptor binding sites.[4,5]

In addition, several investigators have found, using rats with unilateral 6-hydroxydopamine lesions of the substantia nigra pars compacta, that there is an increase in D_2 binding sites in crude membrane preparations from the striatum ipsilateral to the nigral lesion compared to the unlesioned side.[6-8] Using both *in vitro* autoradiographic and *in vivo* labeling methods in the same type of preparation, however, we were not able to detect any asymmetry in D_2 binding sites between the striata ipsi- and contralateral to a unilateral 6-hydroxydopamine lesion of the substantia nigra pars compacta.[9]

These discrepancies raise questions about comparability of *in vivo* and *in vitro* labeling methods as well as of highly disrupted tissue preparations (i.e., crude membrane preparations) vs. relatively intact tissue (i.e., *in vivo* labeling) or tissue sections labeled *in vitro*.

What mechanism(s) might explain these discrepancies? Particulate preparations tend to yield higher B_{max}s for spiperone than do autoradiographic or *in vivo* labeling techniques.[9] Perhaps tissue disruption via homogenization to produce membrane preparations leads to the exposure of newly synthesized but not yet incorporated (i.e., into the neuronal membrane) receptors and/or "used" internalized receptors that are no longer located in the neuronal membrane. If this were the case, then questions should be raised about the physiological significance of these "additional" binding sites that are exposed by tissue disruption, and *in vivo* labeling should represent the "gold standard" for labeling physiologically active and relevant binding sites.

Other technical variables should be considered as well. Frequently, *in vitro* binding studies are carried out under nonphysiological conditions with respect to temperature and ionic composition of buffers. Though departures from physiological conditions are often validated, such departures should be viewed critically.

Finally, with the newly emerging knowledge of the amino acid sequences, tertiary structure, and cellular location of neurotransmitter receptors it is apparent that there are numerous potential sites for regulation of sensitivity to drugs and neurotransmitters other than via changes in receptor number or density.[10] Given the currently available data, it is far from clear that the changes in sensitivity of the striatum to dopamine and dopamine agonists after loss of dopamine afferents, as in PD, are a result of changes in dopamine receptor density or number.

REFERENCES

1. **Rutgers, A. W. F., Lakke, P. W. F., Paans, A. M. J., Vaalburg, W., and Korf, J.,** Tracing of dopamine receptors in hemiparkinsonism with positron emission tomography (PET), *J. Neurol. Sci.,* 80, 237, 1987.

2. **Lindvall, O., Backlund, E.-O., Farde, L., et al.,** Transplantation in Parkinson's disease: two cases of adrenal medullary grafts to the putamen, *Ann. Neurol.,* 22, 457, 1987.

3. **Leenders, K. L., Herold, S., Palmer, A. J., et al.,** Human cerebral dopamine system measured *in vivo* using PET, *J. Cereb. Blood Flow Metab.,* 5, S157, 1985.

4. **Lee, T., Seeman, P., Rajput, A., et al.,** Receptor basis for dopaminergic supersensitivity in Parkinson's disease, *Nature,* 273, 59, 1978.

5. **Rinne, V. K., Lonnberg, P., and Koskinen, V.,** Dopamine receptors in the parkinsonian brain, *J. Neural Transm.,* 51, 97, 1981.

6. **Creese, I., Burt, D., and Snyder, S. H.,** Dopamine receptor binding enhancement accompanies lesion-induced behavioral supersensitivity, *Science,* 197, 596, 1977.

7. **Staunton, D. A., Wolfe, B. B., Groves, P. M., and Molinoff, P. B.,** Dopamine receptor changes following destruction of the nigrostriatal pathway: lack of a relationship to rotational behavior, *Brain Res.,* 211, 315, 1981.

8. **Thal, L., Mishra, R. K., Gardner, E. L., et al.,** Dopamine antagonist binding increases in two behaviorally distinct striatal denervation syndromes, *Brain Res.,* 170, 381, 1979.

9. **Bennett, J. P. and Wooten, G. F.,** Dopamine denervation does not alter *in vivo* ^{3}H-spiperone binding in rat striatum: implications for external imaging of dopamine receptors in Parkinson's disease, *Ann. Neurol.,* 19, 378, 1986.

10. **Bunzow, J. R., van Tol, H. M., Grandy, D. K., et al.,** Cloning and expression of a rat D_2 dopamine receptor cDNA, *Nature,* 336, 783, 1988.

Chapter 5

PARKINSON'S DISEASE AND AGING: PRESYNAPTIC NIGROSTRIATAL FUNCTION

W. R. Wayne Martin

TABLE OF CONTENTS

I. INTRODUCTION

Parkinsonism is a symptom complex which is seen in association with a variety of illnesses, either intrinsic to the nervous system or systemic in nature. The commonest cause is idiopathic Parkinson's disease (PD). This is one of the leading causes of neurologic disability in the elderly with an estimated prevalence of 100 to 150 per 100,000 population.[1] The onset of idiopathic PD is usually after 50 years of age; about 1% of the population over age 65 are thought to be affected. The number of patients with PD may therefore be expected to increase as the number of people in the older age groups continues to increase. The course is slowly, but relentlessly, progressive and often leads to severe disability.

The clinical features include varying combinations of tremor, rigidity, and akinesia. The most common presentation is with tremor affecting the hands. This is characteristically a slow frequency (3 to 6 Hz) tremor present at rest, but disappearing during voluntary movement. Rigidity refers to the increased resistance of the limbs to passive movements, usually felt by the examiner as a relatively uniform resistance throughout the range of movement about a major joint (*plastic rigidity*). The third major feature is a general poverty of movement (*hypokinesia* or *akinesia*), or slow speed of movement (*bradykinesia*). The ability to perform complex or repetitive movements tends to become progressively impaired as the disease progresses. Although the signs and symptoms may be more severe on one side of the body in early stages, in most patients the disease becomes bilaterally symmetric with time. With disease progression, many patients develop the so-called "on-off" phenomenon.[2] This refers to an erratic fluctuation of symptoms in which patients can alternate precipitously between being asymptomatic and being profoundly parkinsonian.

The occurrence of dementia in PD has been controversial. In his original description, James Parkinson suggested that "the senses and intellect are unaffected". It is now generally recognized, however, that about 20 to 40% of patients with PD eventually develop moderate to severe dementia.[3]

The major underlying pathology in Parkinson's disease (PD) is neuronal cell loss in the pigmented nuclei of the brain stem, most notably in the substantia nigra pars compacta. The nigral neurons project to the caudate and putamen and utilize dopamine as a neurotransmitter. As a result of the loss of nigrostriatal dopaminergic neurons, striatal dopamine concentration is markedly depressed in PD. These neurons are thought to exhibit a high degree of plasticity[4] such that mild symptoms in PD are associated with a disproportionately high (about 80%) degree of striatal dopamine loss while a lesser degree of dopamine depletion remains asymptomatic.[5] Extrastriatal dopamine systems are also affected. In particular, decreased dopamine levels have been reported in subcortical limbic regions such as the nucleus accumbens, the medial olfactory area, the lateral hypothalamus, and the amygdaloid nucleus, as well as several limbic cortical and neocortical areas, including parolfactory, frontal, entorhinal, cingulate, and hippocampal cortices.[4] These decreases are most likely due to neuronal degeneration in the ventral tegmental area of the midbrain, the site of origin of the majority of mesolimbic dopaminergic fibers.[6]

Several lines of evidence based on post-mortem studies point to the existence of an asymptomatic functional change in the nigrostriatal pathway occurring with advancing age. These include an age-related decrease in the number of nigral cell bodies[7] and in the striatal content of dopamine[8] and its synthesizing enzymes.[9] Although the underlying cause of death of nigral neurons in PD is unknown, it has been hypothesized to be related to the interplay of external and internal environmental factors acting upon a background of "normal" age-related loss of nigral neurons.[10] The etiology, pathology, and clinical features of PD have been reviewed by Barbeau.[11]

Functional imaging techniques have enabled the *in vivo* assessment of the functional integrity of these nigrostriatal neurons in human subjects by virtue of tracers which act as specific markers for dopaminergic nerve endings. The application of these methods to studies in normal and parkinsonian individuals should help clarify the relationship between presynaptic nigrostriatal dopaminergic function and clinical symptomatology.

II. NEUROCHEMISTRY OF THE DOPAMINERGIC SYSTEM

The enzymatic processes involved in the formation and metabolism of dopamine have been well characterized. Tyrosine hydroxylase is the initial and rate-limiting enzyme in the biosynthetic pathway.[12] This enzyme catalyzes the hydroxylation of tyrosine to form 3,4-dihydroxy-L-phenylalanine (L-DOPA, or levodopa) and is located in dopamine-synthesizing neurons. Levodopa is then decarboxylated to dopamine by aromatic L-amino acid decarboxylase (ALAAD) which is present in highest concentration in the brain within striatal dopaminergic nerve endings.[13] The conversion of tyrosine to levodopa, and levodopa to dopamine occurs within the cytosol and is immediately followed by the uptake of dopamine into storage vesicles in the nerve terminals. When an action potential reaches the nerve terminal, stored dopamine is released into the synaptic cleft. The action of dopamine released in this fashion is terminated primarily by a specific, energy-requiring reuptake process into the presynaptic terminal.[14] In addition, two enzymes are responsible for the catabolism of dopamine. Monoamine oxidase (MAO) is located on the outer layer of mitochondria[15] and plays an important role in the inactivation of free dopamine within the nerve terminal. Catechol O-methyl transferase (COMT) is located on the outer plasma membrane of cells,[16] thus acting on extraneuronal dopamine. The major metabolic products of dopamine are dihydroxyphenylacetic acid (DOPAC) and homovanillic acid (HVA).

The neurochemical mechanisms underlying nigrostriatal plasticity are thought to involve both pre- and postsynaptic mechanisms.[4] Presynaptically, dopamine turnover increases markedly in the remaining nigrostriatal neurons. In PD, this is shown by the shift of the striatal HVA/dopamine ratio in favor of the metabolite suggesting that dopamine is being metabolized, and presumably synthesized, more rapidly in the remaining intact neurons. Postsynaptically, there may be a supersensitivity of striatal dopamine receptor sites,[17] although this is controversial (see Commentary to Chapter 4 by Wooten).

III. *IN VIVO* ASSESSMENT OF DOPAMINERGIC NEURONS

Labeled markers which are specific for the biochemical and physiological processes characteristic of dopaminergic nerve endings have been developed for use with positron emission tomography (PET). These processes include the synthesis of dopamine itself, and the process of dopamine reuptake from the synaptic cleft into the presynaptic nerve ending.

A. DOPA METABOLISM
1. Metabolism of 6-Fluorodopa
The study of presynaptic dopaminergic function with PET has been made possible by the development of the levodopa analog 6-[^{18}F]fluoro-L-dopa (6-FD). Garnett and colleagues have shown that after administration of this compound to human subjects, radioactivity accumulates in areas of the brain which are known to have a high dopamine content.[18]

Because PET visualizes only the presence of positron-emitting isotopes without regard to the identity of the labeled compound, the interpretation of 6-FD/PET data requires some knowledge of the central and peripheral metabolism of 6-FD (Figure 1). Fluorodopamine (FDA) is formed by ALAAD mediated decarboxylation of fluorodopa.[19] FDA is thought to become physiologically ''trapped'' within neuronal vesicles and to be responsible for much of the observed ''specific'' striatal radioactivity. This view is supported by animal studies which have shown by direct measurement that FDA is a major metabolite of 6-FD in the

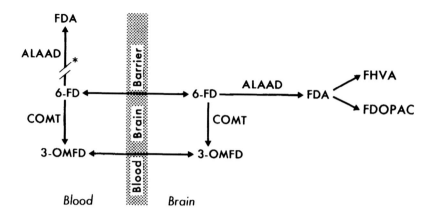

FIGURE 1. Metabolism of 6-fluoro-L-dopa. *, Denotes the reaction blocked by carbidopa. (6-FD = 6-fluoro-L-dopa; FDA = 6-fluorodopamine; 3-OMFD = 3-*O*-methyl-6-FD; FHVA = 6-fluorohomovanillic acid; FDOPAC = 6-fluorodihydroxyphenylacetic acid; ALAAD = aromatic L-amino acid decarboxylase; COMT = catechol-*O*-methyl transferase). (From Martin, W. R. W., et al., *Ann. Neurol.*, 26, 535, 1989. With permission.)

striatum.[20] Support for the presence of vesicular trapping FDA comes from animal studies which showed partial depletion of striatal isotope accumulation in response to reserpine,[21] those which demonstrated release of FDA after depolarization of dopaminergic neurons[22] and by ^{19}F-NMR studies which showed FDA to be present in a synaptosomal preparation.[23] Leenders and colleagues reported that the normal striatum maintains its activity for up to 4 h after 6-FD administration.[24] FDA is visualized with PET by virtue of the ^{18}F label and is likely to be responsible for much of the observed striatal radioactivity.

Further metabolism to radiofluorinated analogs of homovanillic acid (FHVA) and dihydroxyphenylacetic acid (FDOPAC) may occur during the time of a PET study if FDA is released from vesicles. Although direct evidence is not available from human studies, there is evidence of vesicular FDA release in hooded rats, in which appreciable striatal FDOPAC levels are present by 20 min after 6-FD administration,[20] and in monkeys, in which a slowly increasing concentration of striatal FHVA has been reported.[25]

Throughout the brain, there is relatively homogeneous "background" radioactivity formed in part by unmetabolized 6-FD. The neutral amino acid transport system is responsible for the transfer of levodopa[26] and, by analogy, 6-FD across the blood-brain barrier. Evidence for the involvement of this system in 6-FD transport is provided by the competitive inhibition of 6-FD uptake with a concomitant infusion of neutral amino acids.[27]

A second major component, 3-*O*-methyl-6-FD (3-OMFD), also contributes to the background activity. Horne and colleagues have shown that in rats given tritiated levodopa, *O*-methylation occurs rapidly outside the brain by COMT in liver, and other sites.[28] 3-*O*-methyldopa is readily transported across the blood brain barrier and is thought to be responsible for much of the background activity seen in autoradiographic studies.[28,29] 5-Fluorodopa also undergoes rapid *O*-methylation.[30] Although it has been suggested that 6-FD undergoes *O*-methylation much less readily than does 5-FD,[31] our studies show that when 6-FD is given to human subjects pretreated with carbidopa the *O*-methylated form rapidly appears in the blood,[32] possibly because of increased 6-FD availability resulting from peripheral ALAAD inhibition.

Given these factors regarding the distribution of labeled metabolites, the accumulation of ^{18}F in the striatum in excess of background activity is thought to be a function primarily of 6-FD decarboxylation to FDA and, to some extent, of the packaging of FDA within intraneuronal storage vesicles. The roles played by the vesicular release of FDA, by the dopamine re-uptake system, and by further metabolism of FDA are not clear at present. Even if FDA metabolites formed by MAO and/or COMT are present, the striatal radioactivity which is in excess of background activity should give an index of the functional integrity of presynaptic dopaminergic nigrostriatal neurons.

2. Quantitation of 6-Fluorodopa Uptake

The extensive *in vivo* metabolism of 6-FD described above complicates the application of tracer kinetic methods to the analysis of 6-FD/PET data. A comprehensive model requires consideration of multiple factors including the numerous physiological processes which potentially affect striatal tracer uptake, as well as the presence of labeled 6-FD metabolites which are present in peripheral blood and are distributed reversibly throughout the brain. Initial attempts at applying compartmental models to the analysis of 5-fluorodopa uptake measured with a single gamma-ray detector have been reported,[30] and preliminary results from the application of compartmental modeling techniques to 6-FD/PET data have been published.[33,34] Most reported clinical studies, however, have quantified image data with a simple ratio of striatal to nonstriatal activity.

During early times after 6-FD administration, striatal tracer uptake can be considered to be unidirectional. This allows a rate constant for striatal 6-FD uptake to be estimated by analyzing tissue and plasma data obtained following 6-FD administration with a graphical method which is based on the assumption of unidirectional tracer uptake.[35-37] With this approach, the system is assumed to consist of a homogeneous tissue region which is perfused by a known concentration of a test substance. The tissue region may consist of any number of compartments which communicate reversibly with the blood. In addition, there must be at least one compartment that the test substance enters in an irreversible manner. When the test substance is 6-FD, the irreversible compartment is formed by the decarboxylation of 6-FD to FDA and the subsequent physiological "trapping" of FDA within neuronal vesicles. The original approach described by Patlak and colleagues,[35,36] however, cannot be applied directly to the analysis of striatal 6-FD uptake because 3-OMFD, the major peripheral metabolite of 6-FD, is transported into the brain but cannot enter the irreversible compartment. To utilize the graphical analysis, therefore, a correction must be applied for the presence of radioactivity due to 3-OMFD in the striatum.[37] In addition, the true 6-FD input function (in contrast to total plasma activity) must be determined from independent measurements of 6-FD metabolites in plasma.[32,37]

The relationship between normalized "specific" striatal radioactivity (corrected for 3-OMFD activity by subtracting the activity in an equivalent volume of cortex) and the normalized plasma 6-FD input function is illustrated in Figure 2. Since this relationship becomes linear, the "specific" striatal isotope accumulation is considered to be effectively irreversible during the time of the study. The slope of the regression line through the linear portion of this curve is equal to the steady state uptake rate constant of 6-FD from blood to striatum. The relationship between cortical radioactivity and time (Figure 3) shows that the apparent volume of distribution of 6-FD derived activity in cortex becomes constant by about 30 min after 6-FD administration, implying that the amount of tracer in the cortex is in effective steady state with plasma, and that there is no significant irreversible uptake of tracer in this region. At these later times, 6-FD concentration in plasma (and, by assumption, brain) is approaching zero. This apparent volume of distribution in cortex is therefore that of 3-OMFD.

What is the "irreversible" process in striatal 6-FD uptake? In intact nerve endings, enzyme-mediated decarboxylation of levodopa is followed immediately by vesicular trapping of dopamine. This trapping protects dopamine from further metabolism until neuronal stimulation results in its discharge into the synaptic cleft. MAO is present in high concentration within the neuron so that, if vesicular uptake did not occur, rapid intraneuronal oxidation

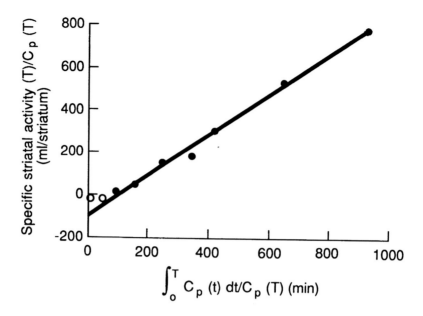

FIGURE 2.   Relationship between "specific" striatal radioactivity and integrated plasma 6-FD activity in a typical normal subject; each value is normalized to plasma 6-FD activity at the appropriate time. "Specific" striatal radioactivity is the total amount of activity in the whole striatum minus nonstriatal activity (from ROIs placed over parietal cortex). The slope of the regression line equals the striatal steady state 6-FD uptake rate constant in (milliliter per striatum per min). (From Martin, W. R. W., et al., *Ann. Neurol.*, 26, 535, 1989. With permission.)

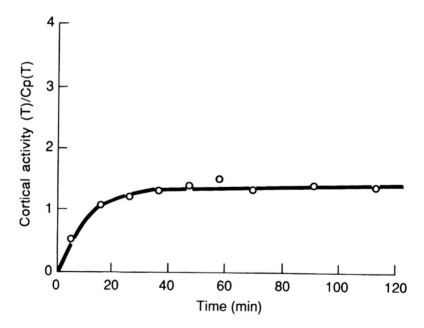

FIGURE 3.   Relationship between normalized cortical activity (apparent volume of distribution) and time in a typical normal subject. Both plasma and tissue activities are measured in CPS per milliliter. (From Martin, W. R. W., et al., *Ann. Neurol.*, 26, 535, 1989. With permission.)

of dopamine to DOPAC would take place. Analogous processes are thought to occur with 6-FD. Although vesicular trapping is an important process in functionally intact nigrostriatal neurons, the linear increase in activity demonstrated with the graphical analysis provides a measurement of the rate constant of the first irreversible process, i.e., the ALAAD mediated decarboxylation of 6-FD to FDA. If the uptake into vesicles failed to occur normally, this analytic method should demonstrate a failure of the striatal activity-plasma activity relationship to maintain linearity at later times. The apparent irreversibility does not rule out vesicular release and subsequent oxidation of FDA during the time of the study, but implies that if oxidation does occur, the labeled compounds so formed remain within the tissue during the study time.

The graphical method described above allows for confirmation of a unidirectional uptake process and quantitation of the rate constant for this process only. The development of more detailed tracer kinetic analyses of 6-FD uptake and metabolism using compartmental modeling techniques is currently under investigation by several groups.[33,34]

B. PRESYNAPTIC DOPAMINE REUPTAKE

Dopamine reuptake sites are present on presynaptic nigrostriatal nerve endings. Drugs which bind to these sites and inhibit dopamine uptake have pharmacological use, and have been used with autoradiography to study the reuptake mechanism.[38,39]

Nomifensine demonstrates high affinity and specificity for catecholamine (including both dopamine and noradrenaline) reuptake sites. Following the administration of [11C]nomifensine, the uptake of radioactivity has been shown to be high in the striatum where there is a high density of dopamine terminals, and much lower in cerebellum, which is almost devoid of dopaminergic innervation.[40] The specificity of [11C]nomifensine for dopamine reuptake sites in the striatum is confirmed by the blockade of nomifensine uptake by mazindol, which also acts at the same site.

The use of nomifensine to study dopamine reuptake sites is complicated by the additional high affinity binding to norepinephrine uptake sites. In contrast to nomifensine, GBR 12935 shows much better selectivity for the dopamine uptake system (although there may be secondary high affinity nonspecific binding sites).[41,42] A fluorinated analog of GBR 12935, GBR 13119, has been labeled with[18]F and has been shown to bind to presynaptic dopamine sites.[43] Since the dopamine reuptake ligands label a different presynaptic site than does 6-FD, data obtained with these compounds should provide complementary information concerning presynaptic dopaminergic function.

IV. AGING AND PRESYNAPTIC NIGROSTRIATAL FUNCTION

Existing evidence for an age-related deterioration in presynaptic nigrostriatal function has been based on post-mortem studies. *In vivo* confirmation of a change occurring as a function of age has been provided by the graphical analysis of 6-FD/PET data obtained in a series of normal subjects.[37] The steady-state striatal 6-FD uptake rate constant decreases by about 50% between the ages of 20 and 80 years (Figure 4). This decrease suggests a decreased capacity for 6-FD decarboxylation and may reflect either neuronal loss, or impaired function in structurally intact nigrostriatal nerve endings.

An age-related decline in [11C]nomifensine-derived radioactivity in caudate and putamen relative to cerebellum in seven healthy volunteers ages 24 to 81 years has also been described, suggesting a loss of functional presynaptic dopamine reuptake sites.[44] In addition, an age-related decline in the thalamus relative to cerebellum was observed, suggesting a loss of noradrenergic reuptake sites. The findings of age-related changes in neuronal function unassociated with clinical evidence of parkinsonism confirm the efficacy of compensatory mechanisms within the dopamine system.

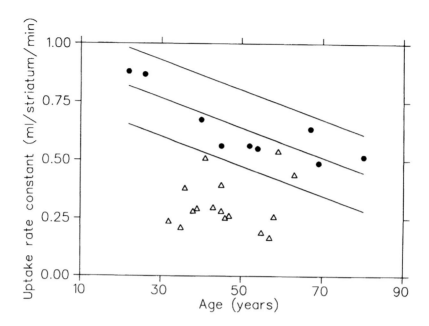

FIGURE 4. Striatal 6-FD uptake as a function of age in normal subjects (●) (n = 9) and patients with Parkinson's disease (△) (n = 16). Each point represents the steady-state uptake rate constant for the entire striatum (average of the two sides) in a single individual. The regression line and two standard errors of prediction above and below this line are shown for the normal subjects. The correlation coefficient for normals is 0.80 (*p* <0.005).

V. PARKINSON'S DISEASE

The 6-FD/PET technique has been applied in several centers to the study of patients with Parkinson's disease (PD) of varying severity (Plate 1*). Most of the published reports have quantified the image data with a simple ratio of striatal activity to nonstriatal ("background") activity. Nahmias et al. reported results in 11 neuropsychologically normal PD patients, nine of whom had strictly unilateral motor abnormalities.[45] In all patients, putamen/background ratios were reduced on the side contralateral to the major motor signs, whereas the caudate/background ratios were normal bilaterally. The reduction in activity was similar in both tremulous and rigid patients.

In patients with slightly more advanced PD, i.e., with bilateral involvement but still significant clinical asymmetry, Martin et al. reported a mild symmetric decrease in caudate/background ratio accompanied by a more marked depression in putamen isotope accumulation.[46] The reduction in putamen activity, although bilateral, was most marked opposite the most severely affected limbs. The observation that the putamen is affected more than the caudate is consistent with neurochemical data concerning the distribution of dopamine depletion in PD.[47] These findings also support the hypothesis that the putamen is more involved in the control of movement than is the caudate.

Patients with more advanced PD characterized by the "on-off" phenomena have a more marked depression of striatal radioactivity than do patients with less advanced disease.[48] This finding suggests a reduced striatal capacity to convert 6-FD into FDA and/or a decreased vesicular storage capacity in the more advanced patients.[49]

By applying the graphical analysis method described above, we have calculated the steady-state striatal 6-FD uptake rate constant in a series of 16 patients with PD (Figure 4).

* Plate 1 appears after page 168.

Fourteen of these patients had rate constants which were more than 2 standard errors of prediction below the regression line for normal controls. We also found a significant negative correlation between the rate constant and the clinical score ($p < 0.05$). Leenders has used a different formulation of this analysis (without background subtraction, and without correction for the presence of labeled 6-FD metabolites in plasma) to show that 6-FD influx correlates with bradykinesia, but not with tremor.[48]

Dopamine reuptake sites in six patients with PD and seven normal controls were studied with [^{11}C]nomifensine and PET.[44] In the PD patients with mainly unilateral involvement, the contralateral putamen exhibited a pronounced decrease. The three younger parkinsonian patients (below age 63) showed markedly less striatal nomifensine-derived activity than age-matched controls, whereas striatal activity in the older patients was essentially similar to those in age-matched controls. These results were obtained with [^{11}C]nomifensine in its racemic form. The authors observe that this hampers a detailed kinetic analysis since inhibition of catecholamine reuptake is related only to the (+)form of the two enantiomers. A large proportion of the ligand administered therefore lacks stereospecificity for the binding sites.[50,51]

The implantation of autologous adrenal medullary tissue into the striatum has been proposed as a treatment for Parkinson's disease. In order to evaluate the efficacy of this procedure, it is essential to have accurate methods of assessing graft function postoperatively. The use of PET has been proposed to determine whether the implanted tissue has functional characteristics similar to those of dopaminergic neurons. Guttman and colleagues have reported that 6-FD/PET scans in five patients did not show a consistent change in striatal uptake when studied 6 weeks postoperatively.[52] [^{68}Ga]EDTA scans performed in two of these patients showed increased permeability of the blood brain barrier at the surgical site. This change in endothelial permeability was still evident 6 months after surgery.[53] These reports suggest that functional imaging studies requiring the assumption of normal endothelial tracer transport in these patients must be interpreted with caution.

VI. CONCLUDING REMARKS

The development of functional imaging techniques utilizing 6-FD and nomifensine has enabled the *in vivo* assessment of the functional integrity of presynaptic nigrostriatal nerve terminals in human subjects. On the basis of post-mortem neurochemical studies, an age-related deterioration in nigrostriatal function has been postulated. PET studies with these tracers have provided *in vivo* confirmation of this change and provide a method to follow these changes with increasing age. Ultimately, with the development of appropriate quantitative techniques, it should be possible to determine the *in vivo* threshold for normal nigrostriatal function, below which the signs and symptoms of parkinsonism appear.

Studies in Parkinson's disease have provided evidence that the impairment in presynaptic dopaminergic function affects nigrostriatal nerve endings in the putamen more than in the caudate, in keeping with the concept that the putamen is more involved with the control of movement than is the caudate. If the caudate is involved in cognitive function, then one might hypothesize that dementia in PD is related to more severe impairment of dopaminergic nerve endings in the caudate than seen in nondemented patients with the same degree of motor deficit. PET studies are currently underway to address this hypothesis.

For these studies of presynaptic nigrostriatal function, the tracer kinetic modeling process which is critical to a proper understanding of PET data is presently in its infancy. With further development of tracer techniques, our ability to quantify the presynaptic function of dopaminergic neurons should improve significantly. It is the development of satisfactory methodology which will make further advances possible because "... we must understand our tools before we can hope to understand our results".[54]

REFERENCES

1. **Kessler, I. I.**, Parkinson's disease in epidemiologic perspective, in *Advances in Neurology,* Vol. 19, Schoenberg, B. S., Ed., Raven Press, New York, 1978, 355.
2. **Marsden, C. D. and Parkes, J. D.**, "On-off" effects in patients with Parkinson's disease on chronic levodopa therapy, *Lancet,* 1, 292, 1976.
3. **Mortimer, J. A., Christensen, K. J., and Webster, D. D.**, Parkinsonian dementia, in *Handbook of Clinical Neurology,* Vol. 2, Frederiks, J. A. M., Ed., Elsevier, Amsterdam, 1985, 371.
4. **Hornykiewicz, O. and Kish, S. J.**, Biochemical pathophysiology of Parkinson's disease, in *Advances in Neurology,* Vol. 45, Yahr, M. D. and Bergmann, K. J., Eds., Raven Press, New York, 1986, 19.
5. **Bernheimer, H., Birkmayer, W., Hornykiewicz, O., Jellinger, K., and Seitelberger, F.**, Brain dopamine and the syndromes of Parkinson and Huntington—clinical, morphological, and neurochemical correlations, *J. Neurol. Sci.,* 20, 415, 1986.
6. **Moore, R. Y. and Bloom, F. E.**, Central catecholamine neuron systems: anatomy and physiology of the dopamine systems, *Annu. Rev. Neurosci.,* 1, 129, 1978.
7. **McGeer, P. L., McGeer, E. G., and Suzuki, J. S.**, Aging and extrapyramidal function, *Arch. Neurol.,* 34, 33, 1977.
8. **Carlsson, A. and Winblad, B.**, Influence of age and time interval between death and autopsy on dopamine and 3-methoxytyramine levels in human basal ganglia, *J. Neural Transm.,* 38, 271, 1976.
9. **Cote, L. J. and Kremzner, L. T.**, Biochemical changes in normal aging in human brain, *Advances in Neurology,* Vol. 38, Raven Press, New York, 1983, 19.
10. **Calne, D. B. and Langston, J. W.**, Aetiology of Parkinson's disease, *Lancet,* 2, 1457, 1983.
11. **Barbeau, A.**, Parkinson's disease: clinical features and etiopathology, in *Handbook of Clinical Neurology,* Vol. 5, (49), Vinken, P. J., Bruyn, G. W., and Klawans, H. L., Eds., Elsevier, Amsterdam, 1986, 87.
12. **Shiman, R., Akino, M., and Kaufman, S.**, Solubilization and partial purification of tyrosine hydroxylase from bovine adrenal medulla, *J. Biol. Chem.,* 246, 1330, 1971.
13. **Lloyd, K. and Hornykiewicz, O.**, Parkinson's disease: activity of L-dopa decarboxylase in discrete brain regions, *Science,* 170, 1212, 1970.
14. **Coyle, J. T. and Snyder, S. H.**, Catecholamine uptake by synaptosomes in homogenates of rat brain: stereospecificity of different areas, *J. Pharmacol. Exp. Ther.,* 170, 221, 1969.
15. **Costa, E. and Sandler, M.**, *Monoamine Oxidase: New Vistas,* Raven Press, New York, 1972.
16. **Nikodejevic, B., Sinoh, S., Daly, J. W., and Creveling, C. R.**, Catechol-O-methyltransferase; 3,5 dihydroxy-4-methoxy benzoic acid and related compounds, *J. Pharmacol. Exp. Ther.,* 174, 83, 1970.
17. **Lee, T., Seeman, P., Rajput, A., Farley, I. J., and Hornykiewicz, O.**, Receptor basis for dopaminergic supersensitivity in Parkinson's disease, *Nature,* 273, 59, 1978.
18. **Garnett, E. S., Firnau, G., and Nahmias, C.**, Dopamine visualized in the basal ganglia of living man, *Nature,* 305, 137, 1983.
19. **Firnau, G., Garnett, E. S., Sourkes, T. L., and Missala, K.**, [18F]FluoroDopa; a unique gamma emitting substrate for dopa decarboxylase, *Experientia,* 31, 1254, 1975.
20. **Cumming, P., Boyes, B. E., Martin, W. R. W., Adam, M., Grierson, J., Ruth, T., and McGeer, E. G.**, The metabolism of [18F]-6-fluoro-L-3,4-dihydroxyphenylalanine in the hooded rat, *J. Neurochem.,* 48, 601, 1987.
21. **Garnett, E. S., Firnau, G., Nahmias, C., and Chirakal, R.**, Striatal dopamine metabolism in living monkeys examined by positron emission tomography, *Brain Res.,* 280, 169, 1983.
22. **Chiueh, C. C., Zukowska-Grjec, Z., Kirk, K. L., and Kopin, I. J.**, 6-Fluorocatecholamines as false adrenergic neurotransmitters, *J. Pharmacol. Exp. Ther.,* 225, 529, 1983.
23. **Diffley, D. M., Costa, J. L., Sokoloski, E. A., Chiueh, C. C., Kirk, K. L., and Creveling, C. R.**, Direct observation of 6-fluorodopamine in guinea pig nerve microsacs by 19F NMR, *Biochem. Biophys. Res. Commun.,* 110, 740, 1983.
24. **Leenders, K., Palmer, A., Turton, D., Quinn, N., Firnau, G., Garnett, S., Nahmias, C., Jones, T., and Marsden, C. D.**, DOPA uptake and dopamine receptor binding visualized in the human brain *in vivo,* in *Recent Developments in Parkinson's Disease,* Fahn, S., Marsden, C. D., Jenner, P., and Teychenne, P., Eds., Raven Press, New York, 1986, 103.
25. **Firnau, G., Sood, S., Chirakal, R., Nahmias, C., and Garnett, E. S.**, Cerebral metabolism of 6-[18F]fluoro-L-3,4-dihydroxyphenylalanine in the primate, *J. Neurochem.,* 48, 1077, 1987.
26. **Pardridge, W. M. and Oldendorf, W. H.**, Kinetic analysis of blood-brain barrier transport of amino acids, *Biochem. Biophys. Acta,* 401, 128, 1975.
27. **Leenders, K. L., Poewe, W. H., Palmer, A. J., Brenton, D. P., and Frackowiak, R. S. J.**, Inhibition of L-[18F]-fluorodopa uptake into human brain by amino acids demonstrated by positron emission tomography, *Ann. Neurol.,* 20, 258, 1986.
28. **Horne, M. K., Cheng, C. H., and Wooten, G. F.**, The cerebral metabolism of L-dihydroxyphenylalanine, *Pharmacology,* 28, 12, 1984.

29. **Miyakoshi, N., Tanaka, M., and Shindo, H.,** Autoradiographic studies on distribution of (L-3,4-dihydroxyphenylalanine (L-dopa) -^{14}C and L-5-hydroxytryptophan (L-5-HTP)-^{14}C in the cat brain, *Jpn. J. Pharmacol.*, 30, 795, 1980.

30. **Garnett, E. S., Firnau, G., Nahmias, C., Sood, S., and Belbeck, L.,** Blood-brain barrier transport and cerebral utilization of dopa in living monkeys, *Am. J. Physiol.*, 238, 318, 1980.

31. **Creveling, C. R. and Kirk, K. L.,** The effect of ring-fluorination on the rate of O-methylation of dihydroxyphenylalanine (DOPA) by catechol-O-methyltransferase: significance in the development of F-18 PETT scanning agents, *Biochem. Biophys. Res. Commun.*, 130, 1123, 1985.

32. **Boyes, B. E., Cumming, P., Martin, W. R. W., and McGeer, E. G.,** Determination of plasma [^{18}F]-6-fluorodopa during positron emission tomography: elimination and metabolism in carbidopa treated subjects, *Life Sci.*, 39, 2243, 1986.

33. **Gjedde, A., Reith, J., Dyve, S., et al.,** Striatal dopamine synthesis in schizophrenia in vivo, *J. Cereb. Blood Flow Metab.*, 9 (Suppl.1), S592, 1989.

34. **Huang, S. C., Barrio, J. R., Hoffman, J. M., et al.,** A compartmental model for 6-[F-18]fluoro-L-dopa kinetics in cerebral tissues, *J. Nucl. Med.*, 30, 735, 1989.

35. **Patlak, C. S., Blasberg, R. G., and Fenstermacher, J. D.,** Graphical evaluation of blood-to-brain transfer constants from multiple-time uptake data, *J. Cereb. Blood Flow Metab.*, 3, 1, 1983.

36. **Patlak, C. S. and Blasberg, R. G.,** Graphical evaluation of blood-to-brain transfer constants from multiple-time uptake data: generalizations, *J. Cereb. Blood Flow Metab.*, 5, 584, 1985.

37. **Martin, W. R. W., Palmer, M. R., Patlak, C. S., and Calne, D. B.,** Nigrostriatal function in man studied with positron emission tomography, *Ann. Neurol.*, 26, 535, 1989.

38. **Hunt, P., Kannengiesser, M. H., and Raynaud, J. P.,** Nomifensine: a new potent inhibitor of dopamine uptake into synaptosomes from rat brain corpus striatum, *J. Pharmacol. Pharm.*, 26, 370, 1974.

39. **Scatton, B., Dubois, A., Dubovich, M. L., Zahniser, N. R., and Fage, D.,** Quantitative autoradiography of ^{3}H-nomifensine binding sites in rat brain, *Life Sci.*, 36, 815, 1985.

40. **Aquilonius, S.-M., Bergstrom, K., Eckernas, S.-A., Harvig, P., Leenders, K. L., Lundquist, H., Antoni, G., Gee, A., Rimland, A., Uhlin, J., and Langstrom, G.,** *In vivo* evaluation of striatal dopamine reuptake sites using ^{11}C-nomifensine and positron emission tomography, *Acta Neurol. Scand.*, 76, 283, 1987.

41. **Andersen, P. J.,** Biochemical and pharmacological characterization of [^{3}H]GBR 12935 binding in vitro to rat striatal membranes: labeling of the dopamine uptake complex, *J. Neurosci.*, 48, 1887, 1987.

42. **Andersen, P. H., Jansen, J. A., and Nielsen, E. B.,** [^{3}H]GBR 12935 binding in vivo in mouse brain: labeling of a piperazine acceptor site, *Eur. J. Pharmacol.*, 144, 1, 1987.

43. **Kilbourn, M. R., Haka, M. S., Ciliax, B. J., and Kuhl, D.,** Syntheses and regional brain uptake of [F-18]GBR 13119, a dopamine uptake blocker, *J. Nucl. Med.*, 29, 767, 1988.

44. **Tedroff, J., Aquilonius, S.-M., Hartvig, P., Lundqvist, H., Gee, A. G., Uhlin, J., and Langstrom, B.,** Monoamine re-uptake sites in the human brain evaluated *in vivo* by means of ^{11}C-nomifensine and positron emission tomography: the effects of age and Parkinson's disease, *Acta Neurol. Scand.*, 77, 192, 1988.

45. **Nahmias, C., Garnett, E. S., Firnau, G., and Lang, A.,** Striatal dopamine distribution in Parkinsonian patients during life, *J. Neurol. Sci.*, 69, 223, 1985.

46. **Martin, W. R. W., Stoessl, A. J., Adam, M. J., Ammann, W., Bergstrom, M., Harrop, R., Laihinen, A., Rogers, J. G., Ruth, T. J., Sayre, C. I., Pate, B. D., and Calne, D. B.,** Positron emission tomography in Parkinson's disease: glucose and dopa metabolism, in *Parkinson's Disease: Advances in Neurology*, Vol. 45, Yahr, M. and Bergmann, K., Eds., Raven Press, New York, 1986, 95.

47. **Hornykiewicz, O.,** Brain neurotransmitter chances in Parkinson's disease, in *Movement Disorders*, Marsden, C. D. and Fahn, S., Eds., Butterworth's, London, 1981, 48.

48. **Leenders, K. L., Palmer, A. J., Quinn, N., Clark, J. C., Firnau, G., Garnett, E. S., Nahmias, C., Jones, T., and Marsden, C. D.,** Brain dopamine metabolism in patients with Parkinson's disease measured with positron emission tomography, *J. Neurol. Neurosurg. Psychiatry*, 49, 853, 1986.

49. **Leenders, K. L.,** PET tracer studies of striatal dopaminergic function, in *Recent Developments in Parkinson's Disease, Volume II*, Fahn, S., Marsden, C. D., Goldstein, M., and Calne, D. B., Eds., Macmillan Healthcare Information, Florham Park, NJ, 1987, 105.

50. **Schact, U. and Leven, M.,** Stereoselective inhibition of synaptosomal catecholamine uptake by nomifensine, *Eur. J. Pharmacol.*, 98, 275, 1984.

51. **Hoyer, D.,** Implications of stereoselectivity in radioligand binding studies, *Trends Pharmacol. Sci.*, 7, 227, 1986.

52. **Guttman, M., Burns, R. S., Martin, W. R. W., et al.,** PET studies of Parkinsonian patients treated with autologous adrenal implants, *Can. J. Neurol. Sci.*, 16, 305, 1989.

53. **Martin, W. R. W., Calne, D. B., Petruk, K., and Burns, R. S.,** Blood-brain barrier abnormalities following autologous adrenal implantation for Parkinson's disease, *Neurology*, 39(Suppl. 1), 203, 1989.

54. **Perlmutter, J. S., and Raichle, M. E.,** *In vitro* or *in vivo* receptor binding: where does the truth lie?, *Ann. Neurol.*, 19, 384, 1986.

Chapter 6

CEREBRAL ENERGY METABOLISM AND BLOOD FLOW IN PARKINSON'S DISEASE

Klaus L. Leenders

TABLE OF CONTENTS

I. INTRODUCTION

In this chapter, a review will be given of the papers dealing with Parkinson's disease and the measurement of cerebral metabolic rate of oxygen (CMRO$_2$), cerebral metabolic rate of glucose (CMRGlu) and cerebral blood flow (CBF) using positron emission tomography (PET). CBF measurements in Parkinson's disease using other methods will also be discussed, as will some animal experiments relevant to the human PET studies. Issues concerning PET methodology are dealt with in the first chapter of this volume.

To date,[*1] the author is aware of only six full papers[1-6] related to the study of CBF and cerebral energy metabolism in parkinsonian patients using PET. These papers appeared in print in 1984 and 1985. Since then it seems that not many studies in this field have been attempted. A number of abstracts and proceedings chapters[7-16] preceded or appeared since the above mentioned full papers providing some additional information. The number of patients described in the six full papers is less than 50. If one considers further that the studied patient populations inevitably must have been clinically heterogeneous and that the five PET units involved employed different methods, it will be clear that conclusions drawn from these results can only be preliminary.

In brain, tissue oxygen utilization and glucose consumption are an expression of energy expenditure and most of this is used for ion transport involved in the generation of trans-membrane potentials. It has been suggested that nerve endings and dendrites have high surface-to-volume ratios and thus a high rate of energy expenditure to pump ions across the neural membranes.[17-19] Brain regions with high densities of nerve endings and dendrites will therefore have high energy requirements and thus high CMRO$_2$, CMRGlu, and CBF. One study[20] reported regional brain glucose utilization measured using PET in 29 children in several stages of development. The anatomical and temporal pattern of glucose utilization paralleled the development of neuronal and synaptic density.

Changing functional activation of brain regions will also be expressed by different levels of energy requirements[21] and be superimposed on that dictated by regional neuronal or synaptic density. Although in the unstimulated state almost all consumed glucose is oxidized to produce ATP, after physiological stimulation there seems to be a mismatch of CMRGlu and CBF increases on the one hand and CMRO$_2$ on the other.[21] The latter was much less than expected from the observed increases of CMRGlu and CBF. The findings are supported by other PET studies[22] comparing uptake of [^{18}F]fluorodeoxyglucose (FDG) with [^{11}C]glucose after physiological stimulation. The former tracer is suggested to reflect total glucose flux from blood to brain whereas the latter relates more to actual oxidative metabolism. How the increase of local CBF and glucose flux after stimulation must be interpreted is still unclear.

All PET studies dealing with cerebral glucose utilization in Parkinson's disease reported so far have used FDG in resting conditions. Although it is generally accepted that global or regional decreases of CMRO$_2$, CMRGlu, or CBF in Parkinson's disease or other neurodegenerative conditions are in most instances the result of neuronal cell loss and thus decrease in synaptic density, interpretation of these measurements must take physiological or other stimulation effects into account.

The situation can be further complicated if in resting state certain brain regions are deactivated due to pathology in other regions. An example may be the "hypometabolism" of the frontal lobe in patients with Steele-Richardson-Olszewski syndrome. In this disease there seems to be little or no cell loss in the frontal lobe whereas CMRO$_2$, CMRGlu, and CBF are all clearly decreased,[23,24] probably reflecting deactivation due to the well established brain stem pathology (see Chapter 8).

---

* December 1988

II. ANIMAL EXPERIMENTAL WORK

A. EFFECTS OF CEREBRAL LESIONS ON ENERGY METABOLISM

Regional glucose utilization has been determined in rat brain using [^{14}C]-2-deoxyglucose autoradiography following a unilateral lesion of the substantia nigra with 6-hydroxydopamine (6-OHDA).[19] The most conspicuous finding was an increased glucose utilization in ipsilateral globus pallidus, maximal at 21 days after the lesion (40% higher than controls). At later times, the response to the lesion was more attenuated (15% higher than controls at 104 days). The authors suggest that a lesion of the substantia nigra with depletion of striatal dopamine content results in disinhibition of striatopallidal pathways. This in turn leads to increased glucose utilization in the terminal fields of the main efferent of the striatum, namely, the globus pallidus. The lateral habenular nucleus also showed an increased uptake of [^{14}C]-2-deoxyglucose. This might have been caused by disinhibition of olfactory cortical efferents since the lesion included the more medially located A-10 dopaminergic neurons resulting in a large reduction of dopamine concentration of the olfactory cortex. No changes in glucose use were found in cortex, striatum, thalamus, or other brain regions. The results of previous animal experiments by other groups using 6-OHDA are discussed by Wooten and Collins.[19]

The neurotoxin 1-methyl-4-phenyl-1,2,3,6-tetrahydropyridine (MPTP) has been used in rats and monkeys to produce syndromes which mimic Parkinson's disease in man (see Chapter 7). In rat and guinea pig, uptake of 2-deoxyglucose was increased in the pars compacta of the substantia nigra, ventral tegmental area, and locus coeruleus following MPTP administration.[25]

In monkeys, increases of glucose use in substantia nigra after MPTP treatment were found in some studies,[26,27] but not in others.[28,29] The varied findings are attributed to differences in severity and duration of the neurotoxic lesion, possibly resulting under certain circumstances in transsynaptic effects. All reports agree about the increase of glucose use, ranging from 25 to 160%, in either both segments or only the external segment of the globus pallidus after MPTP treatment of the monkeys.[26,28-31] One report suggests that the observed increases occur particularly in the putamen-pallidal system and less so in the caudatonigral pathway.[28] This corroborates the notion that the putamen is more involved in the motor symptoms of Parkinson's disease than is the caudate nucleus. Changes in other brain regions seem to be more variable, e.g., decreases in the mediodorsal nucleus in the thalamus[29] and increases in ventral lateral and medial thalamus nuclei[30] have been reported. Diffuse moderate decreases of glucose use in the monkey brain were also seen,[26,27] although the available results seem to indicate that the severe parkinsonian signs and symptoms induced by MPTP are subtended by selective metabolic changes in only a limited number of brain regions.

It is not known through which mechanism the destruction of the dopaminergic nigrostriatal system results in the increased functional activity of the striatopallidal pathway. One possibility might be through the striatal cholinergic system. It seems well established that the dopaminergic input into striatum exerts a local inhibitory influence on the cholinergic system.[32,33] One study reported that ibotenate destruction of the ventromedial globus pallidus, the primary source of cortical cholinergic innervation in the rat, resulted in decreased cortical glucose utilization (on average 15%).[34] On the other hand, blocking acetylcholinesterase in rats caused markedly increased glucose utilization in the dorsal striato-pallido-nigral pathway.[35] On the basis of these findings one might speculate that removal of the nigrostriatal dopaminergic input leads to disinhibition of the intrastriatal cholinergic system, which in turn stimulates the striatal output pathway to the globus pallidus and thus results in increased glucose utilization in the terminal fields of that pathway. It is well known that anticholinergic treatment of parkinsonian patients can alleviate signs and symptoms, although not completely and in the long term not satisfactorily.

B. RESPONSE TO DOPAMINERGIC STIMULATION
1. CBF

CBF can be influenced by levodopa, dopamine, and dopaminergic agonists. In dogs, levodopa was shown to give rise to an initial global increase of CBF followed by a decrease.[36] In that study, global cerebral metabolic rate of oxygen remained unchanged and the authors concluded that the CBF changes were due to primary vascular mechanisms. With dopamine, a dual response was found[37] with CBF decreases after very small doses and pronounced CBF increases after medium doses. The first effect was thought to be due to stimulation of α-adrenergic receptors and the second due to activation of specific dopamine receptors in the cerebral vessels. This was supported by a study,[38] which showed that global CBF increases induced by apomorphine could be abolished by intravenous administration of pimozide, a dopamine antagonist. In this study, $CMRO_2$ did not change. Further work on isolated cerebral arteries of dogs and cats corroborated the finding that dopamine resulted in dose-dependent vasodilation when simultaneous α-adrenoceptor blocking was applied.[39,40]

Regional CBF responses after treatment with the dopamine receptor agonist apomorphine were reported in the dog and rat.[41,42] The responses were heterogeneous but, in general, CBF increased after apomorphine and these increases seemed more pronounced in the frontal brain regions. Cerebellum showed the smallest increase in one of the studies.[41] The regional increases of CBF did not correlate with dopaminergic nerve terminal or receptor density in the brain tissue.[42]

2. CMRGlu

Autoradiographic studies with [14C]-2-deoxyglucose to determine the regional CMRGlu response to dopaminergic drugs in animals with and without nigrostriatal dopaminergic lesions have yielded variable results. Several reports show that dopamine agonists produce specific patterns of increased or decreased CMRGlu in basal ganglia and other brain regions.[43-50] In rat, increased 2-deoxyglucose uptake was seen in the substantia nigra, subthalamic nucleus, globus pallidus, and caudate nucleus.[43] The increases ranged from 15 to 43% and could be prevented by adding haloperidol while the latter substance alone had little effect on glucose use. Intrastriatal administration of dopamine produced patterns of increased 2-deoxyglucose uptake which were comparable to those after systemic dopamine treatment.[44] Levodopa and apomorphine did not produce the same patterns of response.[45] Both drugs increased glucose utilization in the subthalamic and entopeduncular nuclei and substantia nigra. However, in striatum, apomorphine produced an increased CMRGlu while levodopa resulted in a decrease.

A surprising finding in one study[47] was that apomorphine altered glucose utilization in a dose-dependent manner in rat brain even in regions like the cerebellum which are known to contain little or no dopaminergic activity. This casts doubt on the assumption that the 2-deoxyglucose uptake changes reflect changes of regional energy expenditure regulated specifically by the dopaminergic system.

Another study reports increased CMRGlu in monkey brain after levodopa administration in regions outside the nigrostriatal system and its projection fields, particularly in the neocortex.[48] In that study, only monkeys rendered parkinsonian by MPTP showed CMRGlu changes, whereas in normal monkeys levodopa had little if any effect. One communication reports that in unilaterally lesioned (MPTP) monkeys the increase of CMRGlu in the ipsilateral globus pallidus was not reversed by levodopa treatment.[49]

A large range of dopaminergic drugs has been tested to seek "fingerprints" for each class of drugs particularly for dopamine receptor agonists and antagonists.[50] Neuroleptics (D_2 receptor antagonists) tended to reduce glucose use in several brain regions such as thalamus, subthalamus, and neocortex, but had opposite effects elsewhere, such as in nucleus accumbens and substantia nigra. This pattern of modification of CMRGlu was dose dependent, and appeared to follow the rank order of neuroleptics according to their activity on dopamine D_2 receptors. Domperidone, a peripheral dopamine D_2 receptor antagonist, did not produce the same pattern, indicating the involvement of central dopamine receptors in this response. In contrast, dopamine agonists induced an increase in glucose utilization in a large number of structures including neocortex, some thalamic and subthalamic nuclei, red nucleus, and substantia nigra. Here again the responses were dose dependent and corresponded to the capacity of the drugs to activate dopamine receptors. Pretreatment with neuroleptics abolished the effect of the agonists. Further differentiation showed that only compounds which act on dopamine D_2 receptors produced these CMRGlu changes, whereas drugs acting on D_1 receptors had no significant effect. This latter finding was supported by the results of Sharkey and McCulloch.[51]

3. CBF and Energy Metabolism

In several studies CBF and $CMRO_2$ or CMRGlu were investigated simultaneously.[36,38,42,52-54] Global CBF, $CMRO_2$, and CMRGlu were measured in baboons and values after intravenous apomorphine administration compared with baseline.[52] After 0.1 mg/kg apomorphine, CBF increased by 58%, $CMRO_2$ by 36%, and CMRGlu by 72%. As the authors state, the proportionally greater increases in blood flow than in oxygen consumption may be interpreted as evidence of a vascular action. Similar results were obtained by the same group investigating the effect of piribedil, a dopamine agonist, on global CBF and $CMRO_2$ in baboons.[53] After i.v. administration of 0.1 mg/kg piribedil, CBF increased by 40% and oxygen consumption by 13%. Pimozide pretreatment blocked these respective increases. Oxygen consumption did not follow global CBF increases in dogs.[36,38]

Comparisons of regional CBF changes with concomitant CMRGlu changes after apomorphine have also been reported.[42,54] In one study,[54] CBF increased in most of the 36 investigated brain regions but significantly so in only 8. The changes of regional 2-deoxyglucose uptake paralleled rather closely the CBF pattern and the authors take this as evidence that apomorphine acts primarily on tissue energy metabolism to induce CBF changes rather than directly on the vasculature. However, it could equally be that, as in physiological activation studies (see Section I), stimulation of local neuronal activity is associated with increases of CBF and total glucose flux into brain without necessarily increasing local oxidative glucose metabolism. The attenuated or absent increase of oxygen consumption following dopaminergic stimulation of CBF has been mentioned above. A primary pharmacological influence by apomorphine and other agonists on the specific dopaminergic receptors of the cerebral vasculature, resulting in vasodilation of the resistance vessels and thus increased CBF, has been shown and might also lead to increased total glucose flux into brain. The fact that the changes occur in parallel in widespread regions of the brain, including regions like cerebellum which are not related to the dopaminergic system, support this concept.

III. HUMAN *IN VIVO* STUDIES

A. PET STUDIES
1. Global Values

Global CBF, $CMRO_2$, and CMRGlu have been reported to be mildly or moderately reduced in Parkinson's disease in several studies applying PET methods.[1,4-6,11,15,16] Kuhl et al.[1] reported that the CMRGlu reduction in nine patients roughly correlated with severity of bradykinesia and degree of concomitant dementia. However, no decrease of glucose metabolism was found by Rougement et al.[2] in which four patients were compared with seven healthy subjects. In a further study[5] of 11 parkinsonian patients, global CBF was not found to differ significantly from healthy subjects. However, a mild global difference between patients and controls was present (45 ± 11 vs. 49 ± 8 ml/(min/100 g)) and in some cortical regions this difference was more marked. The patients in the latter study were selected for unilaterality and presented with only mild symptoms and signs.

The decrease of CBF in eight bilaterally affected parkinsonian patients was more pronounced than the decrease in $CMRO_2$,[6] e.g., in the basal ganglia region CBF was decreased by 21% compared to normal values of 16 age-matched healthy controls and $CMRO_2$ by only 9%. The authors proposed that impaired dopaminergic innervation of cerebral arterial blood vessels may explain this finding, as dopaminergic stimulation contributes to vasodilatation. This would mean that, in addition to the decrease of regional CBF as the consequence of diminished energy demand by the affected brain tissue, a further decrease is caused by specific vascular mechanisms. Support for this suggestion is the finding of diminished adrenergic receptors on cerebral microvessels in post-mortem brain of parkinsonian patients.[55-57] Alternatively, since Parkinson's disease is characterized by pathology of several brain stem nuclei, diffuse cerebral vasoconstriction as the consequence of disturbed vascular regulation by degenerated brain stem nuclei might contribute to the CBF decrease which follows diminished tissue energy demands. Support for this hypothesis comes from the electrical stimulation studies of brain stem nuclei in rat (parabrachial and fastigial nuclei and dorsal medullary reticular formation) which produce diffuse and marked decreases or increases of CBF, respectively, mostly without influencing energy metabolism.[58,59] A similar and possibly more marked dissociation of CBF and $CMRO_2$ decrease at rest was seen in patients with the Steele-Richardson-Olszewski syndrome studied with PET.[24]

2. Regional Pattern of CBF and Energy Metabolism

Regional differences in oxygen utilization and CBF in parkinsonian brain have also been described using PET.[5-7,8,9,11] Regional "basal ganglia" values on the side contralateral to the affected limbs of predominantly or solely unilateral parkinsonian patients, were significantly higher than the opposite side.[6,7] These findings are illustrated in Figure 1 and Plate 2*. In the first communication reporting basal ganglia asymmetries,[7] in three patients CBF was on average 23% and $CMRO_2$ 17% higher on the side contralateral to the clinically affected side. In a later report[6] on six patients, the mean differences were 14% and 12%, respectively. All six patients had their parkinsonian drug treatment completely withdrawn for 5 to 7 days. In another study, CBF and $CMRO_2$ were measured in one strictly unilateral parkinsonian patient.[10] In the region of the contralateral globus pallidus $CMRO_2$ was 48% higher than on the ipsilateral side, but the values for CBF were not mentioned. This asymmetry of the globus pallidus region was also found in two patients using FDG and PET.[3] Glucose metabolism was 54% higher on the contralateral side in one severely affected unilateral patient and 18% in a moderately affected case. A third patient with mild signs and symptoms showed no side to side differences. Another group reported local cerebral glucose utilization in four severely and probably bilaterally affected parkinsonian patients.[2] Compared to control values, CMRGlu of the basal ganglia was moderately increased.

Regional CBF measurements were reported in 11 patients with hemiparkinsonism.[5] Right-left pallidal blood flow was significantly less tightly coupled in patients than controls, but this coupling improved after levodopa administration. Abnormal basal ganglia CBF asymmetries were found in only 6 of 11 hemiparkinsonian patients and the higher value was not always found on the side contralateral to the affected limbs. This result contrasts with the other reports discussed above, possibly due to interfering effects of dopaminergic treatment. The abnormal asymmetries were found in four of five patients who had not had any dopaminergic drug treatment within 1 month before the PET measurements and in only two of the six patients who had had levodopa within 24 to 72 h before the study. Another study

---

* Plate 2 appears after page 168.

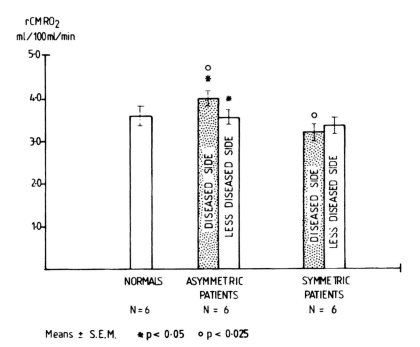

FIGURE 1.   Mean ± SEM of regional oxygen utilization (rCMRO₂) in the basal ganglia region of six predominantly unilaterally and six symmetrically affected parkinsonian patients after 1 week of drug withdrawal. The more diseased basal ganglia regions (contralateral to the more affected limbs) showed on average a higher metabolic rate than the less affected side in the first patient group (*p <0.05; student's paired t-test). (From Leenders, K. L., Wolfson, L., and Jones, T., *Monogr. Neurol. Sci.*, 11, 180, 1984. With permission.)

mentions briefly the results of 11 patients, 5 of whom were clearly lateralized.[15] No asymmetry was found in the basal ganglia regions, although a relative increase of metabolism was found in three patients in caudate and lentiform nucleus.

The mechanism resulting in basal ganglia (globus pallidus) asymmetries, when they occur, is unclear. Striatal disinhibition by impaired nigrostriatal dopaminergic input has been discussed previously in this chapter. It must be stressed again that the number of carefully selected patients studied with PET is still small, and that the effect of clinical condition and dopaminergic treatment on the measurements is difficult to assess.

The question has been raised whether it is the tremor which results in increased contralateral globus pallidus activity.[5] PET studies repeated 1 h after levodopa treatment did not reduce basal ganglia asymmetries even though the tremor had completely disappeared.[4,6] However, voluntary hand or finger movements in normal subjects do give rise to increased CBF in sensorimotor cortical and several subcortical regions.[5,60] In two studies,[5,8] patients with unilateral tremor did not have increased CBF in contralateral sensorimotor cortex, but a third study[15] mentioned a slight increase in metabolism in the contralateral sensorimotor cortex and cerebellum of two patients with lateralized tremor. The effect of voluntary movements on the pattern of CBF changes in patients with Parkinson's disease compared with controls is currently under study.

3. Effect of Levodopa Treatment on CBF and Energy Metabolism

Several PET studies have been performed in order to assess whether the clinical im-

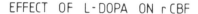

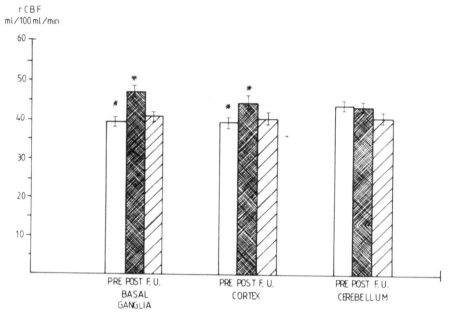

EFFECT OF L-DOPA ON rCBF

Means ± S.E.M. *p<0·005 N=18

A

FIGURE 2.   Mean ± SEM of regional cerebral blood flow (rCBF) (A) and oxygen utilization (rCMRO$_2$) (B) measured in several brain regions of a group of 18 patients with Parkinson's disease before (pre),1 h after a large oral dose of levodopa (post) and several weeks after clinically effective continuous levodopa treatment (follow-up = F.U.). In cortical and sub-cortical regions a significant increase (*p <0.005; student's paired t-test) of CBF was found, but not in cerebellum. (From Leenders, K. L., Wolfson, L., and Jones, T., *Monogr. Neurol. Sci.*, 11, 180, 1984. With permission.)

provement due to the pharmacological action of levodopa is associated with significant global or regional changes in cerebral energy metabolism of CBF.[2,4-8,10,11,14] A moderate dose of levodopa with adequate clinical response (mean dose 195 mg plus carbidopa; range 100 to 250 mg),[5] did not significantly alter CBF.[4,5,8,11] This applies to both acute and chronic administration. However, acute administration of higher doses of levodopa (mean 532 ± 181 mg plus carbidopa; range 300 to 1000 mg)[4] produced a global increase of CBF ranging between 10 and 80% of control. (Figure 2A and Plate 2)[4,7,8] A correlation was found between percentage change of CBF in cortex and plasma levodopa level. There was no correlation of CBF in basal ganglia with plasma levels. No change of oxygen utilization was found corresponding to the CBF increase (Figure 2B and Plate 2). Consequently, there was a compensatory decrease of the fractional oxygen extraction. It was concluded that high doses of levodopa have a vasodilatory effect unrelated to any effect on the parenchymal dopaminergic nervous tissue.

To explore this further, some studies were performed with patients premedicated with domperidone (a peripheral dopamine D$_2$ receptor antagonist). The results showed that the levodopa induced increase of CBF was prevented by the domperidone pretreatment (author's own unpublished data, but see Plate 3*). CMRO$_2$ did not change after those interventions.

* Plate 3 appears after page 168.

EFFECTS OF L-DOPA ON r CMRO$_2$

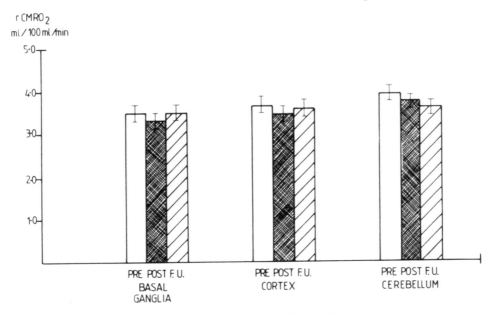

Mean ± S.E.M. N = 18

B

It is suggested that domperidone, which in the dose given does not pass the blood-brain barrier, blocked dopamine D$_2$ receptors in the blood vessel wall, preventing the levodopa-induced D$_2$ receptor-mediated vasodilatation. The vasoactive component of levodopa probably does not play a significant role under normal therapeutic regimes, although occasionally patients report headache after levodopa which might be attributed to global cerebral vasodilation. One study reports a 15% CBF increase 1 h after oral administration of levodopa in one patient. This was accompanied however by a global increase (35%) of CMRO$_2$. No explanation for the mismatch of the magnitude of the CBF and CMRO$_2$ response is given and no mention is made of how the basal ganglia regions responded.

In four patients, glucose metabolism was measured twice with PET, first after withholding levodopa treatment for 2 days, and then 22 h after resuming treatment.[2] No change of glucose utilization was found. However, the daily levodopa dose was moderate (150 to 600 mg).

4. Cortical CBF and Energy Metabolism in Parkinson's Disease

Several studies provide some information on CBF and energy metabolism in cortical regions. An early pioneering study reported the use of the positron emitter oxygen-15 and a gamma camera to investigate 22 patients with Parkinson's disease.[61] There was an indication of diminished oxidative metabolism in the parietal cortex without impairment of blood flow. No signs of dementia were reported but formal neuropsychological testing was not performed. In view of the technical limitations at that time the results could only be interpreted with caution and reservation.

Nine patients with Parkinson's disease and 14 healthy subjects were studied with PET and FDG.[1] A uniform reduction of cerebral glucose metabolism was found throughout the brain (18%). Global CMRGlu correlated inversely with the severity of dementia. One patient was followed for 4 years during which his dementia advanced from mild to moderate. At the same time CMRGlu of the parietal cortex decreased by 39% of the caudate-thalamus only by 16%. As a result, a pattern of CMRGlu had developed similar to that seen in patients with Alzheimer's disease. In a later report[12] of 14 Parkinson's and 28 probable Alzheimer's disease patients, the degree of parietal hypometabolism, expressed as parietocerebellar ratio, was shown to correlate with severity of dementia in both groups. However, as the overlap was considerable and the number of parkinsonian patients small, this finding must be confirmed before such a ratio might be used as an index of cognitive impairment in Parkinson's disease. No explanation exists for why parietal cortex in particular should show impaired energy metabolism in dementia. Whether parietal neuronal and synaptic density has decreased or whether cortical deactivation from degeneration in certain brain stem nuclei has taken place in the affected patients is unclear. Age as such seems to have no effect on the parietocerebellar ratio of $CMRO_2$ or CBF in a group of 34 healthy subjects (author's own data, unpublished).

Similar regional CMRGlu findings in Parkinson's disease with dementia were reported by Peppard et al.[16] In patients without abnormal mental function, only modest widespread glucose hypometabolism was found. Patients with moderate or severe dementia showed a pattern of glucose hypometabolism which resembled that commonly found in patients with Alzheimer's disease, namely, a global decrease with focal additional reductions in the parietal lobes. Glucose utilization in the basal ganglia regions and thalamus was slightly more reduced in patients with parkinsonism compared to patients with Alzheimer's disease. Cortical hypometabolism correlated with the severity of mental changes as graded by their scoring system. There were no demented patients with Parkinson's disease who did not have significant diffuse cortical hypometabolism.

Huber et al. reported FDG/PET studies in 11 patients with Parkinson's disease and showed on average only mild global reductions in cerebral tracer uptake.[15] However, two patients who were moderately and severely demented showed significantly reduced global and cortical glucose utilization. Although the authors did not state which cortical regions were primarily affected, they gave the impression that the findings were similar to those in Alzheimer's disease.

Frontal cortex contralateral to the symptomatic limbs in six unilateral patients had a lower CBF (-12%) and oxygen utilization (-21%) than in healthy subjects.[6] Similar CBF results were obtained by others[5] who found a lower CBF compared to control values particularly in mesocortical regions contralateral to the patients' symptoms. In contrast to the parietal cortex hypometabolism, frontal cortex hypometabolism can be linked to the dopaminergic system.[62-64] In primates, mesocortical dopaminergic projections are present and in Parkinson's disease, decreased dopaminergic input into frontal cortex might result in alterations of local cortical CBF and energy metabolism.

Regional cerebral $CMRO_2$ was measured in ten patients with early untreated Parkinson's disease (author's own data, unpublished). All patients were in the early stages of the disease and had only mild disabilities. None of these patients showed significant cortical atrophy on CT scan and no global impairment of cognitive function was demonstrated on formal testing. Cortical values for $CMRO_2$, however, were on average 10% lower in the patients than in ten age-matched controls.

5. Tumor-Induced Parkinsonism

Pure parkinsonism due to a focal brain lesion is uncommon, but may be caused by brain tumors, particularly frontal meningiomas. One study illustrated the value of longitudinal PET studies to investigate brain pathophysiology. Pure hemiparkinsonism induced by a contralateral frontal meningioma with no sign of paresis, reflex abnormality, or of increased intracranial pressure was investigated in one patient with PET before and after operation.[65] Extensive widespread edema extending from the frontal tumor into the ipsilateral basal ganglia region apparently caused direct striatal dysfunction. CBF was severely impaired locally, but oxygen extraction was raised such that $CMRO_2$ was maintained at 1.3 ml/100 ml/min. The minimum value of $CMRO_2$ for viable cerebral tissue has been estimated elsewhere to be 1.3 ml/100 ml/min according to measurements in 50 subjects using PET.[66] After resection of the frontal meningioma, all values in the basal ganglia region gradually returned to normal and the parkinsonian signs and symptoms disappeared completely. The pathophysiology of CBF and energy metabolism in this case clearly contrasts with that seen in patients with idiopathic Parkinson's disease.

B. OTHER TECHNIQUES (PERFUSION MEASUREMENTS)

Parkinson's disease has also been studied using single photon emitting radionuclides. Until recently, only cortical blood flow measurements could be performed using these methods;[67] all reports concerning Parkinson's disease except two applied the xenon-133 inhalation technique using a limited number of detectors.[68-77] With that method, spatial resolution is restricted, often allowing comparison between left and right hemisphere only. The development of single photon emission computerized tomography (SPECT) constitutes a considerable improvement but to the author's knowledge only two studies devoted to Parkinson's disease using SPECT have been carried out.[72,77] Due to specific physical and technical factors, signals from deep brain structures can be recorded and processed less well than from cortical structures.

A mean global decrease of CBF (-10%) was reported in a study comparing 60 patients with Parkinson's disease with 51 age-matched healthy volunteers using the xenon-133 inhalation method.[68] The decreases became more significant in the elderly patients. No correlation with disease duration was found and decreases were similar in both hemispheres. Another study reported a mean hemispheric decrease of 8% in 30 patients with Parkinson's disease[69] with frontal decreases particularly noted.

Attempts have been made to measure CBF in the deeper brain structures using SPECT and xenon-133 inhalation.[72] Reduced striatal CBF values were found particularly in the left striatum, although there was an equal number of patients with either left- or right-sided symptoms. It is questionable whether the detailed analysis of the deeper structures in this paper is valid in view of the severe limitations inherent to the method used.

The effect of levodopa therapy on CBF was studied using the xenon-133 inhalation technique.[70-72] No effect was seen in one study of mean hemispheric CBF in 26 parkinsonian patients, but the levodopa dose given was low (250 mg) and administered 2 h before measurement.[70] The same group studied ten patients in "on" and "off" phases and found no differences in mean hemispheric CBF.[71] Similar findings were reported by another group in 18 patients using SPECT and xenon-133.[72] However, in two patients, higher levodopa doses were administered resulting in clear CBF increases in all subcortical structures but no values were given.

The dopamine agonist piribedil (0.2 mg/kg) produced a global increase of CBF ($+22\%$) in ten healthy volunteers.[73] Similarly, 2 months after bromocriptine treatment (10 to 30 mg daily), a global CBF increase was seen in 20 parkinsonian patients[74] particularly in frontal regions.

CBF was correlated with cognitive function in 48 patients with Parkinson's disease.[75] Most patients showed a decrease in both CBF (-20%) and intellectual performance, but no direct correlation between the two sets of measurements was found.

SPECT with the flow marker ^{99}Tc-HMPAO was applied to 19 patients with Parkinson's disease.[77] Flow rates in middle frontal regions correlated significantly with several test scores, supporting the concept that specific cognitive impairment seen in parkinsonian patients relates to frontal lobe function.

IV. CONCLUDING REMARKS

At first glance, it may seem that the results concerning CBF and cerebral energy metabolism in patients with Parkinson's disease obtained via PET are somewhat conflicting. However, inspecting the available data in detail and considering the different experimental protocols and clinical conditions of the patients, it becomes clear that general agreement exists concerning several issues, supported by animal studies and, for global measurements, by single photon emission studies.

First, *global* decline of energy metabolism of a mild to moderate degree has been found in almost all studies. It is not clear from PET studies themselves whether this decline is due to neuronal cell loss and thus loss of synaptic density, or to global deactivation from focal subcortical pathological changes.

Second, *regional* changes have been found, the most conspicuous being increased activity of globus pallidus contralateral to the most affected limbs in some asymmetrically affected patients. This finds strong support from several animal experiments. However, it remains unclear under which clinical and pathopysiological circumstances these regional changes occur.

Third, *cognitive* changes appear to be related to the metabolic status of cortex, but the precise relationship is not yet clear. In particular, it remains to be clarified whether frontal cortex has a special role in the mental changes occurring in certain patients with Parkinson's disease.

Fourth, one of the *pharmacological* effects of levodopa or dopamine agonists is, if given in high enough dose, cerebral vasodilatation and thus increased CBF. At the same time, it seems clear that this vascular effect is independent of the influence of levodopa on striatal dopaminergic neurotransmission and thus clinical improvement. It remains unclear whether, in addition to a direct vascular influence, there is regional stimulation of energy metabolism which in turn stimulates CBF after administration of dopamine agonists. The methodological problem of increased total glucose flux vs. changes of oxidative glucose metabolism is discussed in the Introduction and Section II.B.3

It should come as no surprise when cerebral energy metabolism and CBF measurements do not yield immediate or spectacular results in the study of neurodegenerative diseases. Energy metabolism values, even if accurately measured, provide only general indicators for regional brain tissue function, pointing indirectly to the underlying pathophysiology. Only when precisely defined and selected patients (clinically, neurophysiologically, and otherwise) are studied, preferably in longitudinal investigations, may patterns of focal or global disturbances of energy metabolism help clarify disease pathophysiology.

REFERENCES

1. **Kuhl, D. E., Metter, E. J., and Riege, W. H.,** Patterns of local cerebral glucose utilization determined in Parkinson's disease by the (18-F)fluorodeoxyglucose method, *Ann. Neurol.,* 15, 419, 1984.
2. **Rougement, D., Baron, J. C., Collard, P., Bustany, P., Comar, D., and Agid, Y.,** Local cerebral glucose utilisation in treated and untreated patients with Parkinson's disease, *J. Neurol. Neurosurg. Psychiatry,* 47, 824, 1984.
3. **Martin, W. R. W., Beckman, J. H., Calne, D. B., Adam, M. J., Harrop, R., Rogers, J. G., Ruth, T. J., Sayre, C. I., and Pate, B. D.,** Cerebral glucose metabolism in Parkinson's disease, *Can. J. Neurol. Sci.,* 11, 169, 1984.
4. **Leenders, K. L., Wolfson, L., Gibbs, J. M., Wise, R. J. S., Causon, R., Jones, T., and Legg, N. J.,** The effects of L-dopa on regional cerebral blood flow and oxygen metabolism in patients with Parkinson's disease, *Brain,* 108, 171, 1985.

5. **Perlmutter, J. S. and Raichle, M. E.**, Regional blood flow in hemiparkinsonism, *Neurology*, 35, 1127, 1985.

6. **Wolfson, L. I., Leenders, K. L., Brown, L. L., and Jones, T.**, Alterations of regional cerebral blood flow and oxygen metabolism in Parkinson's disease, *Neurology*, 35, 1399, 1985.

7. **Wolfson, L., Leenders, K. L., and Jones, T.**, Regional cerebral blood flow and oxygen metabolism in Parkinson's disease: effects of the disease and treatment, *Neurology*, 33(Suppl. 2), 116, 1983.

8. **Leenders, K. L., Wolfson, L., Gibbs, J., Wise, R., Jones, T., and Legg, N.**, Regional cerebral blood flow and oxygen metabolism in Parkinson's disease and their response to L-Dopa, *J. Cereb. Blood Flow Metab.*, 3(Suppl. 1), S488, 1983.

9. **Kuhl, D. E., Metter, E. J., Riege, W. H., and Markham, C. H.**, Patterns of cerebral glucose utilization in Parkinson's disease and Huntington's disease, *Ann. Neurol.*, 15(Suppl.), S119, 1984.

10. **Raichle, M. E., Perlmutter, J. S., and Fox, P. T.**, Parkinson's disease: metabolic and pharmacological approaches with positron emission tomography, *Ann. Neurol.*, 15 (Suppl.), S131, 1984.

11. **Leenders, K. L., Wolfson, L., and Jones, T.**, Cerebral blood flow and oxygen metabolism measurement with positron emission tomography in Parkinson's disease, *Monogr. Neurol. Sci.*, 11, 180, 1984.

12. **Kuhl, D. E., Metter, E. J., Benson, D. F., Ashford, J. W., Riege, W. H., Fujikawa, D. G., Markham, C. H., Mazziotta, J. C., Maltese, A., and Dorsey, D. A.**, Similarities of cerebral glucose metabolism in Alzheimer's and parkinsonian dementia, *J. Cereb. Blood Flow Metab.*, 5(Suppl. 1), S169, 1985.

13. **Perlmutter, J. S. and Raichle, M. E.**, Reduced blood flow in the frontal mesocortex in parkinsonian patients, *J. Cereb. Blood Flow Metab.*, 59(1), S171, 1985.

14. **Leenders, K. L., Wolfson, L., and Jones, T.**, Positron emission tomography in the study of Parkinson's disease, in *Cerebral Blood Flow and Metabolism Measurement*, Hartmann, A. and Hoyer, S., Eds., Springer Verlag, Berlin, 1985, 459.

15. **Huber, M., Herholz, K., and Heiss, W.-D.**, Positron emission tomography in Parkinson's disease glucose metabolism, in *Early Diagnosis and Preventive Therapy in Parkinson's Disease*, Przuntek, H. and Riederer, P., Eds., Springer Verlag, Wien, 1989, 125.

16. **Peppard, R. F., Martin, W. R. W., Guttman, M., Grochowski, E., Okada, J., McGeer, P. L., Carr, G. D., Phillips, A. G., Steele, J. C., Tsui, J. K. C., and Calne, D. B.**, Cerebral glucose metabolism in Parkinson's disease and the PD complex of Guam, in *Neural Mechanisms in Disorders of Movement*, Crossman, A. and Sambrook, M., Eds., John Libbey, London, 1989, 425.

17. **Schwartz, W. J., Smith, C. B., Davidsen, L., Savaki, H., and Sokoloff, L.**, Metabolic mapping of functional activity in the hypothalamo-neurohypophysial system of the rat, *Science*, 205, 723, 1979.

18. **Mata, M., Fink, D. J., Gainer, H., Smith, C. B., Davidsen, L., Savaki, H., Schwartz, W. J., and Sokoloff, L.**, Activity-dependent energy metabolism in rat posterior pituitary primarily reflects sodium pump activity, *J. Neurochem.*, 34, 213, 1980.

19. **Wooten, G. F. and Collins, R. C.**, Metabolic effects of unilateral lesion of the substantia nigra, *J. Neurosci.*, 1, 285, 1981.

20. **Chugani, H. T., Phelps, M. E., and Mazziotta, J. C.**, Positron emission tomography study of human brain functional development, *Ann. Neurol.*, 22, 487, 1987.

21. **Fox, P. T., Raichle, M. E., Mintun, M. A., and Dence, C.**, Nonoxidative glucose consumption during focal physiologic neural activity, *Science*, 241, 462, 1988.

22. **Blomqvist, G., Widen, L., Stone-Elander, S., Halldin, C., Roland, P. E., Swahn, K. G., Haaparanta, M., Solin, O., Lindqvist, M., Langstrom, B., and Wiesel, F. A.**, Comparison between (1-11C)-D-glucose, (U-11C)-D-glucose and (18F)2-fluoro-2-deoxy-D-glucose as tracers for PET measurements of cerebral glucose utilization, in *Positron Emission Tomography in Clinical Research and Clinical Diagnosis*, Beckers, C., Goffinet, A., and Bol, A., Eds., Kluwer Academic Publishers, Dordrecht, 182, 1989.

23. **D'Antona, R., Baron, J., Samson, Y., Serdary, M., Viader, F., Agid, Y., and Cambier, J.**, Subcortical dementia: frontal cortex hypometabolism detected by positron tomography in patients with progressive supranuclear palsy, *Brain*, 108, 785, 1985.

24. **Leenders, K. L., Frackowiak, R. J. S., and Lees, A. J.**, Steele-Richardson-Olszewski syndrome: brain energy metabolism, blood flow and fluorodopa uptake measured by positron emission tomography, *Brain*, 111, 615, 1988.

25. **Palacios, J. M. and Wiederhold, K. H.**, Acute administration of 1-N-methyl-4-phenyl-1,2,3,6-tetrahydropyridine (MPTP), a compound producing parkinsonism in humans, stimulates (2-14C)deoxyglucose uptake in the regions of the catecholaminergic cell bodies in the rat and guinea-pig brains, *Brain Res.*, 301, 187, 1984.

26. **Schwartzman, R. J. and Alexander, G. M.**, Changes in the local cerebral metabolic rate for glucose in the 1-methyl-4-phenyl-1,2,3,6-tetrahydropyridine (MPTP) primate model of Parkinson's disease, *Brain Res.*, 358, 137, 1985.

27. **Palombo, E., Porrino, L. J., Bankiewicz, K. S., Crane, A. M., Kopin, I. J., and Sokoloff, L.,** Administration of MPTP acutely increases glucose utilization in the substantia nigra of primates, *Brain Res.,* 453, 227, 1988.

28. **Mitchell, I. J., Cross, A. J., Sambrook, M. A., and Crossman, A. R.,** Neural mechanisms mediating 1-methyl-4-phenyl-1,2,3,6-tetrahydropyridine-induced parkinsonism in the monkey: relative contributions of the striatopallidal and striatonigral pathways as suggested by 2-deoxyglucose uptake, *Neurosci. Lett.,* 63, 61, 1986.

29. **Porrino, L. J., Burns, R. S., Crane, A. M., Palombo, E., Kopin, I. J., and Sokoloff, L.,** Changes in local cerebral glucose utilization associated with Parkinson's syndrome induced by 1-methyl-4-phenyl-1,2,3,6-tetrahydropyridine (MPTP) in the primate, *Life Sci.,* 40, 1657, 1987.

30. **Crossman, A. R., Mitchell, I. J., and Sambrook, M. A.,** Regional brain uptake of 2-deoxyglucose in N-methyl-4-phenyl-1,1,3,6,tetrahydropyridine MPTP-induced parkinsonism in the Macaque monkey, *Neuropharmacology,* 24, 587, 1985.

31. **Montgomery, E. G., Buchholz, S., Delitto, A., and Collins, R. C.,** Alterations in basal ganglia physiology following MPTP in monkeys, in *MPTP: A Neurotoxin Producing a Parkinsonian Syndrome,* Markey, S. P., Castagnoli, N., Trevor, A. J., and Kopin, I. J., Eds., Academic Press, Orlando, 1986, 679.

32. **Lehmann, J. and Langer, S. Z.,** The striatal cholinergic interneuron: synaptic target of dopaminergic terminals, *Neuroscience,* 10, 1105, 1983.

33. **Korf, J. and Sebens, J. B.,** Relationship between dopamine receptor occupation by spiperone and acetylcholine levels in the rat striatum after long-term haloperidol treatment depends on dopamine innervation, *J. Neurochem.,* 48, 516, 1987.

34. **London, E. D., McKinney, M., Dam, M., Ellis, A., and Coyle, J. T.,** Decreased cortical glucose utilization after ibotenate lesion of the rat ventromedial globus pallidus, *J. Cerebr. Blood Flow Metab.,* 4, 381, 1984.

35. **Churchill, L., Pazdernik, T. L., Cross, R. S., Giesler, M. P., Nelson, S. R., and Samson, F. E.,** Cholinergic systems influence local cerebral glucose use in specific anatomical areas: diisopropyl phosphorofluoridate versus soman, *Neuroscience,* 20, 329, 1987.

36. **Ekström-Jodal, B., Von Essen, C., Häggendahl, E., and Roos, B. E.,** Effects of L-dopa and L-tryptophane on the cerebral blood flow in the dog, *Acta Neurol. Scand.,* 50, 3, 1974.

37. **Von Essen, C.,** Effects of dopamine on the cerebral blood flow in the dog, *Acta Neurol. Scand.,* 50, 39, 1974.

38. **Von Essen, C. and Roos, B. E.,** Further evidence for the existence of specific dopamine receptors in the cerebral vascular bed of the dog, *Acta Pharmacol. Toxicol.,* 35, 433, 1974.

39. **Toda, N.,** Influence of dopamine and noradrenaline on isolated cerebral arteries of the dog, *Br. J. Pharmacol.,* 58, 121, 1976.

40. **Edvinsson, L., Hardebo, J. E., McCulloch, J., and Owman, Ch.,** Vasomotor response of cerebral blood vessels to dopamine and dopaminergic agonists, in *Advances in Neurology,* Cervos-Navarro, J., Ed., Raven Press, New York, 1978, 85.

41. **Jauzac, P., Blasco, A., Vigoni, F., Valdiguie, P., and Bes, A.,** Cerebral circulatory effects of a dopaminergic agonist (Apomorphine) in the dog, *J. Cereb. Blood Flow Metab.,* 2, 369, 1982.

42. **Ingvar, M., Lindvall, O., and Stenevi, U.,** Apomorphine-induced changes in local cerebral blood flow in normal rats and after lesions of the dopaminergic nigrostriatal bundle, *Brain Res.,* 262, 259, 1983.

43. **Brown, L. L. and Wolfson, L. I.,** Apomorphine increases glucose utilisation in the substantia nigra, subthalamic nucleus and corpus striatum of rat, *Brain Res.,* 140, 188, 1978.

44. **Brown, L. L. and Wolfson, L. I.,** A dopamine-sensitive striatal afferent system mapped with (14-C)deoxyglucose in the rat, *Brain Res.,* 261, 213, 1983.

45. **Warner, C., Brown, L. L., and Wolfson, L. I.,** L-dopa produces regional changes in glucose utilisation which form discrete anatomic patterns in motor nuclei and hypothalamus of rats, *Exp. Neurol.,* 78, 591, 1982.

46. **McMulloch, J., Savaki, H. E., McCulloch, M. C., and Sokoloff, L.,** Specific distribution of metabolic alteration in cerebral cortex following apomorphine administration, *Nature,* 282, 303, 1979.

47. **McMulloch, J., Savaki, H. E., McCulloch, M., Jehle, J., and Sokoloff, L.,** The distribution of alternations in energy metabolism in the rat brain produced by Apomorphine, *Brain Res.,* 243, 67, 1982.

48. **Porrino, L. J., Burns, R. S., Crane, A. M., Palombo, E., Kopin, I. J., and Sokoloff, L.,** Local cerebral metabolic effects of L-dopa therapy in 1-methyl-4-phenyl-1,2,3,6-tetrahydropyridine-induced parkinsonism in monkeys, *Proc. Natl. Acad. Sci. U. S. A.,* 84, 5995, 1987.

49. **Palombo, E., Porrino, L. J., Crane, A. M., Ho, V. W., Bankiewicz, K. S., Kopin, I. J., and Sokoloff, L.,** MPTP-induced hemiparkinsonism in monkeys: effects of L-dopa on local cerebral glucose utilization, *Neurology,* 37(Suppl. 1), 337, 1987.

50. **Palacios, J. M. and Wiederhold, K. H.**, Pharmacological investigation of neurotransmitter mechanisms in the basal ganglia using the 2-deoxyglucose technique: focus on the dopaminergic system, in *Neurotransmitter Interactions in the Basal Ganglia*, Sandler, M., Feuerstein, C., and Scatton, B., Eds., Raven Press, New York, 1987, 183.

51. **Sharkey, J. and McCulloch, J.**, Relationship between local cerebral blood flow and glucose utilization with selective dopamine receptor agonists, *J. Cereb. Blood Flow Metab.*, 5(1), S537, 1985.

52. **McCulloch, J. and Harper, A. M.**, Cerebral circulation: effect of stimulation and blockade of dopamine receptors, *Am. J. Physiol.*, 233(2), H222, 1977.

53. **McCulloch, J. and Edvinsson, L.**, Cerebral circulatory and metabolic effects of piribedil, *Eur. J. Pharmacol.*, 66, 327, 1980.

54. **McMulloch, J., Kelly, P. A., and Ford, I.**, Effect of Apomorphine on the relationship between local cerebral glucose utilisation and local cerebral blood flow (with an appendix on its statistical analysis), *J. Cereb. Blood Flow Metab.*, 2, 487, 1982.

55. **Cash, R., Ruberg, M., Raisman, R., and Agid, Y.**, Adrenergic receptors in Parkinson's disease, *Brain Res.*, 322, 269, 1984.

56. **Cash, R., Raisman, R., Ruberg, M., and Agid, Y.**, Adrenergic receptors in frontal cortex in human brain, *Eur. J. Pharmacol.*, 108, 225, 1985.

57. **Cash, R., Lasbennes, F., Sercombe, R., Seylaz, J., and Agid, Y.**, Modifications in microvascular receptors in parkinsonian subjects, *J. Cereb. Blood Flow Metab.*, 5(1), S163, 1985.

58. **Mraovitch, S., Iadecola, C., and Reis, D. J.**, Vasoconstriction unassociated with metabolism in cerebral cortex elicited by electrical stimulation of the parabrachial nucleus in rat, *J. Cereb. Blood Flow Metab.*, 3(Suppl. 1), 1983, S196.

59. **Iadecola, C., Nakai, M., Mraovitch, S., Ruggiero, D. A., Tucker, L. W., and Reis, D. J.**, Global increase in cerebral metabolism and blood flow produced by focal electrical stimulation of dorsal medullary reticular formation in rat, *Brain Res.*, 272, 101, 1983.

60. **Roland, P. E., Meyer, E., Shibasaki, T., Yamamoto, Y. L., and Thompson, C. J.**, Regional cerebral blood flow changes in cortex and basal ganglia during voluntary movements in normal human volunteers, *J. Neurophysiol.*, 48, 467, 1982.

61. **Lenzi, G. L., Jones, T., Reid, J. L., and Moss, S.**, Regional impairment of cerebral oxidative metabolism in Parkinson's disease, *J. Neurol. Neurosurg. Psychiatry*, 42, 59, 1979.

62. **Javoy-Agid, F. and Agid, Y.**, Is the mesocortical dopaminergic system involved in Parkinson's disease?, *Neurology*, 30, 1326, 1980.

63. **Scatton, B., Rouquier, L., Javoy-Agid, F., and Agid, Y.**, Dopamine deficiency in the cerebral cortex in Parkinson disease, *Neurology*, 32, 1039, 1982.

64. **Bannon, M. J., Wolf, M. E., and Roth, R. H.**, Pharmacology of dopamine neurons innervating the prefrontal cingulate and piriform cortices, *Eur. J. Pharmacol.*, 91, 119, 1983.

65. **Leenders, K. L., Findley, L. J., and Cleeves, L.**, (1986a) PET before and after surgery for tumor-induced parkinsonism, *Neurology*, 36, 1074, 1986.

66. **Powers, W. J., Grubb, R. L., Darriet, D., and Raichle, M. E.**, Cerebral blood flow and cerebral metabolic rate of oxygen requirements for cerebral function and viability in humans, *J. Cereb. Blood Flow Metal.*, 5, 600, 1985.

67. **Lagreze, H. L., and Levine, R. L.**, Quantitative positron emission tomography and single photon emission computed tomography measurements of human cerebral blood flow, *Am. J. Physiol. Imag.*, 2, 208, 1987.

68. **Lavy, S., Melamed, E., Cooper, G., Bentin, S., and Rinot, Y.**, Regional cerebral blood flow in patients with parkinson's disease, *Arch. Neurol.*, 36, 344, 1979.

69. **Bes, A., Guell, A., Fabre, N., Dupui, Ph., Victor, G., and Geraud, G.**, Cerebral blood flow studied by Xenon-133 inhalation technique in parkinsonism: loss of hyperfrontal pattern, *J. Cereb. Blood Flow Metab.*, 3, 33, 1983.

70. **Melamed, E., Lavy, S., Cooper, G., and Bentin, S.**, Regional cerebral blood flow in Parkinsonism, *J. Neurol. Sci.*, 38, 391, 1978.

71. **Melamed, E., Globus, M., and Mildworf, B.**, Regional cerebral blood flow in patients with Parkinson's disease under chronic levodopa therapy: measurements during "on" and "off" response fluctuations, *J. Neurol. Neurosurg. Psychiatry*, 49, 1301, 1986.

72. **Henriksen, L. and Boas, J.**, Regional cerebral blood flow in hemiparkinsonian patients. Emission computerized tomography of inhaled 133-Xenon before and after levodopa, *Acta Neurol. Scand.*, 71, 257, 1985.

73. **Guell, A., Geraud, G., Jauzac, P., Victor, G., and Arne-Bes, M. C.**, Effects of a dopaminergic agonist (piribedil) on cerebral blood flow in man, *J. Cereb. Blood Flow Metab.*, 2, 255, 1982.

74. **Bes, A., Guell, A., Fabre, N., Arne-Bes, M. C., and Geraud, G.**, Effects of dopaminergic agonists (piribedil and bromocriptine) on cerebral blood flow in parkinsonism, *J. Cereb. Blood Flow Metab.*, 3(Suppl. 1), S490, 1983.

75. **Globus, M., Mildworf, B., and Melamed, E.,** Cerebral blood flow and cognitive impairment in Parkinson's disease, *Neurology,* 35, 1135, 1985.

76. **Globus, M., Mildworf, B., and Melamed, E.,** rCBF changes in Parkinson's disease: correlation with dementia, *J. Cereb. Blood Flow Metab.,* 3, 508, 1983.

77. **Goldenberg, G., Podreka, I., Müller, C., and Deecke, L.,** The relationship between cognitive deficits and frontal lobe function in patients with Parkinson's disease: an emission computerized tomography study, *Behav. Neurol.,* 2, 79, 1989.

Chapter 7

MPTP-INDUCED PARKINSONISM

Mark Guttman

TABLE OF CONTENTS

I. INTRODUCTION

Parkinsonism is associated with cell loss and dopamine depletion in the nigrostriatal pathway.[1] The biochemical pathology associated with Parkinson's disease has provided evidence that neurological disorders may be caused by specific neurochemical alterations. The etiology of this neurochemical lesion is currently unknown. Viral, genetic, and environmental factors have been investigated. Patients with toxic exposure to manganese and carbon disulfide also have symptoms of parkinsonism, suggesting that a neurotoxin may be involved in the etiology of Parkinson's disease.[2] In support of this hypothesis, a major breakthrough occurred with the serendipitous finding of parkinsonism associated with the administration of an illicit narcotic in a group of drug addicts.[3] The responsible compound, 1-methyl-4-phenyl-1,2,3,6-tetrahydropyridine (MPTP), has since been shown in animal models to cause histological and biochemical lesions that are similar to Parkinson's disease. This chapter will discuss the use of positron emission tomography (PET) for the *in vivo* evaluation of the dopamine system in MPTP-induced parkinsonism.

Until recently, the biochemical analysis of the nigrostriatal dopamine system has been performed with post-mortem analysis of brain tissue. PET permits the *in vivo* study of this system. As discussed elsewhere in this volume (see Chapters 4 and 5), ligands are available that label the presynaptic and postsynaptic components of this neurotransmitter pathway. The presynaptic system may be examined with 6-[^{18}F]fluoro-L-dopa (6-FD) to obtain a quantitative assessment of the biochemical integrity of the nigrostriatal neuron. Striatal dopamine, which is indirectly assessed by this technique, has a concentration in the micromolar range. Catecholamine nerve terminals may be assessed by nomifensine, which is thought to bind to catecholamine reuptake sites. There are two classes of dopamine receptors in the brain, termed D_1 and D_2[4] which may be studied with a variety of radioactive labeled ligands. These have a concentration in the picomolar range.

II. MPTP

A. MECHANISM OF ACTION

Despite intensive study, the mechanism of the neurotoxicity of MPTP in dopaminergic neurons is not completely known.[2,5,6] After its administration to primates, MPTP rapidly distributes throughout the body and is quickly metabolized to water-soluble compounds. Its high lipid solubility allows for rapid passage across the blood brain barrier. This access to the central nervous system is relatively short lived, however, because of rapid metabolism to hydrophilic charged compounds. The major metabolite appears to be the 1-methyl-4-phenylpyridinium ion (MPP+). This biotransformation takes place in a two-step oxidation process that probably occurs in glial cells in the brain, in the liver, and in other organs. The reaction is mediated primarily by monoamine oxidase B (MAO-B). Blockade of this step by MAO-B inhibitors has been shown to prevent MPTP neurotoxicity in primates.[7] After its formation in the brain, MPP+ enters dopaminergic neurons via the dopamine reuptake system.[8] This is the first of three mechanisms that allows the selective toxicity to dopaminergic neurons. MPP+ is thought to be transported to the dopaminergic cell body in the substantia nigra where it may concentrate further by binding to neuromelanin, thus creating a reservoir of the toxin for prolonged effects. It is then transported into the mitochondria by a specific carrier system, where it interferes with NADP metabolism in the cytochrome oxidase system.[6]

B. THE MPTP MODEL

In 1983, Langston and colleagues described four patients who developed irreversible signs of parkinsonism after intravenous injections of a substance later found to contain

MPTP.[7] Clinically, these patients had signs and symptoms of parkinsonism including tremor, bradykinesia, and rigidity. The symptoms occurred within 4 to 14 days after the initiation of drug administration and the effects progressed for a few days after the drug was stopped.[7] The patients improved clinically with the administration of dopamine agonists and developed side effects similar to those seen in patients with end-stage Parkinson's disease. Pathological studies of a subject who had taken MPTP were reported to show destruction of the substantia nigra with neuromelanin within microglial cells and a structure that resembled a Lewy body.[10]

Extensive studies on the effects of systemically administered MPTP in laboratory animals have shown the drug to have remarkable species-specific effects.[2] In rats, there is relatively little neurotoxicity, possibly due to the biochemical nature of the blood brian barrier. Harik and colleagues report a high level of MAO-B in the endothelial cells of the cerebral circulation in rats.[11] They have postulated that conversion to MPP+ occurs at this level and since this charged molecule does not penetrate the blood brain barrier, there is a relative unresponsiveness of this species to systemic MPTP. In mice, there is biochemical toxicity that is time dependent and is not correlated with a consistent behavioral change.[2]

Primates are the only animals that develop a substantial and enduring syndrome similar to that seen in Parkinson's disease.[2] When MPTP is administered to monkeys, a parkinsonian state develops characterized by bradykinesia, rigidity and, in some cases, tremor. These animals respond to levodopa and have been shown to develop medication related dyskinesias after long-term treatment.[12] Pathologically, there is a reduction in the striatal dopamine content by more thant 70%.[13] The locus coeruleus is also affected by this neurotoxin.[14] Recently, intraneuronal eosinophilic inclusions have been observed and appear to be very similar to Lewy bodies.[15] Marmosets have been studied after administration of MPTP. Behavioral changes appear but they change over time and there may be a biochemical reversal after a subacute time period.[16]

Investigators at the NIH have developed a model for unilateral parkinsonism in cynomolgus monkeys.[17] This model is based on administration of MPTP directly into the cerebral circulation of one hemisphere. In theory, this should produce a unilateral lesion because of the high lipid solubility of the toxin, the efficient uptake of MPP+ via the dopamine reuptake mechanism and the rapid peripheral metabolism to hydrophilic compounds. By giving a slow carotid infusion, the MPTP is extracted by the ipsilateral hemisphere to result in unilateral nigrostriatal damage; the excess MPTP is then detoxified in the periphery. Thus, "first pass" toxic damage is produced, selective to the side of infusion. Using radiographic guidance, the NIH group instilled MPTP directly into the right internal carotid artery.[17] According to their initial report, this produced unilateral dopamine deficiency greater than 90% while leaving the contralateral side unaffected.

The MPTP-induced hemiparkinsonian primate model may be used for the study of parkinsonism with PET. If the contralateral striatum remains intact, there is an internal control for neurochemical and receptor studies. This internal control may allow the study of important biological questions while tracer kinetic models are being designed to enable quantitative analysis of the scans. This animal model is analgous to that of the rat unilaterally lesioned with 6-hydroxydopamine, a very successful model for behavioral analyses of the dopamine system.

III. PET STUDIES

A. MPTP-INDUCED PARKINSONISM IN PRIMATES
1. Presynaptic Studies

Monkeys which have had systemic MPTP administration have been studied with PET and 6-FD.[18,19] The McMaster group studied a monkey with 6-FD scans at the time of MPTP administration, at 2 h, 3 days, and 10 days post administration. The results showed that the

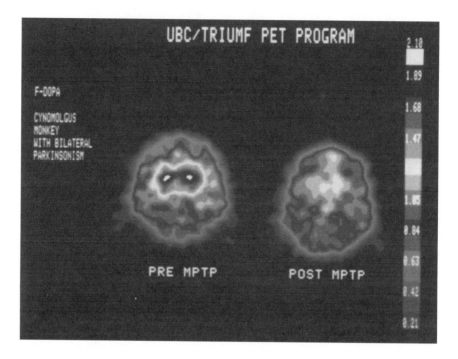

FIGURE 1.   6-Fluorodopa PET scans of a monkey before and after MPTP administration. The animal displayed bilateral symptoms of parkinsonism after the injection.

2-h scan was unchanged; at 3 days the specific striatal radioactivity was increased to 160% and at 10 days the activity was reduced to 45% of the initial value. Clinical correlation was not given. The scan data were compared to post-mortem biochemical analysis in other animals that were given MPTP and sacrificed at similar times; good correlation was found. Another aspect of the McMaster study examined three animals with different stages of parkinsonism. One animal with subclinical damage had a 60% reduction of striatal dopamine measured by HPLC and only a 20% reduction of the 6-FD related specific striatal activity. The mildly affected monkey had 80% reduction of striatal dopamine and 55% reduction of 6-FD related activity. The severely affected animal had good correlation of the dopamine content (97% reduction) to 6-FD related specific activity (100% reduction). One possibility for the poor correlation of the PET data and the HPLC findings in the subclinical and mildly affected animals is that the data from the 6-FD scans were compared to data obtained from other animals. By employing an internal control (the opposite side), as well as using the same animal's scan prior to MPTP administration as a further control it is possible to minimize this potential analytic problem. An example of 6-FD PET scans before and after MPTP administration in a parkinsonian cynomolgus monkey with bilateral symptoms is shown in Figure 1. This animal was studied in Vancouver using the UBC/TRIUMF PETT VI tomograph.[20]

The unilateral MPTP primate model has also been used to assess *in vivo* subclinical dysfunction of the nigrostriatal dopamine system. Clinical symptoms are thought to occur after 80% of this pathway is lesioned; it should be possible to assess lesser degrees of dysfunction with 6-FD/PET. We gave three monkeys repeated injections of MPTP with the end point of clinical hemiparkinsonism.[21] The first monkey had three separate injections into the left internal carotid artery approximately 2 weeks apart and remained asymptomatic. 6-FD/PET scans were performed approximately 10 days after each infusion. There was a stepwise reduction of 6-FD related striatal uptake on the lesioned side of 10, 29, and 60%, respectively, compared to the contralateral side after each of the three infusions. The other two monkeys had single injections. A 6-FD/PET study performed 4 weeks after the MPTP injection in the second animal showed a 40% reduction of 6-FD related striatal activity when clinical signs were absent. The third monkey had a 6-FD PET scan 11 days after the infusion. This showed 34% reduction of striatal activity. The distribution of loss of radioactivity in the 6-FD PET scans was similar to the distribution of dopamine depletion found in parkinsonian patients[22] with the posterior aspect of the striatum being involved earlier than the anterior aspect. This may correspond to earlier and more severe putamenal damage with MPTP, providing further evidence that this toxin provides an appropriate model for the study of Parkinson's disease.

These studies suggest that PET employing 6-FD can provide *in vivo* data on subclinical damage to the nigrostriatal system. The potential value of 6-FD/PET as a preclinical screening tool for Parkinson's disease has significant implications. If it is possible to identify individuals at risk for developing this condition, then there may be a chance of preventing the appearance of symptoms by pharmacological means. The recent report by Birkmayer and colleagues[23] of reduced mortality following the use of MAO-B inhibitors with Parkinson's disease is clearly relevant.

Cynomolgus monkeys that have been made clinically hemiparkinsonian have also been assessed with 6-FD/PET. Four animals given either 1.25 or 2.5 mg of MPTP into the left internal carotid artery have been studied after stable hemiparkinsonism has been established (unpublished data). These monkeys had a reduction of striatal 6-FD related activity of 91, 84, 67, and 86% when compared to the contralateral side. It is possible that the second set of two animals, which received the higher dose of MPTP, had diffusion of the toxic effects of MPTP to the contralateral hemisphere. Results of biochemical analysis of these tissues are currently being analyzed to examine this possibility. If the 7% reduction value is excluded because of possible cross-toxicity, then one may predict a threshold level of dopamine depletion beyond which symptoms may occur. Using the above data, it is apparent that up to 60 to 80% reduction may occur without clinical signs becoming manifest in this unilateral model. When unilateral depletion occurs beyond this threshold, signs of tremor, rigidity, and bradykinesia develop. This is in keeping with the post-mortem observations of Hornykiewicz[1] and has not been previously documented *in vivo*. Animals lesioned with intravenous administration of MPTP with symptoms of bradykinesia, flexed posture and, in some cases, tremor have been studied with post-mortem biochemical analysis.[13] They had approximately 70% depletion of their striatal dopamine content.

6-FD/PET studies have been used to evaluate neural implant viability in parkinsonian monkeys. Miletich and colleagues have shown that after fetal midbrain implantation 6-FD identified the tissue in an animal who displayed clinical improvement.[24] Our group at the University of British Columbia stereotactically implanted sympathetic ganglia and adrenal medulla tissue into the caudate and putamen of four parkinsonian monkeys (unpublished data). 6-FD/PET scans were employed to evaluate the viability of the implants. None of the animals showed improvement in their clinical status or in their PET studies. Further experiments are required to test the usefulness of 6-FD/PET in the assessment of neural implants. Patient studies have identified problems associated with the loss of the integrity of the blood brain barrier which may limit the usefulness of PET in subjects with neurosurgical procedures.[25]

Leenders and colleagues have performed PET scans with [11C]nomifensine to study the presynaptic dopamine reuptake system.[26] They have assessed a single cynomolgus monkey unilaterally lesioned by the intracarotid administration of MPTP and have shown a significant reduction in the uptake of radioactivity in the lesioned striatum. There may be problems with this ligand, however, since there is affinity for other catecholamine neurotransmitter systems. Further *in vitro* studies are necessary for a better understanding of this possible label of nigrostriatal presynaptic nerve terminals.

2. Receptor Studies

Alterations of striatal dopamine receptors secondary to denervation have been studied. The evaluation of D_1 and D_2 receptors *in vivo* has many potential advantages compared to *in vitro* autoradiography or homogenate binding techniques. Assessment will not be confounded by post-mortem artifact and prospective studies should enable the investigation of abnormalities associated with various stages of disease and the effects of treatment. In human studies, post-mortem analysis of striatal D_2 receptors has shown supersensitivity in parkinsonian patients not treated with dopamine agonists.[27] This supersensitivity is reversed if agonists have been administered.[28] Increased D_2 receptor binding has been confirmed in MPTP treated primates by autoradiographic techniques[29] and homogenate binding studies.[30]

Hantraye and colleagues administered MPTP to a baboon and performed sequential PET studies with [76Br]bromospiperone to investigate the alterations of striatal D_2 receptors.[31] The baboon had three series of systemic MPTP injections which resulted in transient parkinsonism. PET studies showed reduction in D_2 binding using a semiquantitative analysis technique. This finding of decreased D_2 sites is difficult to interpret, however, due to the histological alterations found in monkeys that were used as an *in vitro* comparison for the PET studies. These histological studies were performed on another species of monkey that displayed different clinical features compared to the baboon studied with PET. *In vitro* receptor studies on the post-mortem tissue also showed reduction in D_2 sites, likely secondary to the pathological findings in the striatum. Parkinson's disease is not associated with ultrastructural changes in these regions and other investigators have not found evidence of striatal damage in nonhuman primates.[32] Barrio and colleagues at UCLA have employed a spiperone analog to study nemistrina monkeys systemically lesioned with MPTP and report unaltered receptor binding.[33]

Dopamine receptors have also been evaluated in unilaterally lesioned monkeys. Leenders and colleagues used [11C]raclopride to assess a rhesus monkey lesioned with intracarotid administration of MPTP.[26] They performed sequential studies and reported an increase in uptake on the lesioned side compared to the contralateral side. We have confirmed this finding in a cynomolgus monkey lesioned in a similar manner (Figure 2). D_1 receptors have also been assessed in unilaterally lesioned animals and a reduction in the striatal uptake of SCH 23390, a specific D_1 receptor antagonist, has been reported (Figure 2).[34] The loss of D_1 receptors in the striatum is not a consistent finding using *in vitro* analytic techniques after nigrostriatal denervation. Rat studies have shown increased numbers of receptors,[35] no change[36] or reduced binding[37] by various methods of analysis with SCH 23390. If the PET studies in MPTP monkeys are indicative of reduced D_1 receptors in patients with parkinsonism, this may be relevant to the therapeutics of this condition.

In our studies of D_1 receptors with PET, specific binding was evaluated by labeling the active and inactive stereoisomers of SCH 23390.[34,38] Nonspecific binding in the striatum was directly assessed by first performing scans with the inactive enantiomer. Total binding was then measured with the active isomer. Subtraction of the data after normalization was thought to yield an index of the specific D_1 related uptake. A similar subtraction method is also used with both *in vitro* homogenate binding assays and quantitative autoradiographic techniques. The use of direct measurements of nonspecific binding is important because of the potential error involved in employing the assumption that cerebellar regions have similar nonspecific uptake compared to striatal regions. This error has been estimated to be as high as 20 to 30%.[38] *In vitro* results confirm this difference in nonspecific binding with both D_1 and D_2 receptors.

B. HUMAN STUDIES

1. Presynaptic

In a hallmark study, Calne and colleagues studied subjects exposed to MPTP who were clinically asymptomatic with 6-FD and PET.[39] These subjects had reduced striatal uptake

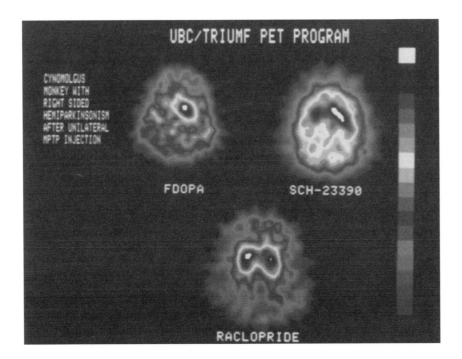

FIGURE 2. 6-Fluorodopa PET scans of a hemiparkinsonian monkey after a single left-sided intracarotid injection of MPTP. Upper left shows 6-FD scan indicating impaired function of the presynaptic nigrostriatal dopamine system ipsilateral to the MPTP injection; upper right shows [¹¹C]SCH 23390 scan revealing reduced uptake on the side of the lesion; lower scan is with [¹¹C]raclopride and shows increased uptake on the side of the lesion. In each case, the lesioned left side is on the left side of the image.

of 6-FD in scans analyzed using a ratio technique. The authors were successful in identifying *in vivo* evidence of subclinical alterations of the nigrostriatal dopamine system with PET. Other examples of subclinical detection of nigrostriatal dysfunction in patients have also been found with PET. Hemiparkinsonian patients have been shown to have reduced striatal uptake of 6-FD on the side contralateral to the unaffected limbs.[40] Guamanian patients with the ALS component of the ALS-PD complex of Guam have been shown to have reduced uptake of 6-FD compared to controls.[41]

Subjects exposed to MPTP who displayed signs of parkinsonism were also studied with 6-FD and PET. The distribution of the reduction in 6-FD derived striatal radioactivity in two subjects was similar to that seen in idiopathic parkinsonism (D. B. Calne, unpublished data).

2. Receptors

Perlmutter and colleagues have performed PET studies with [¹⁸F]spiperone in a clinically symptomatic, untreated subject exposed to MPTP.[42] This ligand binds to D_2 dopamine and S_2 serotonin receptors. The study showed increased association and dissociation rates in the striatum. The dissociation rate was increased to a greater extent than the association rate suggesting an increased number of binding sites present. A direct estimate of the receptor number was not possible because of limitations of the tracer kinetic model used. This study does, however, provide further evidence of the up-regulation of D_2 receptors since this patient had not been treated. The authors suggest that PET may provide insights into rate constants that may be very relevant to clinical pharmacology and therapeutics but are not easily measured *in vitro*

Direct comparison of *in vivo* results from PET studies to *in vitro* data may not be possible because of different experimental conditions. The *in vitro* experiments are performed under equilibrium conditions with saturation analysis in tissue that is either homogenized or sliced. In contrast, PET studies use tracer kinetic methodology to a great extent and do not achieve equilibrium in the same sense as do the *in vitro* experiments. PET has advantages in that the tissue is intact and the kinetics of tracer delivery should be the same as drug delivery in the treatment of patients. It is currently unclear which data (*in vivo* or *in vitro*) are more applicable in answering biological questions in patients.

IV. SUMMARY

The serendipitous discovery of MPTP and its effects on the nigrostriatal dopamine system have enabled the formulation of an animal model that closely parallels human parkinsonism. Nonhuman primates have been lesioned with this toxin and the effects have been studied with PET. The pre- and postsynaptic dopamine system has been investigated, providing *in vivo* evidence concerning presymptomatic and symptomatic parkinsonism. This work has been extended to human PET studies with subjects exposed to MPTP being studied with 6-FD and [^{18}F]spiperone. These techniques show great promise for the elucidation of basic mechanisms involved in the neural alterations of Parkinson's disease; they may also have a tremendous impact on the direction of therapy for this condition.

REFERENCES

1. **Hornykiewicz, O.,** Dopamine (3-hydroxytyramine) and brain function, *Pharmacol. Rev.,* 18, 925, 1966.
2. **Langston, J. W. and Irwin, I.,** MPTP: current concepts and controversies, *Clin. Neuropharmacol.,* 9, 485, 1986.
3. **Langston, J. W., Ballard, P., Tetrud, J. W., and Irwin, I.,** Chronic parkinsonism in humans due to a product of meperidine-analog synthesis, *Science,* 219, 979, 1983.
4. **Kebabian, J. W. and Calne, D. B.,** Multiple receptors for dopamine, *Nature,* 277, 93, 1979.
5. **Schultz, W.,** MPTP-induced parkinsonism in monkeys: mechanism of action, selectivity and pathophysiology, *Gen. Pharmacol.,* 19, 153, 1988.
6. **Singer, T. P., Castagnoli, N., Jr., Ramsay, R. R., and Trevor, A. J.,** Biochemical events in the development of parkinsonism induced by 1-methyl-4-phenyl-1,2,3,6-tetrahydropyridine, *J. Neurochem.,* 49, 1, 1987.
7. **Langston, J. W., Irwin, I., and Langston, E. B.,** Pargyline prevents MPTP-induced parkinsonism in primates, *Science,* 225, 1480, 1984.
8. **Javitch, J. A., D'Amato, R. J., Strittmatter, S. M., and Snyder, S. H.,** Parkinsonism-inducing neurotoxin, N-methyl-4-phenyl-1,2,3,6-tetrahydropyridine: uptake of the metabolite N-methyl-4-phenylpyridine by dopamine neurons explains selective toxicity, *Proc. Natl. Acad. Sci. U.S.A.,* 83, 2173, 1985.
9. **D'Amato, R. J., Alexander, G. M., Schwartzmann, R. J., Kitt, C. A., Price, D. L., and Snyder, S. H.,** Evidence for neuromelanin involvement in MPTP-induced neurotoxicity, *Nature,* 327, 324, 1987.
10. **Davis, G. C., Williams, A. C., Markey, S. P., Ebert, M. H., Caine, E. D., Reichert, C. M., and Kopin, I. J.,** Chronic parkinsonism secondary to intravenous injection of meperidine analogues, *Psychiatry Res.,* 1, 249, 1979.
11. **Harik, S. I., Mitchell, M. J., and Kalaria, R. N.,** Human susceptibility and rat resistance to systemic 1-methyl-4-phenyl-1,2,3,6-tetrahydropyridine (MPTP) neurotoxicity correlate with blood-brain barrier monoamine oxidase B activity, *J. Cereb. Blood Flow Metab.,* 7(Suppl. 1), S369, 1987.
12. **Bedard, P. J., Dipaolo, T., Falardeau, P., and Boucher, R.,** Chronic treatment with levodopa, but not bromocriptine induces dyskinesia in MPTP-parkinsonian monkeys, correlation with [^{3}H]spiperone binding, *Brain Res.,* 379, 294, 1986.
13. **Dipaolo, T., Bedard, P., Daigle, M., and Boucher, R.,** Long-term effects of MPTP on central and peripheral catecholamine and indolamine concentrations in monkeys, *Brain Res.,* 379, 286, 1986.
14. **Mitchell, I. J., Cross, A. J., Sambrook, M. A., and Crossman, A. R.,** Sites of the neurotoxic action of 1-methyl-4-phenyl-1,2,3,6-tetrahydropyridine in the macaque monkey include the ventral tegmental area and the locus ceruleus, *Neurosci. Lett.,* 61, 195, 1985.

15. **Forno, L. S., Langston, J. W., DeLanney, L. E., Irwin, I., and Ricaurte, G. A.,** Locus ceruleus lesions and eosinophillic inclusions in MPTP-treated monkeys, *Ann. Neurol.,* 20, 449, 1986.
16. **Jenner, P., Rose, S., Nomoto, M., and Marsden, C. D.,** MPTP-induced parkinsonism in the common marmoset: behavioral and biochemical effects, *Adv. Neurol.,* 45, 183, 1986.
17. **Bankiewicz, K. S., Oldfield, E. H., Chieuh, C. C., Doppman, J. L., Jacobowitz, D. M., and Kopin, I. J.,** Hemiparkinsonism in monkeys after unilateral internal carotid artery infusion of 1-methyl-4-phenyl-1,2,3,6-tetrahydropyridine (MPTP), *Life Sci.,* 39, 7, 1986.
18. **Chieuh, C. C., Firnau, G., Burns, R. S., Nahmias, C., Chirakal, R., Kopin, I. J., and Garnett, E. S.,** Determination and visualization of damage to striatal dopaminergic terminals in 1-methyl-4-phenyl-1,2,3,6-tetrahydropyridine-induced parkinsonism by [^{18}F]-labeled 6-fluoro-L-dopa and positron emission tomography, *Adv. Neurol.,* 45, 167, 1986.
19. **Chieuh, C. C., Burns, R. S., Kopin, I. J., Kirk, K. L., Firnau, G., Nahmias, C., Chirakal, R., and Garnett, E. S.,** 6-^{18}F-dopa/positron emission tomography visualized degree of damage to brain dopamine in basal ganglia of monkeys with MPTP-induced parkinsonism, in *MPTP: A Neurotoxin Producing a Parkinsonian Syndrome,* Markey, S. P., Castagnoli, N., Jr., Trevor, A. J., and Kopin, I. J., Eds., Academic Press, Orlando, 1986, 327.
20. **Evans, B., Harrop, R., Heywood, D., Mackintosh, J., Moore, R. W., Pate, B. D., Rogers, J. G., Ruth, T. J., Sayre, C., Sprenger, H., Van Oers, N., and Guang, Yao Xiao,** Engineering developments on the UBC-TRIUMF modified PETT VI positron emission tomography, *IEEE Trans. Nucl. Sci.,* NS-30, 707, 1983.
21. **Guttman, M., Yong, V. Y. W., Kim, S. U., Calne, D. B., Martin, W. R. W., Adam, M. J., and Ruth, T. J.,** Asymptomatic striatal dopamine depletion: PET scans in unilateral MPTP monkeys, *Synapse,* 2, 469, 1988.
22. **Bernheimer, H., Birkmayer, W., Hornykiewicz, O., Jellinger, K., and Seitelberger, F.,** Brain dopamine and the syndromes of Parkinson and Huntington: clinical, morphological and neurochemical correlations, *J. Neurol. Sci.,* 20, 415, 1973.
23. **Birkmayer, W., Knoll, J., Riederer, P., Youdim, M. B. H., Hars, V., and Marton, J.,** Increased life expectancy resulting from addition of L-deprenyl to Madopar treatment in Parkinson's disease: a long term study, *J. Neural Transm.* 64, 113, 1985.
24. **Miletich, R. S., Bankiewicz, K., Plunkett, R., Finn, R., Jacobs G., Baldwin, P., Adams, R., Kopin, I., DiChiro, G., and Oldfield, E.,** L-[^{18}F]-fluorodopa PET imaging of catecholaminergic tissue implants in hemiparksinonian monkeys, *Neurology,* 38(Suppl. 1), 145, 1988.
25. **Guttman, M., Peppard, R. F., Martin, W. R. W., Adam, M. J., Ruth, T. J., Calne, D. B., Walsh, E., Allen, G., and Burns, R. S.,** PET studies of parkinsonian patients treated with autologous adrenal implants, *Neurology,* 38(Suppl. 1), 144, 1988.
26. **Leenders, K. L., Aquilonius, S.-M., Bergstrom, K., Bjurling, P., Crossman, A. R., Eckernas, S.-A., Gee, A. G., Harvig, P., Lundqvist, H., Langstrom, B., Rimland, A., and Tedroff, J.,** Unilateral MPTP lesion in a rhesus monkey: effects on the striatal dopaminergic system measured in vivo with PET using various novel tracers, *Brain Res.,* 445, 61, 1988.
27. **Guttman, M. and Seeman, P.,** L-dopa reverses the elevated density of D2 dopamine receptors in Parkinson's diseased striatum, *J. Neural Transm.,* 64, 93, 1985.
28. **Guttman, M., Seeman, P., Reynolds, G. P., Riederer, P., Jellinger, K., and Tourtellotte, W. W.,** Dopamine D2 receptor density remains constant in treated Parkinson's disease, *Ann. Neurol.,* 19, 487, 1986.
29. **Joyce, J. N., Marshall, J. F., Bankiewicz, K. S., Kopin, I. J., and Jacobowitz, D. M.,** Hemiparkinsonism in a monkey after unilateral internal carotid artery infusion of 1-methyl-4-phenyl-1,2,3,6-tetrahydropyridine (MPTP) is associated with regional ipsilateral change in striatal dopamine D2 receptor density, *Brain Res.,* 382, 360, 1985.
30. **Alexander, G. M., Schwartzman, R. J., and Ferraro, T. N.,** Spiperone binding and dopamine levels in the straitum of MPTP-treated monkeys, *Ann. Neurol.,* 22, 149, 1987.
31. **Hantraye, P., Loc'h, C., Tacke, U., Riche, D., Stulzaft, O., Doudet, D., Guibert, B., Naquet, R., Maziere, B., and Maziere, M.,** In vivo visualization by positron emission tomography of the progressive striatal dopamine receptor damage occurring in MPTP-intoxicated nonhuman primates, *Life Sci.,* 39, 1375, 1986.
32. **Gibb, W. R. G., Lees, A. J., Wells, F. R., Barnard, R. O., Jenner, P., and Marsden, C. D.,** Pathology of MPTP in the marmoset, *Adv. Neurol.,* 45, 187, 1986.
33. **Barrio, J. R., Huang, S. C., Schneider, J. S., Hoffman, J. M., Luxen, A., Satyamurthy, N., Bahn, M., Keen, R. E., Nissenson, C., Mazziotta, J. C., and Phelps, M. E.,** Pre- and postsynaptic striatal dopamine neurotransmission in MPTP-treated primates, *Soc. Neurosci. Abstr.,* 13, 566, 1987.
34. **Guttman, M., Adam, M., Ruth, T., Calne, D. B., Kebabian, J., and Schoenleber, R.,** SCH 23390 PET scans show reduced D-1 receptor binding in unilaterally MPTP-lesioned monkeys, *Neurology,* 38(Suppl. 1), 259, 1988.

35. **Porceddu, M. L., Giorgi, O., De Montis, D., Mele, S., Cocco, L., Ongini, E., and Biggio, G.,** 6-hydroxydopamine-induced degeneration of nigral dopamine neurons: differential effect on nigral and striatal D-1 dopamine receptors, *Life Sci.*, 41, 697, 1987.

36. **Filloux, F. M., Walmsley, J. K., and Dawson, T. M.,** Presynaptic and postsynaptic D-1 dopamine receptors in the nigrostriatal system of the rat brain: a quantitative autoradiographic study using the selective D-1 antagonist [³H]SCH 23390, *Brain Res.*, 408, 205, 1987.

37. **Marshall, J. F., Navarrete, and Joyce, J. N.,** Decreased [³H]SCH 23390 labeling of striatal D-1 sites after nigrostriatal injury, *Soc. Neurosci. Abstr.*, 13, 1344, 1987.

38. **Guttman, M., Adam, M. J., Ruth, T., Calne, D. B., Kebabian, J. W., and Schoenleber, R.,** D-1 dopamine receptor PET scans using SCH-23390 show different nonspecific uptake in striatum compared to background, *Neurology*, 38(Suppl. 1), 364, 1988.

39. **Calne, D. B., Langston, J. W., Martin, W. R. W., Stoessl, A. J., Ruth, T. J., Adam, M. J., Pate, B. D., and Schulzer, M.,** Positron emission tomography after MPTP: observations relating to the cause of Parkinson's disease, *Nature*, 317, 246, 1985.

40. **Garnett, E. S., Nahmias, C., and Firnau, G.,** Central dopaminergic pathways in hemiparkinsonism examined by positron emission tomography, *Can. J. Neurol. Sci.*, 11, 174, 1984.

41. **Guttman, M., Steele, J. C., Stoessl, J., Peppard, R. F., Martin, W. R. W., Walsh, E. M., Ruth, T., Adam, M. J., Pate, B. D., Tsui, J. K. C., Schoenberg, B., Spencer, P. S., Iacolucci, J. P., and Calne, D. B.,** 6-[¹⁸F]fluorodopa PET scanning in the ALS-PD complex of Guam, *Neurology*, 37(Suppl. 1), 113, 1987.

42. **Perlmutter, J. S., Kilbourn, M. R., Raichle, M. E., and Welch, M. J.,** MPTP-induced up-regulation of in vivo dopaminergic radioligand-receptor binding in humans, *Neurology*, 37, 1575, 1987.

Chapter 8

POSITRON EMISSION TOMOGRAPHY IN PROGRESSIVE SUPRANUCLEAR PALSY

Jerôme Blin, Jean-Claude Baron, and Yves Agid

TABLE OF CONTENTS

I. CLINICOPATHOLOGIC OVERVIEW

A. INTRODUCTION

Progressive supranuclear palsy (PSP), originally described by Steele, Richardson, and Olszewski,[1,2] is a degenerative disease characterized clinically by four main features: (1) atypical parkinsonism with extrapyramidal rigidity, bradykinesia, unsteady gait, abrupt falls, postural abnormalities, axial dystonia in extension, and lack of tremor; (2) pseudobulbar palsy with dysarthria and dysphagia; (3) supranuclear ophthalmoplegia (particularly of vertical gaze); and (4) intellectual decline.[3-5] The clinical impairment progresses steadily over the years. The combination of symptoms and signs is variable and even the most typical sign, supranuclear ophthalmoplegia, may not appear until late in the course of the disease.[6-8]

The clinical diagnosis can receive some support from ancillary investigations but the abnormalities seen are not diagnostic. The electroencephalogram shows only minor abnormalities on a well-organized background rhythm, but prolonged polygraphic recording has shown a marked disturbance of sleep, consisting of hyposomnia, disorganization of nonrapid eye movement and absent or markedly reduced rapid eye movement sleep.[9-11] Computed tomography often shows enlargement of the third ventricle without conspicuous cortical atrophy,[12] and atrophy of the midbrain,[13] better visualized by magnetic resonance imaging.[14] Hence the diagnosis relies on the association of the characteristic clinical features, especially the ophthalmoplegia. However, there are no published diagnostic criteria specific for PSP, and sometimes the diagnosis can be confirmed only post mortem.

This explains why the diagnosis is often made only about 4 to 5 years after the onset of the disease. The typical onset is around age 62 and the mean overall duration is 5.7 to 6.9 years.[15-17] The contribution of PSP to parkinsonism and dementia is almost certainly underestimated; the true incidence is unknown, although much lower than Parkinson's disease (PD). Duvoisin[18] suggested that PSP may constitute "the second most important cause of parkinsonism, exceeded only by Parkinson's disease".

B. PATHOLOGY

The histopathological alterations of PSP consist of neuronal cell loss, gliosis, and neurofibrillary tangles made of straight filaments. Their distribution and severity appear relatively constant from one patient to another (Figure 1). Four brain regions are severely involved in all patients: (1) the substantia nigra; (2) the pallido-subthalamic complex (with a predominant lesion of the internal pallidum); (3) the mesencephalic tegmentum, particularly the superior colliculus, pretectal area (implicated in ocular motricity), and periacqueductal gray; and (4) the substantia innominata and pedunculopontine tegmental nucleus.[19] By contrast, several structures are constantly spared: the cerebellar cortex, amygdala, and cerebral cortex (except for frontal cortex which may be mildly affected in some cases). Among the moderately and/or inconsistently affected areas are the hippocampus, striatum, thalamus, septum, locus coeruleus, reticular formation, and dentate nucleus.[20]

C. CLINICAL FEATURES

Two clinical features are of particular interest: the lack of response to levodopa, and the cognitive impairment. In contrast to PD, patients with PSP often do not benefit from levodopa[21,22] despite a similar nigrostriatal dopaminergic deficiency.[23-26] The intellectual deterioration is classically characterized by memory disturbances without aphasia, apraxia, or agnosia, and by features that suggest frontal lobe impairment.[27] In a detailed neuropsychological study, Cambier et al.[28] reported the following frontal lobe features: mental slowing, impaired attention, reduced verbal fluency, poor abstract thinking and reasoning, dynamic apraxia, grasping, motor impersistence, and imitation and utilization behavior. Language

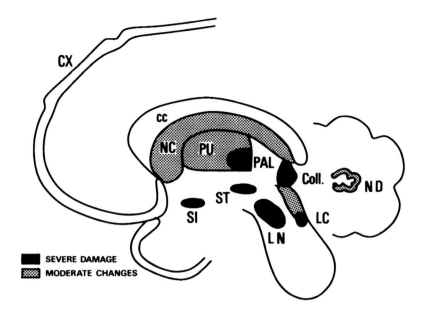

FIGURE 1. Histopathological changes in progressive supranuclear palsy: (cc) corpus callosum; (Coll) superior colliculus; (CX) cerebral cortex; (ND) dentate nucleus; (LC) locus coeruleus; (NC) caudate nucleus; (PAL) pallidum; (PUT) putamen; (SI) substantia innominata; (LN) substantia nigra; (ST) subthalamus. (From Hirsch, E. D., Graybiel, A. M., Duyckaerts, C., and Javoy-Agid, F., *Proc. Natl. Acad. Sci. U.S.A.*, 84, 5976, 1987. With permission.)

tests showed impairment of word-finding, verbal fluency, word definition, and comprehension of complex orders; there was no paraphasia and repetition was not impaired. Similar findings have been reported by Maher et al.[29] Psychiatric manifestations also occur, particularly in the early stage.[30] Pillon et al.,[31] comparing neuropsychological features of PSP with Alzheimer's and Parkinson's disease, found no significant differences on tests of language, calculation, ideomotor apraxia, or visuomotor activity, but performance on tests believed to reflect frontal lobe dysfunction was considerably impaired in PSP. These neuropsychological findings are surprising since in most patients frontal cortex pathology is minimal or absent, although many subcortical and brainstem nuclei are severely affected. This pattern of cognitive impairment, so characteristic of PSP, has been termed "subcortical dementia" by Albert et al.[27]

II. CEREBRAL ENERGY METABOLISM IN PSP

A. INITIAL FINDINGS

D'Antona et al.[32] studied six patients with presumed PSP using the ^{18}F-fluoro-2-deoxy-D-glucose (FDG) method and the ECAT II camera. Each patient had a history of falls, nuchal rigidity, bradykinesia, supranuclear impairment of vertical gaze, mild to severe cognitive impairment, and minimal clinical effect of levodopa and/or dopaminergic agonists; disease duration ranged from 1 to 8 years. These patients were compared to eight controls of similar age.

Visual inspection of the PET images revealed a marked symmetric decrease of the cerebral metabolic rate of glucose (CMRGlu) in the frontal cortex, somewhat variable in magnitude from one patient to another, but present in all (Figure 2). Compared with control values, whole cortex glucose utilization was lower in PSP (19.7% lower at the basal ganglia level, 14.6% at the corona radiata level) but the difference did not reach statistical significance. Regional CMRGlu values were lower than control values in all areas but preferentially

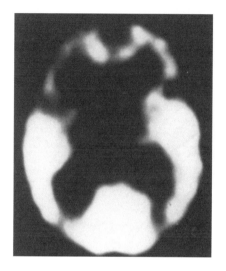 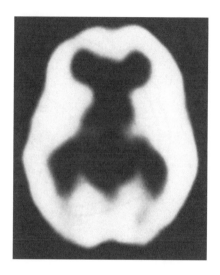

PSP PATIENT   CONTROL SUBJECT

FIGURE 2.   Regional cerebral metabolic rate of glucose studied by positron emission tomography and 18F-fluoro-2-deoxyglucose in a control subject and a patient suffering from progressive supranuclear palsy. Note the marked prefrontal hypometabolism in the patient with PSP. (From Hirsch, E. C., Graybiel, A. M., Duyckaerts, C., and Javoy-Agid, F., *Proc. Natl. Acad. Sci. U.S.A.*, 84, 5976, 1987. With permission.)

so in lateral and medial frontal regions: -21.7% and -29.7%, respectively, compared to -20.7% in temporal, -19.6% in temporoparietal, -15.7% in parietal, -9% in parietooccipital, and around -8% in occipital regions. The difference was significant only in the frontal regions of the lower plane ($p < 0.05$).

Analysis of the relative CMRGlu values, obtained by dividing each regional absolute value by the mean cortical value in the same plane, revealed a highly significant reduction in both medial and lateral frontal regions ($p < 0.01$) of both the low and the high planes and an increase in occipital regions ($p < 0.01$) of both cuts as compared to controls. There was no significant right-left asymmetry for any of the cortical regions studied.

B. SUBSEQUENT STUDIES

The findings of reduced mean CMRGlu of cerebral cortex were confirmed by Foster et al.[33] in nine PSP patients compared to six normal subjects ($p = 0.003$). These authors reported that "analysis of individual brain regions indicated that significant declines in cerebral glucose utilization were present in most regions throughout the cortex" and that "values normalized to average metabolic rates indicated that anterior brain regions, particularly those in the superior half of the cortex, were more impaired".

In four patients with disease duration from 3 to 6 years, Leenders et al.[34] reported a significant decrease in the cerebral metabolic rate of oxygen (CMRO$_2$) suggesting that the decrease in cortical glucose utilization is accompanied by a proportional fall in CMRO$_2$ (although this proportionality has not yet been firmly established by combined CMRGlu-CMRO$_2$ measurement). The decrease was present in all cortical regions, with lower values in frontal cortex (-20 to -24% compared to normals) than in posterior cortex (-3 to -19%). These authors reported also a significant decrease in the CMRO$_2$ of basal ganglia (-22%) and white matter (-20%). The ratio of frontal regions to occipital cortex was reduced from normal but more so in the higher plane (-17.8%, $p < 0.025$) than in the lower plane (-5%, nonsignificant).

TABLE 1
Cerebral Energy Metabolism in PSP
Patients (Group I, N = 23)

Reduction in metabolic rate relative to age-
matched controls (N = 15)

Whole cortex	− 21.2%**
Prefrontal cortex	− 25.4%***
Nonfrontal cortex	− 16.9%*
Caudate nucleus	− 19.1%*
Lentiform nucleus	− 20.7%***
Thalamus	− 25.7%***
Cerebellum	− 23.9%***

Note: Student's t test
*: $p <0.01$
**: $p <0.001$
***: $p <0.0001$

We have now studied cerebral energy metabolism in 35 patients with presumed PSP (Blin et al., in preparation). These patients presented with at least eight of the following nine clinical criteria for PSP: progressive onset, disease duration less than 10 years, parkinsonism, no significant improvement with levodopa, vertical voluntary gaze palsy, falls, pseudobulbar palsy, absence of focal neurological signs, and normal standard blood tests. There were 23 patients with all nine criteria (definite PSP, group I) and 12 with 8 criteria (probable PSP, group II). The PET studies consisted of either the FDG or the steady state ^{15}O method, carried out on either the ECAT II or the LETI-TTVO1-TOF PET camera. To allow comparison of the patients' data despite different tracers and different PET devices, and assuming a proportional effect of PSP on $CMRO_2$ and CMRGlu (see above), the data were normalized by calculating ratios of each patient's regional metabolic value to the mean value of the corresponding regions in a group of age-matched controls for the considered method.

The results of the normalized metabolic values of group I patients were compared to a control group (n = 15) of similar age (66.7 ± 1.6 and 61.7 ± 1.8 years, mean ± SEM, respectively). We found a highly significant decrease in the metabolic rate in all brain regions (Table 1). In cerebral cortex, the reduction in metabolic rate was most prominent in frontal regions although other cortical regions were also affected. The basal ganglia, the thalamus, and the cerebellum were abnormal. The metabolic ratio (regional value divided by nonfrontal cortical value) was significantly decreased for frontal cortex, more so for the superior frontal cortex ($p <0.01$) than for inferior frontal cortex ($p <0.05$) (Figure 3). In contrast, the ratio of nonfrontal cortex to whole cerebral cortex was significantly increased ($p <0.0001$). The corresponding ratios of the subcortical structures (Figure 3) showed a trend for a relative increase in the caudate and lenticular nuclei (+ 3.4%) and for a decrease in the thalamus and cerebellum, but these differences were not statistically significant.

C. SUMMARY OF METABOLIC ABNORMALITIES
The pattern of brain metabolic abnormalities in PSP that emerges from these studies is strikingly consistent. This pattern consists of:

1. A diffuse metabolic depression affecting all cortical regions, subcortical structures, and cerebellum.
2. Within the cerebral cortex, depression maximal in the prefrontal cortex (− 22 to − 27%), with a slight predominance for the upper prefrontal cortex. Among nonfrontal

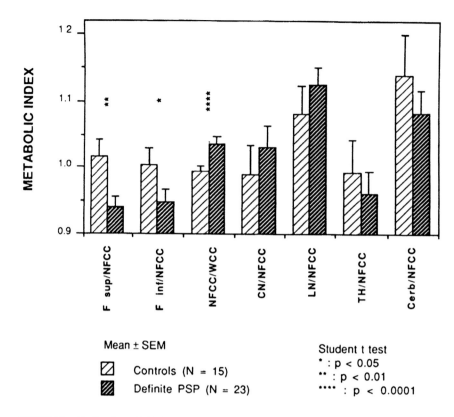

FIGURE 3.   Regional metabolic index, in 23 definite PSP patients and 15 age-matched controls, calculated as regional metabolic rate divided by nonfrontal cerebral cortex (NFCC) value, for the superior frontal cortex (F sup), inferior frontal cortex (F inf), caudate nucleus (CN), lentiform nucleus (LN), thalamus (TH), and cerebellum (Cerb); for the NFCC index, the whole cerebral cortex (WCC) value was the denominator.

cortical areas, the least affected is the occipital cortex (-8 to -12%), followed by parietal (-4 to -16%) and temporal (-21%) cortex. The result is a marked antero-posterior gradient of effects, as depicted in the PET images (Figure 2) and the metabolic ratios (Figure 3).

3.   Among the subcortical structures, metabolic depression most marked in the thalamus and cerebellum, and least in the caudate and lenticular nuclei (Figure 3). Although the latter differences are not very prominent, they tend to further distinguish the PSP patients from the controls in terms of metabolic ratios.

D. SPECIFICITY OF PREFRONTAL CORTEX HYPOMETABOLISM
The issue of specificity is important if prefrontal hypometabolism is to be used as an additional criterion for the diagnosis of PSP. If this observation is specific to PSP, it provides a clue to help better understand its pathophysiology.

In nondemented patients with PD, cortical energy metabolism has been found to be largely normal except for some inconsistent changes in basal ganglia.[35-38] Reduction of whole brain CMRGlu (-18%) has been reported, however, in a group of PD patients with variable severity, cognitive deficit and disease duration.[37,38] In unilateral PD, regional $CMRO_2$ was found to be increased in the basal ganglia ($+13\%$) and marginally decreased in the frontal cortex (-8%) contralateral to the motor deficit.[36] All of these minor changes were inde-pendent of levodopa therapy.[35,36,39] In demented patients with PD, Kuhl et al.[40] reported a reduction in cortical glucose utilization which was most severe in the parietal cortex, similar to that seen in Alzheimer's disease. On the whole, therefore, the pattern of prefrontal cortex hypometabolism in PSP has not been observed in PD patients with or without dementia.

In patients with olivo-ponto-cerebellar atrophy (OPCA), Gilman et al.[41] reported a significant decrease of CMRGlu in the cerebellum and brainstem, but not in the thalamus in contrast to our findings in PSP.

In other degenerative diseases of basal ganglia, reduction of frontal cortex metabolism has not been specifically reported. In Wilson's disease, Hawkins et al.[42] observed a marked decrease in cortical CMRGlu (-47% in frontal, -50% in parietal, and -37% in occipital cortex) and the basal ganglia (-51% in lenticular nucleus, -41% in caudate nucleus) but a lesser change in thalamus (-16%). In symptomatic Huntington's disease, the striata are markedly hypometabolic (lenticular nucleus: -21 to -41%, caudate nucleus: -37 to -61%) but the cerebral cortex and thalamus show no clear-cut metabolic changes,[38,43-46] although slight frontal cortex hypometabolism was noted in patients with disease duration greater than 6 years.[44]

In presumed Alzheimer's disease (AD), numerous PET studies have demonstrated cortical hypometabolism that begins and predominates in the temporoparietal cortex (-12 to -57%), with later and smaller decreases in frontal (-3 to -41%) and occipital (-3 to -36%) cortices.[47,53] A striking feature of the cortical hypometabolism in AD is the frequent asymmetry in parietal, temporal, and frontal cortex correlated with lateralized cognitive changes. The subcortical structures exhibit a less marked metabolic reduction than cerebral cortex, similar for caudate nucleus (-11 to -26%), lenticular nucleus (-8 to -27%), thalamus (-10 to -29%), and cerebellum (-10 to -27%).[49,51-53]

In the single published case of necropsy-proven Pick's disease studied by PET, Kamo et al.[49] observed a marked decrease in CMRGlu in frontal cortex (-60%) and a much less marked decrease in other cortical regions (mean decrease: -21%) and in subcortical structures (-33% in basal ganglia, -36% in thalamus, -20% in cerebellum).

Thus, both AD and advanced Pick's disease display a different pattern of cerebral hypometabolism than that seen in PSP. In AD, the cortical hypometabolism exhibits a posteroanterior gradient inverse to that of PSP, while in Pick's disease the cortical gradient is similar to PSP but considerably exaggerated. In addition, in both AD and Pick's disease, the subcortical structures are less affected than cortical regions, accentuating the distinctive patterns of brain hypometabolism among AD, Pick's disease, and PSP.

A predominantly frontal cortex hypometabolism has been occasionally reported in primary degenerative dementias.[54-56] The lack of detailed accounts of quantitative regional data in these reports makes comparison with PSP difficult, but visual inspection of the published images suggests a close resemblance to the pattern seen in PSP. In the absence of pathologically established diagnoses, some of these cases have been categorized as AD.[54-56] Frakowiack et al.[54] have indicated that this pattern occurred in advanced AD cases. Cases of AD with predominantly frontal pathology seem very rare.[57] In a series of 158 neuropathologically studied cases of dementia, only 26 disclosed mainly frontal or frontotemporal abnormalities, among which were 4 cases of Pick's disease, 3 of Creutzfeld-Jacob disease, 2 of AD, 1 of bilateral thalamic infarction, and 16 constituting a separate group with histological features of neither AD nor Pick's disease. In other cases of "anterior" dementia with predominantly cognitive dysfunction (changes mainly in personality and social behavior), Chase et al.[58] recently published PET images of CMRGlu which are similar to PSP images. Until further information is available on these cases, particularly a quantitative report of CMRGlu and a clear-cut pathological diagnosis, the specificity of the symmetrical prefrontal cortex hypometabolism for PSP remains uncertain.

Nevertheless, at present, this pattern of cerebral metabolism does appear to be specific for PSP as opposed to other diseases with dementia, parkinsonism or lesions of basal ganglia. The cortical hypometabolism predominates in frontal regions in accord with the neuropsychological finding that clinical manifestations refereable to frontal cortex are more marked in PSP than in PD or AD.[31]

E. INTERPRETATION OF RESULTS

In PSP, the cerebral cortex is largely spared by the degenerative process. In only a few patients does the frontal cortex display mild histological changes (which could not be clearly distinguished from age-matched controls).[59] Therefore, neither the metabolic depression of the entire cortex seen in PSP, nor preferential hypometabolism of prefrontal cortex can be explained by direct neuronal lesions, in contrast to AD where cortical pathology presumably accounts for most of the observed reduction in glucose utilization.[51] D'Antona et al.[32] suggested a mechanism of cortical deafferentation in accordance with the concept of subcortical dementia. Among the subcorticocortical systems that are affected, the reticular formation, serotonergic raphe complex, noradrenergic locus coeruleus system, dopaminergic mesocortical system, cholinergic innominatocortical system, and the striato-pallido-thalamocortical circuit are potential candidates to explain the cortical hypometabolism. All of these systems have projections to the prefrontal cortex, some preferentially so. D'Antona et al.,[32] reviewing experimental 2-deoxyglucose autoradiographic studies in animals, favored lesions of the reticular, cholinergic, and pallidothalamic systems, but suggested that combined lesions were probably responsible for the metabolic changes. It is well established that thalamic damage depresses cortical energy metabolism.[60] However, the histological involvement of the thalamus in PSP is minimal and inconsistent, although detailed analysis of specific thalamic nuclei is not yet available.

Recent data on the biochemical changes in PSP and the metabolic sequelae of subcortical lesions shed new light on the problem. Medial raphe lesions in rats do not depress cerebral cortex glucose utilization.[61] Lesions of the nucleus basalis of Meynert in baboons, however, result in a marked, diffuse but predominantly frontal cortical hypometabolism which is linearly correlated to the severity of the depression in cortical ChAT activity.[62,63] Interestingly, this cortical metabolic depression recovers with time despite sustained cholinergic deficiency. Ruberg et al.[25] found a mild but significant depression in ChAT (up to 40%) in frontal and cingulate cortex of eight patients, while Kish et al.[26] found no change in two patients. There were no significant noradrenergic, serotonergic, or dopaminergic cortical deficits.[25,26] These data tend to lessen the role of the monoaminergic systems in the cortical hypometabolism of PSP, except to some extent the cholinergic system. The reticular formation, however, remains a possible candidate.

In addition to lesions of monoaminergic systems projecting to frontal cortex, dysfunction of the basal ganglia requires consideration as a cause for the cortical changes. A review of the available PET literature on pathology of the basal ganglia reveals some association between metabolic abnormalities in the caudate and/or lenticular (including the pallidum) nucleus and frontal cortex hypometabolism, although extensive degeneration of the striatum as in Huntington's disease appears not to result in cortical hypometabolism (a marginal reduction in glucose utilization of the frontal cortex has been mentioned in advanced cases only[44]). In Wilson's disease, where damage involves mainly the striatum and the pallidum, a conspicuous cortical metabolic reduction without preferential frontal localization has been reported.[42] In hemiparkinsonism, a mild metabolic reduction in the frontal cortex contralateral to the affected limbs has been observed,[36] in agreement with cerebral blood flow findings.[64] Bilateral pallidal lesions, which result in behavioral disturbances reminiscent of frontal cortex malfunction,[65] are associated with mild prefrontal cortex hypometabolism without reduction in thalamic CMRGlu.[66] In PSP, prominent histological lesions are present in the pallidum and the dopamine deficiency in the caudate nucleus reaches the same severity as in the putamen (at variance with PD); there is also a cholinergic deficiency in the striatum where the histological lesions are mild and inconsistent. These findings suggest that the basal ganglia may be implicated in the pathogenesis of cortical hypometabolism in PSP.

Our recent study of 35 PSP patients (Blin et al., in preparation) also indicates a marked CMRGlu decrease (-25.7%) in the thalamus. In unilateral thalamic stroke, Baron et al.[60] have demonstrated cortical hypometabolism most marked in anterior regions secondary to lesions of the anterior thalamus. Interestingly, thalamic glucose utilization is only marginally reduced in most degenerative diseases of the basal ganglia (PD, Huntington's disease, Wilson's disease) as well in OPCA. The involvement of striatum, pallidum, and possibly thalamus in PSP could disrupt the striato-pallido-thalamo-cortical pathway and cause the observed frontal cortex hypometabolism. Further dysfunction of the thalamofrontal pathways could result from involvement of other nuclei which project to thalamus, such as the dentate nucleus and the substantia nigra. This hypothesis could be an alternative or additive explanation to the speculative effects of minor lesions of monoaminergic and reticular systems.

III. CEREBRAL BLOOD FLOW

The depression of cerebral energy metabolism in PSP is accompanied by a similar reduction of cerebral blood flow (CBF).[34] The same regional pattern of decrease in CBF as with $CMRO_2$ has been described. The CBF reduction was larger in all structures, possibly because of hypocapnia, and was counterbalanced by an increased oxygen extraction ratio.

IV. CLINICOMETABOLIC CORRELATIONS

Few studies of the correlations between metabolic and clinical data in PSP have appeared in the literature. D'Antona et al.[32] found no clear-cut correlation between frontal signs and relative frontal hypometabolism, but a trend was apparent when absolute frontal CMRGlu values were considered. Leenders et al.[34] reported a good correlation between the duration of the disease and the upper frontal cortex $CMRO_2$. Foster et al.[67] observed a tendency for average cortical CMRGlu to negatively correlate to WAIS full-scale IQ.

In our study of 35 patients, we have attempted to correlate PET data with the following clinical parameters:

Disease duration (Figure 4)—Despite the nonlongitudinal nature of the study, we found significant correlations. Energy metabolism decreased linearly with disease duration in both frontal ($r = -0.352$, $p < 0.05$) and nonfrontal cortex ($r = -0.336$, $p < 0.05$). Cortical metabolic depression was present at the time of diagnosis and progressed over the years; the frontal cortex metabolism was consistently below that of the posterior cortex at all stages of the disease so that the frontal cortex/nonfrontal cortex ratio values showed no significant time-related decline ($r = -0.191$, NS). The lenticular nucleus/nonfrontal cortex ratio was above normal initially and remained so throughout the duration of the disease ($r = -0.093$, NS). These findings suggest that the hypofrontal pattern is already present in the initial stages of the disease and that it may constitute an early marker of PSP. In addition, the typical pattern of brain metabolism in PSP remains stable as the disease evolves.

Frontal score—The "frontal score" was obtained in each patient by summation of four quantitative neuropsychological tests (a simplified version of the Wisconsin card-sorting test, a test of verbal fluency, a graphic series, and a frontal behavior score) known to be sensitive to frontal lobe dysfunction.[31] In group I (definite PSP) ($n = 17$), there was a positive linear correlation between this score and the CMRGlu of the frontal cortex, posterior cortex and subcortical structures. These data suggest that in addition to a causal relationship between frontal score and frontal metabolism, there are incidental correlations related to the diffuse brain hypometabolism found in PSP. Cortical hypometabolism and clinical symptoms are both dependent on the duration of the disease. Conversely, neuropsychological "nonfrontal" items are not entirely preserved, particularly in the late stages of the disease.

Parkinsonian basal score (Figure 5)—The parkinsonian basal score evaluated the parkinsonian disability while off levodopa[68] using the modified Columbia rating scale.[69] In

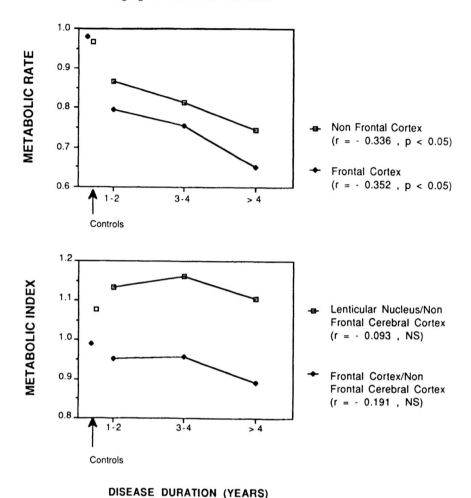

FIGURE 4.   Regional metabolic PET data as a function of disease duration in 35 PSP patients. The data were averaged by duration intervals 1 to 2 years, 3 to 4 years, and more than 4 years to facilitate the representation of the results, but linear correlations on all 35 data were performed for statistical assessment. On the top graph are shown the metabolic rates in the frontal cortex and the nonfrontal cortex for both the patients (lines) and the corresponding values in 15 controls matched for age (arrow); the values are expressed relative to slightly younger controls (53 years, mean age, N = 27). There was a linear decline in metabolic rates of both cortical areas, statistically significant for each, and of similar slope, but the frontal cortex value was already lower than the nonfrontal value in the initial stages of the disease, as compared to controls. The lower graph shows the metabolic index (region metabolic rate/nonfrontal cortex value) for the frontal cortex and the lenticular nucleus; the corresponding values in 15 age-matched controls are also shown for comparison. The frontal index is depressed initially and remains stable for the whole duration (no significant correlation), while the lenticular index remains elevated and similarly stable (NS).

group I patients (n = 15), this score was linearly correlated with basal ganglia CMRGlu as well as with other subcortical structures and the various cortical regions.

V. INVESTIGATIONS OF THE NIGROSTRIATAL DOPAMINERGIC PATHWAY

Only two studies of dopaminergic pathways have appeared in the literature. Leenders et al.[34] investigated the striatal uptake and kinetics of 6-[^{18}F]fluoro-L-dopa (6-FD), a marker

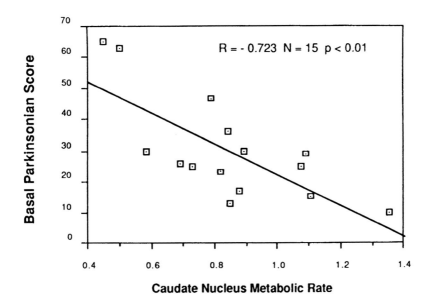

FIGURE 5. Relationship between the basal parkinsonian score (see text) and the caudate nucleus metabolic rate (expressed relative to control values), measured in the same patients (N = 15 definite PSP). The parkinsonian score is such that the higher values indicate severe parkinsonism. There was a significant negative linear correlation.

of the presynaptic dopamine metabolism, while Baron et al.[70,71] studied the dopaminergic D_2 receptors in the striatum using [^{76}Br]bromospiperone (BSP).

Leenders et al.[34] reported a significant decrease in striatal 6-FD accumulation between the second and third hours after tracer injection, similar to that observed in PD. The average striatum/surrounding brain ratio was significantly lower in the five PSP patients compared to five slightly younger controls (1.59 ± 0.17 and 1.83 ± 0.11, mean $\pm$ SD, respectively, $p = 0.025$). This reduced capacity of the nigrostriatal dopaminergic nerve terminals to form and store [^{18}F]fluorodopamine in PSP is concordant with post-mortem analyses which have shown a decrease of dopamine and homovanillic acid in the striatum.[25,26] Leenders et al. also reported that this decrease was correlated with both the frontal cortex $CMRO_2$ and the frontal/occipital CBF ratio but not with the clinical parkinsonism score.

Baron et al.[70,71] studied seven patients (mean age 66.4 ± 6 years; disease duration 1 to 10 years) with BSP to assess postsynaptic striatal D_2 receptors. Five of these patients did not respond to levodopa, while the response in the remaining two was minimal. Although there was no significant difference in either cerebellar or striatal uptake at 4.5 h post injection between patients and a group of seven age- and sex-matched controls, a highly significant decrease in the striatum/cerebellum (S/C) ratio was observed (1.32 ± 0.23 in patients and 1.74 ± 0.17 in controls, mean $\pm$ 1SD, $p < 0.02$) (Figure 6). The S/C ratio is a reliable measure of specific binding of BSP in the striatum if, as is the case with BSP, the amount of injected ligand is both negligible (i.e., a tracer dose) and consistent from subject to subject, and the measure is performed after essentially stable ligand concentrations are reached in striatum and cerebellum.[72] The lack of difference in cerebellar uptake at 4.5 hours indicated a similar nonspecific binding of BSP in patients and controls; in addition, no difference was observed in the early cerebellar uptake (5 to 20 min after injection), suggesting similar penetration of ligand in brain among patients and controls. Under these conditions, it was felt that the reduced S/C ratio in PSP indicated a loss of D_2 receptor density (or a diminished affinity), estimated at 60%. This compares well with the figure of 45% found post-mortem by Ruberg et al.[25]

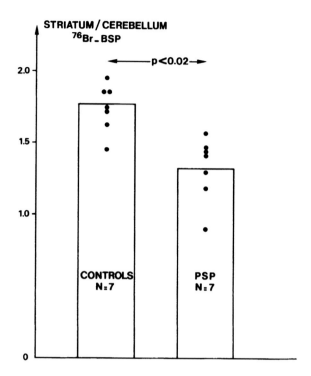

FIGURE 6.   Striatum/cerebellum radioactive concentration ratios obtained in seven PSP patients and seven age- and sex-matched control subjects; 4.5 to 5 h after intravenous injection of trace amounts of the dopamine D_2 receptor antagonist ^{76}Br-Bromospiperone. The significant decrease in this ratio in PSP reflects a loss of postsynaptic D_2 receptors in the striatum.

This loss of D_2 postsynaptic receptors in the striatum may explain the lack of response to levodopa and dopamine agonists in PSP and may also contribute to some of the extrapyramidal features. In the study of Baron et al.,[72] no correlations were attempted between the individual S/C ratios and the clinical data (e.g., disease duration, parkinsonism, response to levodopa) because of the limited patient sample. These investigations would be of obvious value to better understand the clinical significance of the loss of striatal D_2 receptors.

REFERENCES

1. **Richardson, J. C., Steele, J. C., and Olszewski, J.,** Supranuclear ophthalmoplegia, pseudobulbar palsy, nuchal dystonia and dementia: a clinical report on eight cases of "heterogenous system degeneration", *Trans. Am. Neurol. Assoc.,* 88, 25, 1963.
2. **Steels, J. C., Richardson, J. C., and Olszewski, J.,** Progressive supranuclear palsy, *Arch. Neurol.,* 10, 333, 1964.
3. **Steele, J. C.,** Progressive supranuclear palsy, *Brain,* 95, 693, 1972.
4. **Steele, J. C.,** Progressive supranuclear palsy, in *Handbook of Clinical Neurology,* Vol. 22, Vinken, P. J., Bruyn, G. W., and Klawans, H. L., Eds., Elsevier, Amsterdam, 1975, 217.
5. **Brusa, A., Mancardi, G. L., and Bugiani, O.,** Progressive supranuclear palsy: an overview, *Ital. J. Neuro. Sci.,* 4, 205, 1980.
6. **Jellinger, K., Riederer, P., and Tomonaga, M.,** Progressive supranuclear palsy: clinico-pathological and biochemical studies, *J. Neural Transm.,* (Suppl.), 16, 111, 1980.

7. **Dubas, F., Gray, F., and Escourolle, R.,** Maladie de Steele-Richardson-Olszewski sans ophtalmoplegie, *Rev. Neurol.,* 139, 407, 1983.
8. **Davis, P. H., Bergeron, C., and McLachlan, D. R.,** Atypical presentation of progressive supranuclear palsy, *Ann. Neurol.,* 17, 337, 1985.
9. **Gross, R. A., Spehlmann, R., and Daniels, J. C.,** Sleep disturbances in progressive supranuclear palsy, *Electroencephalogr. Clin. Neurophysiol.,* 45, 16, 1978.
10. **Leygonie, F., Thomas, J., Degos, J. D., Bouchareine, A., and Barbizet, J.,** Troubles du sommeil dans la maladie de Steele-Richardson. Etude polygraphique de 3 cas, *Rev. Neurol.,* 132, 125, 1976.
11. **Mouret, J.,** Differences in sleep in patients with Parkinson's disease, *Electroencephalogr. Clin. Neurophysiol.,* 38, 653, 1975.
12. **Morariu, M. A.,** Progressive supranuclear palsy and normal pressure hydrocephalus, *Neurology,* 29, 1544, 1979.
13. **Ambrosetto, P., Michelucci, R., Forti, A., and Tassinari, C. A.,** CT findings in progressive supranuclear palsy, *J Comput. Assist. Tomogr.,* 8, 406, 1984.
14. **Polsby, M., Patronas, N. J., Dwyer, A., Weinberger, D., Chase, T. N., and Di Chiro, G.,** Progressive supranuclear palsy and magnetic resonance imaging, *Neurology,* 35(Suppl. 1), 136, 1985.
15. **Kristensen, M. O.,** progressive supranuclear palsy — 20 years later, *Acta Neurol. Scand.,* 71, 177, 1985.
16. **Maher, E. R. and Lees, A. J.,** The clinical features and natural history of the Steele-Richardson-Olszewski syndrome (progressive supranuclear palsy), *Neurology,* 36, 1005, 1986.
17. **Golbe, L. I., Davis, P. H., Schoenberg, B. S., and Duvoisin, R. C.,** Prevalence and natural history of progressive supranuclear palsy, *Neurology,* 37(Suppl. 1), PP326, 1987.
18. **Duvoisin, R. C., Golbe, L. I., and Lepore, F. E.** Progressive supranuclear palsy, *Can. J. Neurol. Sci.,* 14, 547, 1987.
19. **Hirsch, E. C., Graybiel, A. M., Duyckaerts, C., and Javoy-Agid, F.,** Neuronal loss in the pedunculopontine tegmental nucleus in Parkinson disease and in progressive supranuclear palsy, *Proc. Natl. Acad. Sci. U.S.A.,* 84, 5976, 1987.
20. **Agid, Y., Javoy-Agid, F., Ruberg, M., Pillon, B., Dubois, B., Duyckaerts, C., Hauw, J.-J., Baron, J. C., and Scatton, B.,** Progressive supranuclear palsy: anatomoclinical and biochemical considerations, *Adv. Neurol.,* 45, 191, 1986.
21. **Klawans, H. L. and Ringel, S. P.,** Observations on the efficacy of L-dopa in progressive supranuclear palsy, *Eur. Neurol.,* 5, 115, 1971.
22. **Jackson, J. A., Jankovic, J., and Ford, J.,** Progressive supranuclear palsy: clinical features and response to treatment in 16 patients, *Ann. Neurol.,* 13, 273, 1983.
23. **Hornykiewicz, O.,** Biochemical abnormalities in some extrastriatal neuronal systems in Parkinson's disease, in *Parkinson's Disease — Current Progress. Problems and Management,* Rinne, U.K., Klinger, M., and Stamm, G., Eds., Elsevier, Amsterdam, 1980, 109.
24. **Bokobza, B., Ruberg, M., Scatton, B., Javoy-Agid, F., and Agid, Y.,** [³H]spiperone binding, dopamine and HVA concentrations in Parkinson's disease and supranuclear palsy, *Eur. J. Pharmacol.,* 99, 167, 1984.
25. **Ruberg, M., Javoy-Agid, F., Hirsch, E., Scatton, B., Lheureux, R., Hauw, J.-J., Duyckaerts, C., Gray, F., Morel-Maroger, A., Rascol, A., Serdaru, M., and Agid, Y.,** Dopaminergic and cholinergic lesions in progressive supranuclear palsy, *Ann. Neurol.,* 18, 523, 1985.
26. **Kish, S. J., Chang, L. J., Mirchandani, L., Shannak, K., and Hornykiewicz, O.,** Progressive supranuclear palsy: relationship between extrapyramidal disturbances, dementia, and brain neurotransmitter markers, *Ann. Neurol.,* 18, 530, 1985.
27. **Albert, M. L., Feldman, R. G., and Willis, A. L.,** The 'subcortical dementia' of progressive supranuclear palsy, *J. Neurol. Neurosurg. Psychiatry.,* 37, 121, 1974.
28. **Cambier, J., Masson, M., Viader, F., Limodin, J., and Strube, A.,** Le syndrome frontal de la paralysie supranucleaire progressive, *Rev. Neurol.,* 141, 528, 1985.
29. **Maher, E., Smith, E. M., and Lees, A. J.,** Cognitive deficits in the Steele-Richardson-Olszewski syndrome (progressive supranuclear palsy), *J. Neurol. Neurosurg. Psychiatry,* 48, 1234, 1985.
30. **Janati, A. and Appel, A. R.,** Psychiatric aspects of progressive supranuclear palsy, *J. Nerv. Ment. Dis.,* 172, 85, 1984.
31. **Pillon, B., Dubois, B., Lhermitte, F., and Agid, Y.,** Heterogeneity of cognitive impairment in progressive supranuclear palsy, Parkinson's disease, and Alzheimer's disease, *Neurology,* 36, 1179, 1986.
32. **D'Antona, R., Baron, J. C., Samson, Y., Serdaru, M., Viader, F., Agid, Y., and Cambier, J.,** Subcortical dementia. Frontal cortex hypometabolism detected by positron tomography in patients with progressive supranuclear palsy, *Brain,* 108, 785, 1985.
33. **Foster, N. L., Gilman, S., Berent, S., Brown, M. B., and Hichwa, R. D.,** Glucose hypometabolism in progressive supranuclear palsy is not limited to frontal cortex, *Ann. Neurol.,* 22, 123, 1987.
34. **Leenders, K. L., Frakowiak, R. S. J., and Lees, A. J.,** Steele-Richardson-Olszewski syndrome: brain energy metabolism, blood flow and fluorodopa uptake measured by positron emission tomography, *Brain,* 111, 615, 1988.

35. **Rougemont, D., Baron, J. C., Collard, P., Bustany, P., Comar, D., and Agid, Y.,** Local cerebral glucose utilization in treated and untreated patients with Parkinson's disease, *J. Neurol. Neurosurg. Psychiatry,* 47, 824, 1984.

36. **Wolfson, L. I., Leenders, K. L., Brown, L. L., and Jones, T.,** Alterations of regional cerebral blood flow and oxygen metabolism in Parkinson's disease, *Neurology,* 35, 1399, 1985.

37. **Kuhl, D. E., Metter, E. J., and Riege, W. H.,** Patterns of local cerebral glucose utilization determined in Parkinson's disease by the [^{18}F]Fluorodeoxyglucose method, *Ann. Neurol.,* 15, 419, 1984.

38. **Kuhl, D. E., Metter, E. J., Riege, W. H., and Markham, C. H.,** Patterns of cerebral glucose utilization in Parkinson's disease and Huntington's disease, *Ann. Neurol.,* 15(Suppl.), S119, 1984.

39. **Leenders, K. L., Wolfson, L., Gibbs, J. M., Wise, R. J. S., Causon, R., Jones, T., and Legg, N. J.,** The effects of L-dopa on regional cerebral blood flow and oxygen metabolism in patients with Parkinson's disease, *Brain,* 108, 171, 1985.

40. **Kuhl, D. E., Metter, E. J., Benson, D. F., Ashford, J. W., Riege, W. H., Fujikawa, D. G., Markham, C. H., Mazziotta, J. C., Maltese, A., and Dorsey, D. A.,** Similarities of cerebral glucose metabolism in Alzheimer's and Parkinsonian dementia, *J. Cereb. Blood Flow Metab.,* 5(Suppl. 1), S169, 1985.

41. **Gilman, S., Markel, D. S., Koeppe, R. A., Junck, L., Gebarski, S. S., and Hichwa, R.,** A comparison of computed tomographic and positron emission tomographic findings in Olivopontocerebellar atrophy, *Ann. Neurol.,* 20, 121, 1986.

42. **Hawkins, R. A., Mazziota, J. C., and Phelps, M. E.,** Wilson's disease studied with FDG and positron emission tomography, *Neurology,* 37, 1707, 1987.

43. **Hayden, M. R., Martin, W. R. W., Stoessl, A. J., Clark, C., Holloenberg, S., Adam, M. J., Ammann, W., Harrop, R., Rogers, J., Ruth, T., Sayre, C., and Pate B. D.,** Positron emission tomography in the early diagnosis of Huntington's disease, *Neurology,* 36, 888, 1986.

44. **Kuhl, D. E., Phelps, M. E., Markham, C. H., Metter, E. J., Riege, W. H., and Winter, J.,** Cerebral metabolism and atrophy in Huntington's disease determined by 18FDG and computed tomographic scan, *Ann. Neurol.,* 12, 425, 1982.

45. **Young, A. B., Penney, J. B., Starosta-Rubinstein, S., Markel, D. S., Berent, S., Giordani, B., Ehrenkaufer, R., Jewett, D., and Hichwa, R.,** PET scan investigations of Huntington's disease: cerebral metabolic correlates of neurological features and functional decline, *Ann. Neurol.,* 20, 296, 1986.

46. **Mazziotta, J. C., Phelps, M. E., Pahl, J. J., Huang, S.-C., Baxter, L. R., Riege, W. H., Hoffman, J. M., Kuhl, D. E., Lanto, A. B., Wapenski, J. A., and Markham, C. H.,** Reduced cerebral glucose metabolism in asymptomatic subjects at risk for Huntington's disease, *N. Engl. J. Med.,* 316, 357, 1987.

47. **Haxby, J. V., Duara, R., Grady, C. L., Cutler, N. R., and Rapoport, S. I.,** Relations between neuropsychological and cerebral metabolic asymmetries in early Alzheimer's disease, *J. Cereb. Blood Flow Metab.,* 5, 193, 1985.

48. **Duara, R., Grady, C., Haxby, J., Sundaram, M., Cutler, N. R., Heston, L., Moore, A., Schlageter, N., Larson, S., and Rapoport, S. I.,** Positron emission tomography in Alzheimer's disease, *Neurology,* 36, 879, 1986.

49. **Kamo, H., McGeer, P. L., Harrop, R., McGeer, E. G., Calne, D. B., Martin, W. R. W., and Pate, B. D.,** Positron emission tomography and histopathology in Pick's disease, *Neurology,* 37, 439, 1987.

50. **Chase, T. N., Foster, N. L., Fedio, P., Brooks, R., Mansi, L., and Di Chiro, G.,** Regional cortical dysfunction in Alzheimer's disease as determined by positron emission tomography, *Ann. Neurol.,* 15(Suppl.), S170, 1984.

51. **McGeer, E. G., Harrop, R., McGeer, P. L., Martin, W. R. W., Pate, B. D., and Li, D. K. B.,** Comparison of PET, MRI, and CT with pathology in a proven case of Alzheimer's disease, *Neurology,* 36, 1569, 1986.

52. **Horwitz, B., Grady, C. L., Schageter, N. L., Duara, R., and Rapoport, S. I.,** Intercorrelations of regional cerebral glucose metabolic rates in Alzheimer's diseases, *Brain Res.* 407, 294, 1987.

53. **Cutler, N. R., Haxby, J. V., Duara, R., Grady, C. L., Kay, A. D., Kessler, R. M., Sundaram, M., and Rapoport, S. I.,** Clinical history, brain metabolism, and neuropsychological function in Alzheimer's disease, *Ann. Neurol.* 18, 298, 1985.

54. **Frakowiack, R. S. J., Pozzilli, C., Legg, N. J., Du Boulay, G. H., Marshall, J., Lenzi, G. L., and Jones, T.,** Regional cerebral oxygen supply and utilization in dementia. A clinical and physiological study with oxygen-15 and positron tomography, *Brain,* 104, 753, 1981.

55. **Benson, D. F., Kuhl, D. E., Hawkins, R. A., Phelps, M. E., Cummings, J. L., and Tsai, S. Y.,** The fluorodeoxyglucose 18F scan in Alzheimer's disease and multi-infarct dementia, *Arch. Neurol.* 40, 711, 1983.

56. **Metter, E. J., Riege, W. H., Benson, D. F., Phelps, M. E., and Kuhl, D. E.,** Variability of regional cerebral glucose metabolism in Alzheimer's disease patients as compared to normal subjects, *J. Cereb. Blood Flow Metab.* 5 (Suppl. 1), S127, 1985.

57. **Brun, A.,** Frontal lobe degeneration of non-Alzheimer type I. Neuropathology, *Arch. Gerontol. Geriatr.* 6, 193, 1987.

58. **Chase, T. N., Burrows, H., and Mohr, E.**, Cortical glucose utilization patterns in primary degenerative dementias of the anterior and posterior type, *Arch. Gerontol. Geriatr.* 6, 289, 1987.
59. **Ishino, H., Ikeda, H., and Otsuki, S.**, Contribution to clinical pathology of progressive supranuclear palsy (Subcortical argyrophilic dystrophy). On the distribution of neurofibrillary tangles in the basal ganglia and brain-stem and its clinical significance, *J. Neurol. Sci.* 24, 471, 1975.
60. **Baron, J. C., D'Antona, R., Pantano, P., Serdaru, M., Samson, Y., and Bousser, M. G.**, Effects of thalamic stroke on energy metabolism of the cerebral cortex, *Brain,* 109, 1243, 1986.
61. **Cudennec, A., Duverger, D., Nishikata, T., McReeDegueurce, A., MacKenzie, E. T., and Scatton, B.**, Influence of ascending serotoninergic pathways on integrated functional activity in the conscious rat brain. I. Effects of electrolytic or neurotoxic lesions of the dorsal and/or median raphe nucleus, *Brain Res.,* 444, 214, 1988.
62. **Kiyosawa, M., Baron, J. C., Hamel, E., Pappata, S., Duverger, D., Riche, D., Mazoyer, B., Naquet, B., and MacKenzie, E. T.**, Time-course of effects of unilateral lesions of the nucleus basalis of Meynert on glucose utilization of the cerebral cortex: positron tomography in baboons, *Brain,* 112, 435, 1989.
63. **Kiyosawa, M., Pappata, S., Duverger, D., Riche, D., Cambon, H., Mazoyer, B., Samson, Y., Crouzel, C., Naquet, R., MacKenzie, E., and Baron, J.-C.**, Cortical hypometabolism and its recovery following nucleus basalis lesions in baboons: a PET study, *J. Cereb. Blood Flow Metab.* 7, 812, 1987.
64. **Bès, A., Güell, A., Fabre, N., Dupui, P., Victor, G., and Géraud, G.**, Cerebral blood flow studies by Xenon-133 inhalation technique in Parkinsonism: loss of hyperfrontal pattern, *J. Cereb. Blood Flow Metab.,* 3, 33, 1983.
65. **Laplane, D., Baulac, M., Wildlöcher, D., and Dubois, B.**, Pura psychic akinesia with bilateral lesions of basal ganglia, *J. Neurol. Neurosurg. Psychiatry,* 47, 377, 1984.
66. **Laplane, D., Levasseur, M., Pillon, B., Dubois, B., Baulac, M., Mazoyer, B., Tran Dinh, S., Sette, G., Dánze, F., and Baron, J. C.**, Obsession-compulsions and other behavioral changes with bilateral basal ganglia lesions: a neuropsychological, magnetic resonance imaging, and positron emission tomography, *Brain,* 112, 699, 1989.
67. **Foster, N. L., Gilman, S., Berent, S., and Hichwa, R. D.**, Distinctive patterns of cerebral cortical glucose metabolism in progressive supranuclear palsy and Alzheimer's disease studied with positron emission tomography, *Neurology,* 36 (Suppl. 1), 338, 1986.
68. **Esteguy, M., Bonnet, A. M., Lhermitte, F., and Agid, Y.**, "Le test à la L-dopa" dans la maladie de Parkinson, *Rev. Neurol.* 141, 413, 1985.
69. **Lhermitte, F., Agid, Y., and Signoret, J.-L.**, Onset and end-of-dose levodopa induced dyskinesias, *Arch. Neurol.* 35, 621, 1978
70. **Baron, J. C., Mazière, B., Loc'h, C., Sgouropoulos, P., Bonnet, A. M., and Agid, Y.**, Progressive supranuclear palsy: loss of striatal dopamine receptors demonstrated in vivo by positron tomography, *Lancet,* 1, 1163, 1985.
71. **Baron, J. C., Mazière, B., Loc'h, C., Sgouropoulos, P., Bonnet, A. M., and Agid Y.**, Loss of striatal [76Br]Bromospiperone binding sites demonstrated by positron tomography in progressive supranuclear palsy, *J. Cereb. Blood Flow Metab.,* 6, 131, 1986.
72. **Mazière, B., Loc'h, C., Baron, J.-C., Sgouropoulos, P., Duquesnoy, N., D'Antona, R., and Cambon, H.**, In vivo quantitative imaging of dopamine receptors in human brain using positron emission tomography and (76Br)Bromospiperone, *Eur. J. Pharmacol.,* 114, 267, 1985.

Chapter 9

OLIVOPONTOCEREBELLAR ATROPHY

Sid Gilman

TABLE OF CONTENTS

I. INTRODUCTION

Olivopontocerebellar atrophy (OPCA) is a chronic progressive neurological disease characterized pathologically by degeneration of neurons in the inferior olives, pons, and cerebellum.[1-4] Degeneration can occur also in other sites within the central nervous system, and in some cases, OPCA is associated with multisystem degeneration.[5,6] The disease occurs both sporadically and with hereditary transmission.[3,4,6] When hereditary, the disease is usually expressed as an autosomal dominant trait, but at times as an autosomal recessive trait.[4] A locus on chromosome 6 has been identified in dominantly inherited OPCA.[7]

A. CLINICAL CHARACTERISTICS

The age of onset of OPCA varies widely, but most patients become symptomatic in middle age. The presenting complaints are usually related to ataxia of gait and disorders of speech. Difficulty with coordination of the upper extremities commonly occurs soon afterwards. The disease often progresses to the point that the patient is wheelchair bound. Neurological examination of symptomatic patients usually reveals ocular dysmetria, ataxic speech, and ataxia of limb movements and gait. Many patients show involvement of corticobulbar and corticospinal systems with spasticity of speech, spasticity of the limbs, hyperactive deep tendon reflexes, and extensor plantar responses in addition to their signs of ataxia. Dementia has been reported, but the frequency of dementia in OPCA is unclear. In Berciano's[6] review of the literature, dementia was found in 22% of familial cases and 11% of sporadic cases. Higher rates of occurrence have been recorded, with values as high as 40% in one series,[4] and some authors claim that chronic progressive dementia may be a uniform part of OPCA.[8]

B. NEUROPATHOLOGICAL CHANGES

At autopsy, typical cases of OPCA show gross shrinkage of the ventral part of the pons, the inferior olives, the middle cerebellar peduncles, and the cerebellar cortex.[9,10] Both light and electron microscopy reveal shrinkage and loss of neurons in the pons and inferior olives with corresponding loss of pontocerebellar (mossy) fibers and olivocerebellar (climbing) fibers, respectively.[11,12] Purkinje cells are severely reduced but not completely lost, and granule cells are reduced. Golgi cells are probably unaffected and basket cells are relatively preserved. Dentate neurons also are preserved. The distribution and severity of the neuropathological changes in OPCA vary considerably between cases. In many patients, the long tracts of the spinal cord are affected. There may also be degeneration of neurons in the striatum and substantia nigra. In cases involving multisystem degeneration, there may be extensive involvement of the central nervous system. Recently, neuronal loss in the basal nucleus of Meynert was described in a patient with hereditary OPCA and mental deterioration.[13]

C. NEUROCHEMICAL CHANGES

Studies of post-mortem brain tissue in OPCA have revealed abnormalities of neurotransmitter levels and of neurotransmitter receptor densities.[14-19] Perry and colleagues have detected several different biochemical profiles in dominantly inherited OPCA from studies of amino acid levels in post-mortem brain tissues.[20,21] One set of cases is characterized by decreased glutamate, aspartate, and GABA levels in the cerebellar cortex and by decreased GABA levels in the dentate nucleus. Taurine content is increased in the cerebellar cortex. In a second group, there are decreased levels of glutamate, aspartate, and GABA in the cerebellar cortex and decreased levels of GABA in the dentate nucleus. Taurine levels in the cerebellar cortex are within normal limits. In a third group, the levels of glutamate, aspartate, and GABA are within normal limits in the cerebellar cortex, but the GABA content of the dentate nucleus is reduced. In a fourth group, glutamate, aspartate, and GABA levels are decreased in the cerebellar cortex, and GABA levels are decreased in the dentate nucleus. Unlike the other disorders, however, glutamate is decreased in other brain regions, notably the cerebral cortex and striatum.

The groups described above may not represent distinctive biochemical subtypes of OPCA, but only differences in the degree of degeneration of particular types of neurons among different cases of OPCA. Evidence supporting this comes from correlative studies of neurotransmitters and neuronal cell densities in OPCA. Kanazawa et al.[14] found that the concentrations of glutamate and aspartate in the cerebellar cortex varied markedly from case to case. Glutamate concentrations in the anterior vermis were correlated with the density of granule cells there, and aspartate concentrations in the anterior vermis were correlated with the density of neurons in the inferior olives. GABA concentrations in the dentate nucleus were decreased in all cases of OPCA and were correlated with the degree of loss of Purkinje cells.

Only a few studies of neurotransmitter receptor binding in OPCA have been reported.[17-19] Using [³H]GABA as a ligand, Kish et al.[17] found a marked increase of GABA neurotransmitter receptor binding in the cerebellar cortex at post-mortem of patients with a dominantly inherited form of OPCA. A marked decrease of dentate nucleus GABA levels was found, suggesting a considerable loss of Purkinje cells. Receptor binding in the deep cerebellar nuclei was not examined. In a later study using methyl [³H]flunitrazepam as a ligand, Kish et al.[18] found that benzodiazepine receptor binding was either normal or slightly elevated in the cerebellar cortex. Binding in the deep cerebellar nuclei was not studied. Whitehouse et al.[19] using [³H]flunitrazepam in an autoradiographic study, found that benzodiazepine receptor binding was unchanged in the cerebellar cortex, but increased in the dentate nucleus.

Other neurochemical abnormalities have been found in post-mortem tissues of OPCA patients, including a reduction of noradrenaline levels in the cerebellar cortex;[22] decreased levels of choline acetyltransferase in the cerebral cortex and hippocampus;[23] and changes in the concentrations of immunoreactive thyrotropin releasing hormone in the cerebellar cortex, dentate nuclei, and olivary nuclei.[24]

D. GLUTAMATE DEHYDROGENASE DEFICIENCY

A deficiency in the specific activity of the enzyme glutamate dehydrogenase (GDH) in fibroblasts and leukocytes has been reported in autosomal recessive and autosomal dominant forms of OPCA,[25-31] but abnormality of GDH activity has not been found in post-mortem tissue.[32]

E. THE DIAGNOSIS OF OPCA

There is no specific diagnostic laboratory test for OPCA; the diagnosis depends upon the exclusion of other disorders that may cuase a progressive ataxia in middle life. These disorders include demyelinative disease, neoplasms, paraneoplastic processes, vascular diseases, toxic/metabolic disorders, infectious diseases, malformations, and other degenerative diseases. A positive family history, of course, is helpful in the diagnosis of OPCA. The demonstration of brainstem and cerebellar atrophy through anatomical imaging with CT or MR is helpful, but a sizeable number of patients with OPCA show no evidence of atrophy, especially early in the course. CSF protein may be slightly elevated and the EEG may show an excessive amount of slow activity.[32] Auditory evoked potentials are abnormal in some patients,[33] and impaired sensory nerve conduction has been reported.[34,35]

II. CEREBRAL GLUCOSE METABOLISM IN OPCA

Positron emission tomography (PET) with ¹⁸F-2-fluoro-2-deoxy-D-glucose (FDG) has

TABLE 1
Average Ages of the Subjects Studied[a]

	Control Subjects		Patients with OPCA[b]	
	n	Age	n	Age
Male	18	52 ($\pm$ 16)	18	55 ($\pm$ 13)
Female	17	50 ($\pm$ 10)	22	53 ($\pm$ 14)
All subjects	35	51 ($\pm$ 13)	40	54 ($\pm$ 13)

[a]   Values given are the mean $\pm$ SD.
[b]   OPCA = olivopontocerebellar atrophy.

TABLE 2
Local Cerebral Metabolic Rates for Glucose (in mg/100 g/ min) in all Subjects[a]

Structure	Control subjects[b]	Patients with OPCA[c]
Cerebellar vermis	5.35 $\pm$ 1.05	3.77 $\pm$ 0.99[d]
Left cerebellar hemisphere	5.96 $\pm$ 1.27	4.20 $\pm$ 1.15[e]
Right cerebellar hemisphere	5.84 $\pm$ 1.24	4.21 $\pm$ 1.11[e]
Brainstem	4.36 $\pm$ 0.81	3.42 $\pm$ 0.79[e]
Thalamus	6.93 $\pm$ 1.14	6.56 $\pm$ 1.34
Cerebral cortex	5.73 $\pm$ 0.98	5.64 $\pm$ 1.08

[a]   Values given are the mean $\pm$ SD.
[b]   n = 35.
[c]   n = 40; OPCA = olivopontocerebellar atrophy.
[d] $p < 0.05$.
[e] $p < 0.0005$.

been used to study the pattern of metabolic activity in patients with OPCA. These studies were undertaken to determine whether PET might prove to be a helpful diagnostic test for adult onset cerebellar degeneration. Thus far, 40 patients with OPCA and 35 age- and sex-matched normal controls have been studied (Tables 1 and 2), and the results from 30 of these patients and 30 of the normal controls have been published.[36-38] The normal controls had no history of neurological disease and no significant abnormalities on neurological or general physical examination. The subjects were taking no medications known to affect central nervous system function or to cause CNS side effects. The diagnosis of OPCA was made on the basis of the history, physical examination, neurological examination, laboratory tests to exclude other diseases, and the findings on CT scans. None of the patients had a history of chronic alcoholism or of exposure to medications such as phenytoin that might cause cerebellar ataxia. None of the patients had disorders of sensory function adequate to cause ataxia of movement.

The studies were performed in the University of Michigan Cyclotron/P.E.T. Facility with the subjects lying supine, awake, and blindfolded in a quiet room. Scans were performed 30 to 75 min after injection of 5 to 10 mCi of FDG. PET scans were performed with a TCC PCT4600A tomograph having an in-plane resolution of 11 mm FWHM and a z-axis resolution of 9.5mm FWHM. Five planes with 11.5 mm center-to-center separation were imaged simultaneously. Four sets of scans were taken per patient, including two interleaved sets through lower brain levels and two interleaved sets through higher brain levels for a total of 20 slices, each separated by 5.75 mm.

Blood samples were collected from the radial artery. Local cerebral metabolic rate for glucose (LCMRG) was calculated using a three-compartment model and single scan ap-

TABLE 3
Local Cerebral Metabolic Rates for Glucose Normalized to the Cerebral Cortex in all Subjects[a]

Structure	Control subjects[b]	Patients with OPCA[c]
Cerebellar vermis	0.93 ± 0.08	0.67 ± 0.15[d]
Left cerebellar hemisphere	1.04 ± 0.11	0.75 ± 0.16[d]
Right cerebellar hemisphere	1.02 ± 0.11	0.75 ± 0.16[d]
Brainstem	0.76 ± 0.05	0.61 ± 0.10[d]
Thalamus	1.22 ± 0.10	1.17 ± 0.10[e]

[a] Values given are the mean ± SD.
[b] n = 35.
[c] n = 40; OPCA = olivonpontocerebellar atrophy.
[d] $p < 0.0005$.
[e] $p < 0.05$.

proximation described by Phelps et al.[39] with gray matter kinetic constants derived from normals.[40] Regions of interest (ROIs) were studied in the cerebellar hemispheres, vermis, brainstem, thalamus, and cerebral cortex. Data were collected from the ROIs by placing a 22×11 mm parallelogram over each cerebellar hemisphere, an 11×18 mm rectangle over the vermis, an 11×15 mm rectangle over the brainstem, and an 11×11 mm square over each thalamus. Each ROI was centered over a local peak in LCMRG. Data were obtained from two slices containing the cerebellum and brainstem and from one slice containing the thalamus. Data from the cerebral cortex were obtained by measuring LCMRG in the cortical ribbon from five consecutive slices beginning with the lowest slice containing the basal ganglia.

The scans of patients with OPCA revealed a marked decrease of LCMRG in the cerebellar hemispheres, vermis, and brainstem (Plate 4*), with no obvious abnormality in other parts of the brain. Statistical testing of the data revealed significant differences in LCMRG between OPCA patients and controls in the cerebellar hemispheres, cerebellar vermis, and brainstem (Table 2). No significant difference in LCMRG was found between controls and OPCA patients in the thalamus or cerebral cortex. With the data normalized to the cerebral cortex, LCMRG again was significantly decreased in OPCA patients compared to controls in the cerebellar hemispheres, cerebellar vermis, and brainstem, and differences in LCMRG between groups in the thalamus reached significance (Table 3). Both males and females with OPCA showed significant differences from sex-matched controls (Tables 4 and 5).

LCMRG normalized to the cerebral cortex was plotted for each of the structures studied in 30 OPCA patients and in 30 normal controls (Figure 1). This revealed that LCMRG in the OPCA patients is below two standard deviations from the normal controls in 19 of 30 cases for the brainstem, 21 for the vermis, and 17 (right) to 19 (left) for the cerebellar hemispheres. At least one cerebellar or brainstem region had LCMRG values decreased below two standard deviations from the means of the controls in 24 of 30 patients. Accordingly, 80% of OPCA patients had at least one markedly hypometabolic region detected with PET. In only two control subjects were one or more regions below two standard deviations from the mean of the normal group, demonstrating a false positive rate of 6.7%.

LCMRG was examined in patients with sporadic as compared with familial OPCA (Tables 6 and 7). Mean LCMRG was consistently lower in the sporadic than the familial cases, a difference that reached statistical significance for the cerebellar hemispheres and vermis, but not the brainstem. The differences between sporadic and familial cases probably reflects differences in the stages of the disease between groups. The familial cases had a

* Plate 4 appears after page 168.

TABLE 4
Local Cerebral Metabolic Rates for Glucose (in mg/100 g/min) in Males[a]

Structure	Control subjects[b]	Patients with OPCA[b]
Cerebellar vermis	5.22 ± 1.02	3.58 ± 1.05[c]
Left cerebellar hemisphere	5.80 ± 1.15	3.96 ± 1.14[c]
Right cerebellar hemisphere	5.67 ± 1.15	3.93 ± 1.11[c]
Brainstem	4.27 ± 0.70	3.34 ± 0.78[c]
Thalamus	6.81 ± 1.01	6.47 ± 1.38
Cerebral cortex	5.67 ± 0.86	5.53 ± 1.03

[a] Values given are the mean ± SD.
[b] n = 18; OPCA = olivopontocerebellar atrophy.
[c] $p < 0.001$.

TABLE 5
Local Cerebral Metabolic Rates for Glucose (in mg/100 g/min) in Females[a]

Structure	Control subjects[b]	Patients with OPCA[c]
Cerebellar vermis	5.49 ± 1.10	3.94 ± 0.92[d]
Left cerebellar hemisphere	6.12 ± 1.40	4.40 ± 1.14[d]
Right cerebellar hemisphere	6.02 ± 1.34	4.44 ± 1.09[d]
Brainstem	4.47 ± 0.92	3.48 ± 0.81[d]
Thalamus	7.05 ± 1.29	6.64 ± 1.32
Cerebral cortex	5.78 ± 1.11	5.72 ± 1.15

[a] Values given are the mean ± SD.
[b] n = 17.
[c] n = 22; OPCA = olivopontocerebellar atrophy.
[d] $p < 0.001$.

younger average age (Table 6) and were less severely affected than the sporadic cases. The familial group included many cases that the investigators recruited into the study after evaluating an afflicted relative. Thus, many of these patients were evaluated earlier than the sporadic cases.

OPCA is known to be associated with atrophy of the cerebellum and brainstem, and this can influence measurement of tissue metabolic rates through partial volume averaging. In the present study, CT scans were performed on the OPCA patients and these showed variable degrees of atrophy within the cerebellum and brainstem (Figure 2). In some cases, the atrophy was within normal limits for the patient's age. In most, however, the cerebellum showed focal or generalized atrophy of the folia with enlargement of the sulci and the fourth ventricle. Often the brainstem was smaller than normal for the patient's age.

The degree of atrophy in the cerebellum and brainstem was quantitated by a neuroradiologist with rating scales (Table 8) and the resulting data were plotted against LCMRG.[36] Figure 3 shows LCMRG averaged between the two cerebellar hemispheres and normalized to the cerebral cortex plotted against the CT ratings for atrophy in the cerebellar hemispheres for 30 patients with OPCA. As shown in the illustration, there is a significant relationship between metabolic rate and CT measures of atrophy. The shaded region in the illustration indicates the range of two standard deviations of LCMRG in the normal controls. This shows that several patients with OPCA have marked hypometabolism but only minor degrees of atrophy and that some have normal metabolic rates despite moderate atrophy.

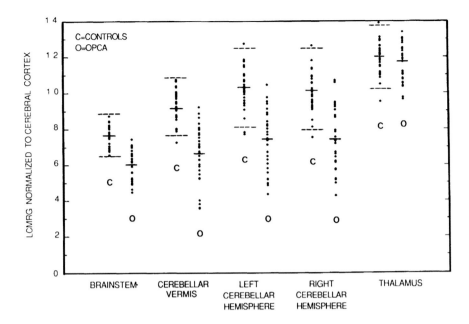

FIGURE 1. Graphs of local cerebral metabolic rate for glucose (LCMRG) normalized to the cerebral cortex in normal control subjects as compared to patients with olivopontocerebellar atrophy. Each point represents the average value for each case in the structure specified. The solid horizontal lines depict the mean value for each group and the broken horizontal lines indicate the limits of two standard deviations of the means for the normal volunteers. (From Gilman, S. et al., *Ann. Neurol.*, 213, 223, 1988. With permission.)

TABLE 6
Comparison of Patients with Sporadic and
Familial OPCAᵃ

	Sporadic	Familial
Age (years)	58 ± 11	49 ± 14
Males	11	7
Females	12	10
Duration of symptoms (years)	6 ± 5	7 ± 6
Age of onset of symptoms	50 ± 16	41 ± 15

ᵃ Values given are the mean ± SD; OPCA = olivopontocerebellar atrophy.

The metabolic rate of the cerebellum and brainstem has been correlated with the degree of impairment in clinical neurological function, including the speech, cranial, and somatic motor disorders.[37,38] Speech was evaluated by oral motor assessment and perceptual speech analysis. The severity of the ataxic and spastic dysarthric components of speech were assessed from video tape or audio tape samples of spontaneous speech, expository speech, oral reading, diadochokinetic rates, duration of sustaining vowels, and counting from 1 to 75. The deviant speech dimensions of Darley et al.[41] were used. A quantitative rating scale was developed extending from 0 (unaffected) to 3 (severely affected), and each deviant speech dimension was assigned a number.

To quantitate the ataxic and spastic components of speech separately, it was necessary to modify the Mayo Clinic rating system.[37] The modification was needed because the Mayo Clinic lists include many of the same deviant speech dimensions in both ataxic and spastic

TABLE 7

Local Cerebral Metabolic Rates for Glucose (in mg/100 g/min) in Sporadic and Familial OPCA[a]

Structure	Sporadic[b]	Familial[c]
Cerebellar vermis	3.43 ± 0.75	4.24 ± 1.09[d]
Left cerebellar hemisphere	3.81 ± 0.86	4.74 ± 1.29[d]
Right cerebellar hemisphere	3.87 ± 0.84	4.67 ± 1.29[d]
Brainstem	3.26 ± 0.64	3.64 ± 0.93
Thalamus	6.40 ± 1.31	6.78 ± 1.38
Cerebral cortex	5.35 ± 0.86	6.02 ± 1.25

[a] Values given are the mean ± SD; OPCA = olivopontocerebellar atrophy.
[b] n = 23.
[c] n = 17.
[d] $p < 0.05$.

dysarthria (Table 9). In addition, some of the deviant dimensions in these lists do not match our clinical experience with ataxic and spastic dysarthria. Accordingly, we reorganized the deviant dimensions and assigned weighting values to indicate the relative importance of the individual deviant dimensions (Table 10). We computed a total ataxic dysarthria rating and a separate spastic dysarthria rating for each patient by summing the ratings of the individual speech dimensions.

A significant inverse correlation was found between the degree of ataxia of speech and the absolute level of LCMRG within the cerebellar vermis, both cerebellar hemispheres (Figure 4), brainstem, and cerebral cortex, but not the thalamus (Table 11). A significant inverse correlation was also found between the degree of spasticity of speech and the absolute level of LCMRG within the cerebellar vermis, both cerebellar hemispheres, brainstem, and cerebral cortex, but not thalamus (Table 11). The metabolic data were normalized to the cerebral cortex and a significant inverse correlation still remained between the degree of ataxia of speech and LCMRG within the cerebellar vermis, cerebellar hemispheres, and brainstem, but not thalamus (Table 11). The normalized data revealed no significant correlation between the severity of spasticity in speech and LCMRG in any of the structures studied (Table 11).

The partial correlations method was used to determine the relationship of each speech characteristic, i.e., ataxic and spastic dysarthria, to LCMRG without the contribution of the other speech characteristic.[37] This method revealed that when the effects due to variations in spastic speech were accounted for, a significant inverse correlation remained between the degree of ataxia in speech and LCMRG normalized to the cerebral cortex (Table 12). In contrast, when the effects due to variations in ataxic speech were accounted for, no significant correlations were found between the degree of spasticity in speech and LCMRG in any of the structures studied.

We have also studied the relationship between the severity of cranial and somatic motor dysfunction and the metabolic rate of the cerebellum and brainstem. A rating scale was devised to quantitate the severity of the clinical motor disorders in OPCA (Table 13). The signs chosen for inclusion in the scale were selected because of their importance in the diagnosis of OPCA. The scale was based upon our clinical experience with this disorder and was devised prior to analysis of data from PET scans. We found a significant relationship between the overall severity of the clinical disturbance and the level of decline in LCMRG normalized to the cerebral cortex for the cerebellar vermis, left and right cerebellar hemispheres (Figure 5), and the brainstem of OPCA patients (Table 14). No correlation between clinical score and LCMRG was noted for the thalamus.

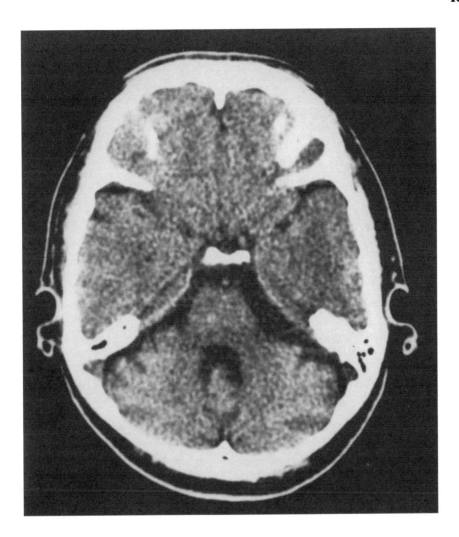

A

FIGURE 2.   CT scans of the three patients depicted in Figure 1. The image on the left (A) corresponds to the left-most PET image and shows mild atrophy in the cerebellum and brainstem. The middle image (B) corresponds to the middle PET image. A moderate degree of atrophy affects the posterior fossa structures. The image on the right (C) corresponds to the right-most PET scan. Severe atrophy is evident in the cerebellum and brainstem. Note that the right-most image is taken at a different angle than the other two, showing more of the vermal regions of the cerebellum and a more rostral level of the brainstem.

The severity of tissue atrophy in the posterior fossa assessed by CT was also evaluated with respect to clinical severity.[38] A statistically significant relationship was found for the cerebellar vermis and both cerebellar hemispheres, but not for the thalamus (Table 15). The correlations were slightly less strong than those noted between LCMRG and clinical score. The amount of tissue atrophy as determined by CT correlates significantly with the decline in LCMRG measured by PET in the cerebellum and brainstem (Table 16). Clinical score also correlates significantly with both PET and CT. Since all three measures correlate with each other, the partial correlations method was used to assess the relationship of PET and CT to clinical score independently of each other (Table 17). The method revealed that when the effects due to variations in LCMRG were accounted for, the degree of tissue atrophy

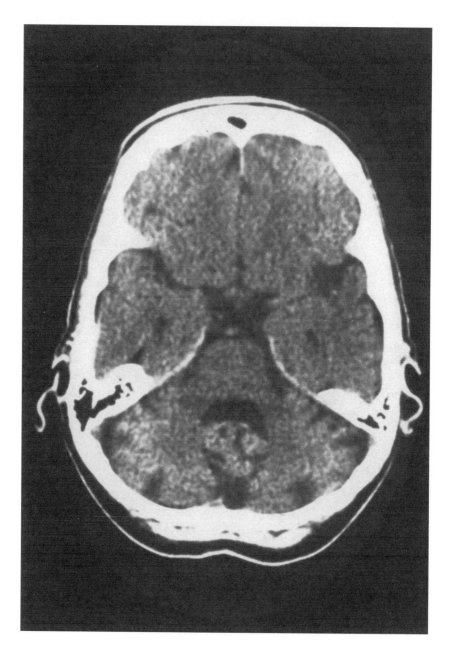

B

no longer correlated significantly with the severity of motor disturbances in OPCA. In contrast, when the effects due to variations in atrophy were accounted for, the degree of hypometabolism still correlated significantly with clinical severity.

III. SUMMARY

Olivopontocerebellar atrophy is a chronic progressive neurological disease of undetermined cause characterized pathologically by degeneration of neurons in the inferior olives, pons, and cerebellum. The disease occurs both sporadically and with hereditary transmission.

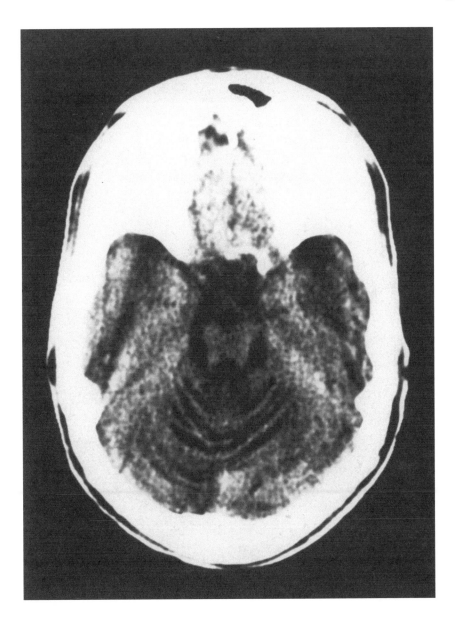

C

The presenting complaints are usually related to ataxia of gait and disorders of speech, with difficulty in coordination of the upper extremities commonly occurring soon afterward. Positron emission tomography with ^{18}F-2-fluoro-2-deoxy-D-glucose was used to study 40 patients with OPCA and 35 age-matched normal controls. The studies revealed significant hypometabolism in the cerebellar hemispheres, cerebellar vermis, and brainstem in OPCA patients in comparison with the normal controls. A significant relationship was found between the degree of atrophy as measured by CT scans and the level of LCMRG in the cerebellum and brainstem. Nevertheless, several patients had minimal atrophy and substantially reduced LCMRG, suggesting that atrophy does not fully account for the finding of hypometabolism.

The severity of the ataxic and spastic components of dysarthria in OPCA patients was studied in relation to LCMRG. Perceptual analysis was used to characterize the speech disorders, and rating scales were used to quantitate the degree of ataxia and spasticity of

TABLE 8
Rating Scales for Evaluating the
Degree of Atrophy in CT Scans

Cerebellum

0	Normal
1	Atrophy in a single folium
2	Atrophy in two folia
3	Mild atrophy in all folia
4	Moderate atrophy in all folia
5	Severe atrophy in all folia

Brainstem

0	Normal
1	Mild atrophy
2	Moderate atrophy
3	Severe atrophy

From Gilman, S. et al., *Ann. Neurol.*, 23, 223, 1988. With permission.

CEREBELLAR HEMISPHERES

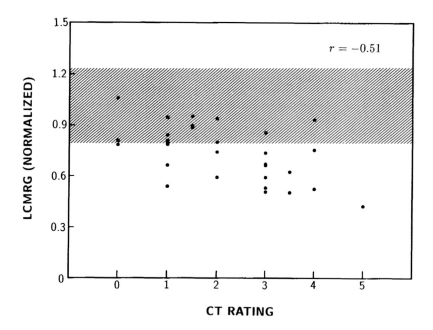

FIGURE 3.   Graph of the mean local cerebral metabolic rate for glucose (LCMRG) normalized to the cerebral cortex in the left and right cerebellar hemispheres plotted against the degree of atrophy observed in the CT scans. The criteria used to rate the amount of atrophy in CT scans are depicted in Table 8. A significant relationship ($p < 0.005$) is seen between LCMRG and the degree of atrophy in the cerebellar tissue. The shaded region indicates the range of two standard deviations of LCMRG in the normal control group. (From Rosenthal, G. et al., *Ann. Neurol.*, 24, 414, 1988. With permission.)

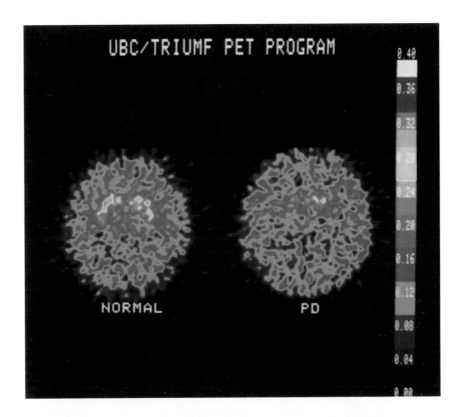

Plate 1. Images obtained following 6-FD administration to a normal subject (left) and a patient with Parkinson's disease (right). Both images are at the same axial level through the basal ganglia and represent 30 min of emission data acquired during the second hour after tracer administration. Figures on the color scale refer to radioactivity concentration in CPS per milliliter.

LEFT SIDED PARKINSONISM
PRE AND POST L-DOPA

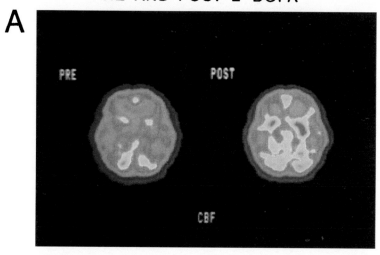

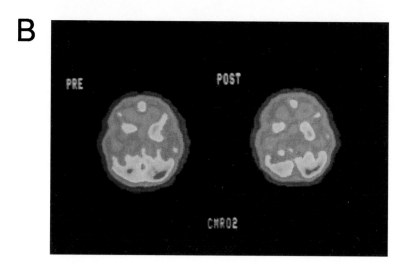

Plate 2.   PET (ECAT-II) brain images of a patient with predominantly unilateral (left body side) signs and symptoms of Parkinson's disease. The patient is viewed from above and frontal is up. In the right basal ganglia region (right side of the image) a higher CBF (Panel A) and oxygen utilization (CMRO$_2$) (Panel B) is found both before (left image = pre) and 1 h after (right image = post) oral levodopa administration. CBF increases globally after levodopa (Panel A).

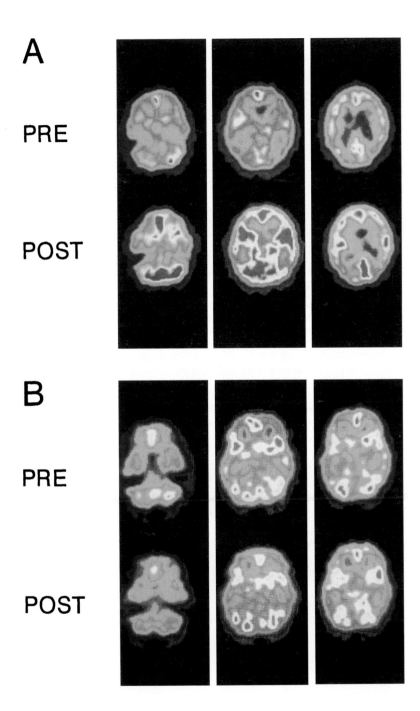

Plate 3. Panel A—PET (ECAT-II) brain images representing CBF in a healthy volunteer before (upper row) and 1 h after oral levodopa administration (lower row). Position of the head as in Plate 2. The left-hand-side image (for both rows) represents a cross-section through a lower (cerebellar) level of the brain, the middle image cuts through the insula and basal ganglia regions, and the right through the planum temporale. After levodopa administration a global increase of CBF is seen. Panel B—Similar to panel A, but now oral domperidone (60 mg) was given as premedication 1 h before the oral levodopa dose. No CBF increase is seen under these circumstances.

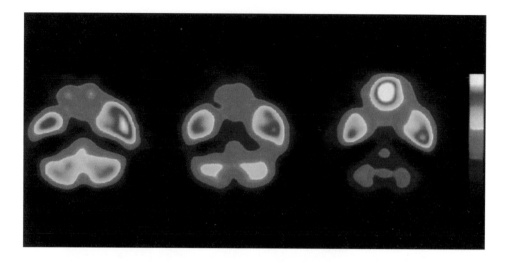

Plate 4. Positron emission tomography (PET) scans from three patients with olivopontocerebellar atrophy (OPCA) showing cerebral glucose utilization as detected with ^{18}F-2-fluoro-2-deoxy-D-glucose. The data in all three scans are normalized to the mean metabolic rate of the cerebral cortex. Relative rates of glucose utilization are shown in the colored bar. The scans are at the level of the cerebellum and the base of the temporal and frontal lobes. The PET scan on the left is from a 53-year-old woman with OPCA who presented mild clinical signs. The reduction in glucose utilization in the cerebellum and brainstem is mild in this patient. The middle image is the PET scan of a 71-year-old woman with OPCA who showed moderately severe clinical signs. A moderate reduction in metabolic rate for glucose in the posterior fossa structures is noted. The image on the right is a PET scan of a 25-year-old woman with OPCA who was severely affected. A severe decline in metabolic rate is evident in the cerebellum and brainstem of this patient.

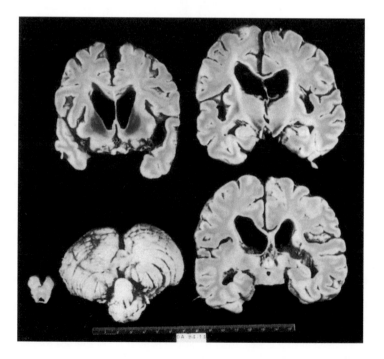

Plate 5. Perls' stain for ferric iron. Prominent ventriculomegaly, caudate atrophy, and striatal iron accumulation consistent in a patient who died of Huntington's disease. (From Drayer, B. P., *BNIQ.*, 3, 15, 1987. With permission.)

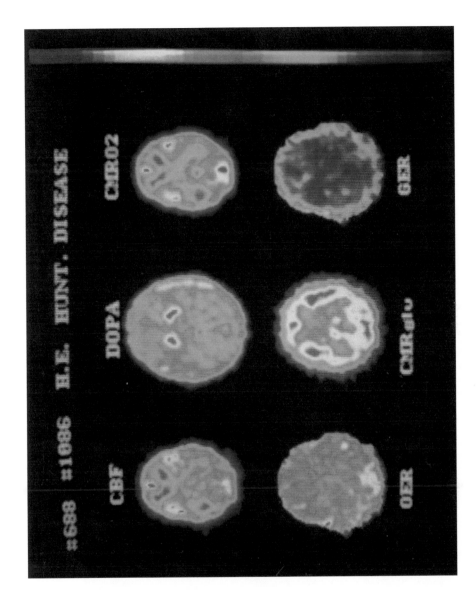

Plate 6. Blood flow, metabolism, and dopamine systems in Huntington's disease. Note that while the striatal blood flow (CBF), oxygen (CMRO$_2$) and glucose (CMRGlu) metabolism are all low, nigrostriatal input to the striatum remains intact (DOPA). (From Leenders, K. L., et al., *Movement Disorders*, 1, 69, 1986. With permission.)

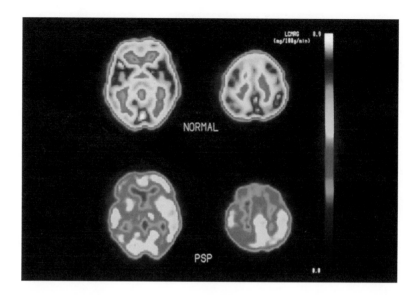

Plate 7.   Positron emission tomographic scan images following ^{18}F-FDG administration in a typical normal subject (top images) and a typical patient with progressive supranuclear palsy (bottom images). Each is a horizontal section in a plane parallel to and approximately 4 cm (left images) or 8 cm (right images) above the canthomeatal line. The front of the head is to the top of the image and the right of the head is to the right of the image. The color bar is the scale used to indicate rates of glucose utilization in mg/100 g/min with the highest values at the top and the lowest values at the bottom of the bar. (From Foster, N. L., et al., *Ann. Neurol.*, 24, 399, 1988. With permission.)

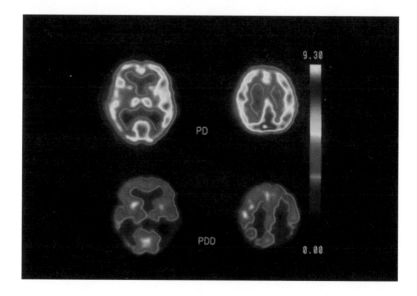

Plate 8.   Positron emission tomographic scan images following ^{18}F-FDG administration in a patient with Parkinson's disease and normal mentation (top images) and a demented patient with Parkinson's disease (bottom images). These horizontal sections are approximately 4 cm (left) or 8 cm (right) above the canthomeatal line. Note the similarity of the top image to that of the normal in Plate 7. By contrast the metabolic rate in the patient with dementia is diffusely hypometabolic with especially low metabolic rates in the posterior (parietal and temporal) regions of cerebral cortex. This study performed in collaboration with Dr. David E. Kuhl and other members of the Division of Nuclear Medicine at the University of Michigan.

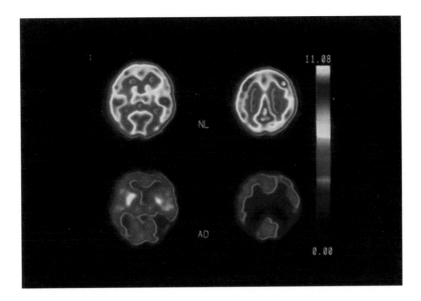

Plate 9. Positron emission tomographic scan images following ^{18}F-FDG administration in a typical normal subject (top images) and a typical patient with Alzheimer's disease (bottom images). Images are approximately 4 cm (left) or 8 cm (right) above the canthomeatal line. Like the demented patient with Parkinson's disease in Figure 4 of Chapter 13, the patient with Alzheimer's disease demonstrates diffuse hypometabolism, most profound in posterior regions of the cerebral cortex. This study performed in collaboration with Dr. David E. Kuhl and other members of the Division of Nuclear Medicine at the University of Michigan.

TABLE 9
Deviant Dimensions Found in Ataxic and Spastic Speech According to the Mayo Clinic Lists

Ataxic	Spastic
Imprecise consonants	Imprecise consonants
Monopitch	Monopitch
Monoloudness	Monoloudness
Slow rate	Slow rate
Harsh voice	Harsh voice
Excess and equal stress	Excess and equal stress
Irregular articulatory breakdown	Reduced stress
Distorted vowels	Low pitch
Prolonged phonemes	Hypernasality
Prolonged intervals	Strained-strangled quality
	Short phrases
	Distorted vowels
	Pitch breaks
	Breathy voice — continuous

From Kluin, K. J. et al., *Ann. Neurol.*, 23, 547, 1988. With permission.

TABLE 10
Deviant Dimensions Important in Ataxic and Spastic Speech According to the University of Michigan Lists

Ataxic	Spastic
Excess and equal stress (3)	Strained-strangled quality (3)
Irregular articulatory breakdown (2)	Reduced stress (2)
Alternating loudness (2)	Harsh voice — continuous (2)
Variable rate (2)	Slow rate (2)
Fluctuating Pitch (2)	Low pitch (2)
Harsh voice — transient (1)	Imprecise phonemes (1)
Breathy voice — transient (1)	Monoloudness (1)
Altered Nasality — transient (1)	Hypernasality — continuous (1)
Voice tremors (1)	Monopitch (1)
Audible inspiration (1)	Prolonged phonemes and/or intervals (1)

Note: The numbers in parentheses indicate the relative weight used for each deviant dimension in determining each patient's dysarthria rating

From Kluin, K. J. et al., *Ann. Neurol.*, 23, 547, 1988. With permission.

speech in each patient. A significant correlation was found between the severity of ataxia in speech and LCMRG within the cerebellar vermis, cerebellar hemispheres, and brainstem, but not the thalamus. No significant correlation was found between the severity of spasticity in speech and LCMRG in any of these structures.

The severity of cranial and somatic motor dysfunction in OPCA patients was studied in relation to LCMRG. A scale was devised to quantitate the degree of ataxia in the neurological examinations. A significant correlation was found between the severity of motor impairment and LCMRG within the cerebellar vermis, both cerebellar hemispheres, and the brainstem. A significant but weaker relationship was noted between the degree of tissue atrophy as measured by CT in the same regions and clinical severity. A partial correlation analysis revealed that LCMRG and not the amount of atrophy is the more important correlate of motor dysfunction in OPCA.

CEREBELLAR HEMISPHERES

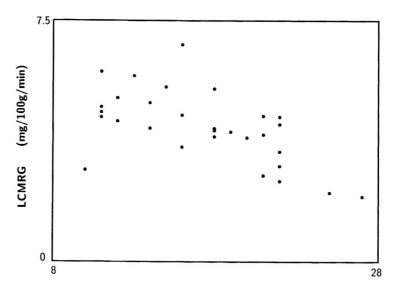

University of Michigan Ataxic Dysarthria Rating

FIGURE 4. Graph of local cerebral metabolic rate for glucose (LCMRG) in mg/ 100 g/min for the cerebellar hemispheres plotted against the severity of ataxic dysarthria. There is a significant inverse correlation between the degree ataxia in speech and the level of LCMRG within the cerebellar hemispheres. There is no difference in the results between the left and right cerebellar hemispheres and thus the two are shown together. (From Kluin, K. J. et al., *Ann. Neurol.*, 23, 547, 1988. With permission).

TABLE 11
Correlation Coefficients Between LCMRG in Various Regions of the CNS and Dysarthria Ratings for Ataxic Speech and Spastic Speech

	LCMRG (absolute)[a]		LCMRG (normalized)[b]	
Brain region	**Ataxic**	**Spastic**	**Ataxic**	**Spastic**
Cerebellar vermis	−0.57[e]	−0.45[c]	−0.40[c]	−0.24
Cerebellar hemispheres	−0.59[e]	−0.51[d]	−0.48[d]	−0.30
Brainstem	−0.56[e]	−0.47[d]	−0.42[c]	−0.10
Thalamus	−0.24	−0.27	−0.10	−0.13
Cerebral cortex	−0.34[c]	−0.44[c]	—	—

[a] Absolute local cerebral metabolic rate for glucose in mg/100 g/min.
[b] Local cerebral metabolic rate for glucose normalized to the cerebral cortex.
[c] $p < 0.05$.
[d] $p < 0.005$.
[e] $p < 0.001$.

From Kluin, K. J. et al., *Ann. Neurol.*, 23, 547, 1988. With permission.

TABLE 12
Results of the Partial Correlations Method of Examining the Relationships Between LCMRG and Dysarthria Ratings for Ataxic and Spastic Speech Characteristics

Brain region	LCMRG (absolute)[a]		LCMRG (normalized)[b]	
	Ataxic (given spastic)	Spastic (given ataxic)	Ataxic (given spastic)	Spastic (given ataxic)
Cerebellar vermis	-0.47^d	-0.28^c	-0.34^c	-0.09
Cerebellar Hemispheres	-0.48^d	-0.36^c	-0.41^c	-0.12
Brainstem	-0.45^d	-0.30^c	-0.42^c	-0.09
Thalamus	-0.14	-0.19	-0.05	-0.10
Cerebral cortex	-0.19	-0.35^c	—	—

Note: When the relationship of spastic speech and LCMRG is eliminated, the severity of ataxia in speech is inversely correlated with absolute LCMRG in the cerebellum and brainstem (first column). When the relationship of ataxic speech and LCMRG is eliminated, the severity of spasticity in speech is inversely correlated with absolute LCMRG in the cerebellum, brainstem, and cerebral cortex (second column). With LCMRG data normalized to the cerebral cortex, the severity of ataxia in speech is inversely correlated with LCMRG in the cerebellum and brainstem (third column). With LCMRG data normalized to the cerebral cortex, the severity of spasticity in speech is not correlated with LCMRG in any of the structures studied.

[a] Absolute local cerebral metabolic rate for glucose in mg/100 g/min.
[b] Local cerebral metabolic rate for glucose normalized to the cerebral cortex.
[c] $p < 0.05$.
[d] $p < 0.01$.

From Kluin, K. J. et al., *Ann. Neurol.*, 23, 547, 1988. With permission.

TABLE 13
Rating Scale for Clinical Motor Disorders in OPCA

Somatic Motor Signs

Ataxia of gait
  0 No deficit
  1 Ataxic but able to walk in tandem
  2 Unable to walk in tandem
  3 Unable to walk without assistance
  4 Unable to walk
Heel-knee-shin
  0 No deficit
  1 Mild to moderate deficit
  2 Severe deficit
Finger-nose-finger
  0 No deficit
  1 Mild to moderate deficit
  2 Severe deficit
Rapid alternating movements
  0 No deficit
  1 Mild to moderate deficit
  2 Severe deficit

TABLE 13 (continued)
Rating Scale for Clinical Motor
Disorders in OPCA

Cranial Motor Signs

Nystagmus
 0 Not present
 1 Present
Ocular Dysmetria
 0 Not present
 1 Present
Ataxia of speech
 0 No perceptible deficit
 1 Mild deficit
 2 Moderate deficit
 3 Severe deficit
Impaired tongue movements
 0 Not present
 1 Present

From Rosenthal, G. et al., *Ann. Neurol.*, 24, 414, 1988.
With permission.

CEREBELLAR HEMISPHERES

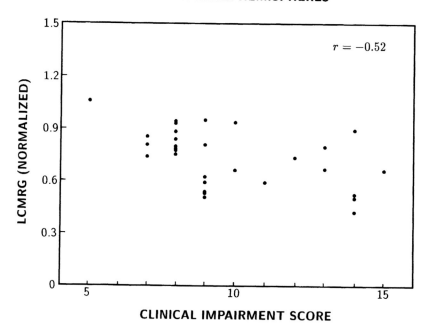

FIGURE 5.   Severity of clinical impairment plotted against the mean local cerebral metabolic
rate for glucose (LCMRG) normalized to the cerebral cortex in the left and right cerebellar
hemispheres. A significant relationship (p <0.005) is seen between clinical severity and
LCMRG. (From Rosenthal, G. et al., *Ann. Neurol.*, 24, 414, 1988. With permission.)

TABLE 14
Spearman Rank Correlation Coefficients of the Relationship Between the Clinical Impairment Score and the Local Cerebral Metabolic Rates for Glucose Normalized to the Metabolic Rate of the Entire Cerebral Cortex

Cerebellar vermis	−0.53[a]
Left cerebellar hemisphere	−0.53[b]
Right cerebellar hemisphere	−0.48[a]
Brainstem	−0.39[b]
Thalamus	−0.02

Note: Clinical Impairment score was determined from the neurological examination and perceptual analysis of speech.

[a] $p < 0.005$.
[b] $p < 0.05$.

From Rosenthal, G. et al., *Ann. Neurol.*, 24, 414, 1988. With permission.

TABLE 15
Spearman Rank Correlation Coefficients of the Relationship Between the Clinical Impairment Score and Tissue Atrophy as Determined by Visual Rating of Computed Tomograph Scans

Cerebellar vermis	0.42[a]
Left cerebellar hemisphere	0.36[a]
Right cerebellar hemisphere	0.42[a]
Brainstem	−0.04

[a] $p < 0.05$.

From Rosenthal, G. et al., *Ann. Neurol.*, 24, 414, 1988. With permission.

TABLE 16

**Spearman Rank Correlation
Coefficients of the Relationship
Between Tissue Atrophy and Local
Cerebral Metabolic Rates for
Glucose Normalized to the
Metabolic Rate of the Entire
Cerebral Cortex**

Cerebral vermis	−0.47[a]
Left cerebellar hemisphere	−0.45[b]
Right cerebellar hemisphere	−0.54[a]
Brainstem	−0.38[b]

[a] $p < 0.005$.
[b] $p < 0.05$.

From Rosenthal, G. et al., *Ann. Neurol.*, 24, 414, 1988. With permission.

TABLE 17

**Results of the Partial Correlations Method of
Examining the Relationship Between Clinical
Impairment, LCMRG, and Tissue Atrophy**

	LCMRG given tissue atrophy	Tissue atrophy given LCMRG
Cerebellar vermis	−0.42[a]	0.22
Left cerebellar hemisphere	−0.44[b]	0.16
Right cerebellar hemisphere	−0.33[a]	0.22
Brainstem	−0.44[b]	−0.12

Note: When the effect of the relationship between LCMRG and tissue atrophy is eliminated, the clinical impairment score remains significantly correlated with LCMRG in all regions of interest in the cerebellum and brainstem (first column). When the effect of the relationship between LCMRG and tissue atrophy is eliminated, the amount of tissue atrophy no longer correlates with the clinical impairment score (second column). LCMRG = local cerebral metabolic rate for glucose.

[a] $p < 0.05$.
[b] $p < 0.01$.

From Rosenthal, G. et al., *Ann. Neurol.*, 24, 414, 1988. With permission.

ACKNOWLEDGMENTS

This work was supported in part by NIH Grant 15655 and the Campbell Foundation. I am indebted to my colleagues for their participation in this work: Drs. Stephen S. Gebarski, Larry Junck, and Robert Koeppe; Ms. Karen Kluin and Dorene Markel; Mr. Guy Rosenthal; and the staff of the Division of Nuclear Medicine.

REFERENCES

1. **Eadie, M. J.**, Olivo-ponto-cerebellar atrophy (Dejerine-Thomas type), in *Handbook of Clinical Neurology*, Vol. 21, Vinken, P. J. and Bruyn, G. W., Eds., Elsevier/North Holland, Amsterdam, 1975, 415.

2. **Eadie, M. J.**, Olivo-ponto-cerebellar atrophy (Menzel type), in *Handbook of Clinical Neurology*, Vol. 21, Vinken, P. J. and Bruyn, G. W., Eds., Elsevier/North Holland, Amsterdam, 1975, 433.

3. **Gilman, S., Bloedel, J. R., and Lechtenberg, R.**, *Disorders of the Cerebellum*, F. A. Davis, Philadelphia, 1981.

4. **Harding, A. E.**, *The Hereditary Ataxias and Related Disorders*, Churchill Livingstone, London, 1984.

5. **Duvoisin, R. C.**, An apology and an introduction to the olivopontocerebellar atrophies, in *The Olivopontocerebellar Atrophies*, Duvoisin, R. C. and Plaitakis, A., Eds., Raven Press, New York, 1984, 5.

6. **Berciano, J.**, Olivopontocerebellar atrophy. A review of 117 cases, *J. Neurol. Sci.*, 53, 253, 1982.

7. **Rich, S. S., Wilkie, P., Schut, L., Vance, G., and Orr, H. T.**, Spinocerebellar ataxia: localization of an autosomal dominant locus between two markers on human chromosome 6, *Am. J. Hum. Genet.*, 41, 524, 1987.

8. **Cummings, J. L. and Benson, D. F.**, *Dementia: A Clinical Approach*, Butterworths, Boston, 1983.

9. **Oppenheimer, D. R.**, Diseases of the basal ganglia, cerebellum and motor neurons, in *Greenfield's Nueropathology*, 4th ed., Adams, J. H., Corsellis, J. A. N., and Duchen, L. W., Eds., John Wiley & Sons, New York, 1984, chap. 15.

10. **Koeppen, A. H. and Barron, K. D.**, The neuropathology of olivopontocerebellar atrophy, in *The Olivopontocerebellar Atrophies*, Duvoisin, R. C. and Plaitakis, A., Eds., Raven Press, New York, 1984, 13.

11. **Landis, D. M. D., Rosenberg, R. N., Landis, S. C., Schut, L., and Nyhan, W. L.**, Olivopontocerebellar degeneration. Clinical and ultrastructural abnormalities, *Arch. Neurol.*, 31, 295, 1974.

12. **Petito, C. K., Hart, M. N., Porro, R. S., and Earle, K. M.**, Ultrastructural studies of olivopontocerebellar atrophy, *J. Neuropathol. Exp. Neurol.*, 32, 503, 1973.

13. **Tagliavini, F. and Pilleri, G.**, Neuronal loss in the basal nucleus of Meynert in a patient with olivopontocerebellar atrophy, *Acta Neuropathol. (Berlin)*, 66, 127, 1985.

14. **Kanazawa, I., Kwak, S., Sasaki, H., Mizusawa, H., Muramoto, O., Yoshizawa, K., Nukina, N., Kitamura, K., Kurisaki, H., and Sugita, K.**, Studies on neurotransmitter markers and nueronal cell density in the cerebellar system in olivopontocerebellar atrophy and cortical cerebellar atrophy, *J. Neurol. Sci.*, 71, 193, 1985.

15. **Perry, T. L., Hansen, S., Currier, R. D., and Berry, K.**, Abnormalities in nuerotransmitter amino acids in dominantly inherited cerebellar disorders, in *Advances in Nuerology*, Vol. 21, Kark, R. A. P., Rosenberg, R. N., and Schut, L. J., Eds., Raven Press, New York, 1978, 303.

16. **Perry, T. L., Kish, S. J., Hansen, S., and Currier, R. D.**, Neurotransmitter amino acids in dominantly inherited cerebellar disorders, *Neurology*, 31, 237, 1981.

17. **Kish, S. J., Perry, T. L., and Hornykiewicz, O.**, Increased GABA receptor binding in dominantly-inherited cerebellar ataxias, *Brain Res.*, 269, 370, 1983.

18. **Kish, S. J., Perry, T. L., and Hornykiewicz, O.**, Benzodiazepine receptor binding in cerebellar cortex: observations in olivopontocerebellar atrophy, *J. Neurochem.*, 42, 466, 1984.

19. **Whitehouse, P. J., Muramoto, O., Troncoso, J. C., and Kanazawa, I.**, Neurotransmitter receptors in olivopontocerebellar atrophy: an autoradiographic study, *Neurology*, 36, 193, 1986.

20. **Perry, T. L.**, Four biochemically different types of dominantly inherited olivopontocerebellar atrophy, in *The Olivopontocerebellar Atrophies*, Duvoisin, R. C. and Plaitakis, A., Eds., Raven Press, New York, 1984, 205.

21. **Perry, T. L.**, Neurotransmitter abnormalities in dominantly inherited olivopontocerebellar atrophies, *Ital. J. Neurol. Sci.*, 4, 79, 1984.

22. **Kish, S. J., Shannak, K. S., and Hornykiewicz, O.**, Reduction of noradrenaline in cerebellum of patients with olivopontocerebellar atrophy, *J. Neurochem.*, 42, 1476, 1984.

23. **Kish, S. J., Currier, R. D., Schut, L., Perry, T. L., and Morito, C. L.**, Brain choline acetyltransferase reduction in dominantly inherited olivopontocerebellar atrophy, *Ann. Neurol.*, 22, 272, 1987.

24. **Mitsuma, T., Nogimori, T., Adachi, K., Mukoyama, M., Ando, K., and Sobue, I.**, Concentrations of immunoreactive thryrotropin-releasing hormone in the brain of patients with olivopontocerebellar atrophy, *J. Neurol. Sci.*, 71, 369, 1985.

25. **Plaitakis, A., Berl, S., and Yahr, M. D.**, Abnormal glutamate metabolism in an adult onset degenerative neurological disorder, *Science*, 216, 193, 1982.

26. **Plaitakis, A., Berl, S., and Yahr, M. D.**, Neurological disorders associated with deficiency of glutamate dehydrogenase, *Ann. Neurol.*, 115, 144, 1984.

27. **Duvoisin, R. C., Chokroverty, S., Lepore, F., and Nicklas, W. J.**, Glutamate dehydrogenase deficiency in patients with olivopontocerebellar atrophy, *Neurology*, 33, 1322, 1983.

28. **Konagaya, Y., Konagaya, M., and Takayanagi, T.**, Glutamate dehydrogenase and its isozyme activity in olivopontocerebellar atrophy, *J. Neurol. Sci.*, 74, 231, 1986.

29. **Sorbi, S., Tonini, S., Giannini, E., Piacentini, S., Marini, P., and Amaducci, L.,** Abnormal platelet glutamate dehydrogenase activity and activation in dominant and nondominant olivopontocerebellar atrophy, *Ann. Neurol.,* 19, 239, 1986.

30. **Finocchiaro, G., Taroni, F., and DiDonato, S.,** Glutamate dehydrogenase in olivopontocerebellar atrophies: leukocytes, fibroblasts, and muscle mitochondria, *Neurology,* 36, 550, 1986.

31. **Yamaguchi, T., Hayashi, K., Murakami, H., Ota, K., and Maruyama, S.,** Glutamate dehydrogenase deficiency in spinocerebellar degenerations, *Neurochem. Res.,* 7, 627, 1982.

32. **Grossman, A., Rosenberg, R. N., and Warmoth, L.,** Glutamate and malate dehydrogenase activities in Joseph disease and olivopontocerebellar atrophy, *Neurology,* 37, 106, 1987.

33. **Gilroy, J. and Lynn, G. E.,** Computerized tomography and auditory evoked potentials: use in the diagnosis of olivopontocerebellar degeneration, *Arch. Neurol.,* 35, 143, 1978.

34. **Wadia, N. H., Irani, P., Mehta, L., and Purohit, A.,** Evidence of peripheral neuropathy in a variety of heredo-familial olivo-ponto-cerebellar degeneration frequently seen in India, in *Spinocerebellar Degenerations,* Sobue, I., Ed., University of Tokyo Press, Tokyo, 1980.

35. **McLeod, J. G. and Evans, W.,** Peripheral neuropathy in spinocerebellar degenerations, *Muscle Nerve,* 4, 51, 1981.

36. **Gilman, S., Markel, D. S., Koeppe, R. A., Junck, L., Kluin, K. L., Gebarski, S. A. and Hichwa, R. D.,** Cerebellar and brainstem hypometabolism in olivopontocerebellar atrophy studied with positron emission tomography, *Ann. Neurol.,* 23, 223, 1988.

37. **Kluin, K. J., Gilman, S., Markel, D. S., Koeppe, R. A., Rosenthal, G., and Junch, L.,** Speech disorders in olivopontocerebellar atrophy correlate with positron emission tomography findings, *Ann. Neurol.,* in press.

38. **Rosenthal, G., Gilman, S., Koeppe, R. A., Kluin, K. J., Markel, D. S., Junck, L., and Gebarski, S. A.,** Motor dysfunction in olivopontocerebellar atrophy is related to cerebral metabolic rate studied with positron emmission tomography *Ann. Neurol.,* 24, 414, 1988.

39. **Phelps, M. E., Huang, S. C., Hoffman, E. J., Selin, C., Sokoloff, L, and Kuhl, D. E.,** Tomographic measurement of local cerebral glucose metabolic rate in humans with (F-18) 2-fluoro-2-deoxy-D-glucose: validation of method, *Ann. Neurol.,* 6, 371, 1979.

40. **Hawkins, R. A., Mazziotta, J. C., Phelps, M. E., Huang, S. C., Kuhl, D. E., Carson, R. E., Metter, E. J., and Riege, W. H.,** Cerebral glucose metabolism as a function of age in man: influence of the rate constants in the fluorodeoxyglucose method, *J. Cereb. Blood Flow Metab.,* 3, 250, 1983.

41. **Darley, F. L., Aronson, A. E., and Brown, J. R.,** *Motor Speech Disorders,* W. B. Saunders, Philadelphia, 1975.

Chapter 10

PET AND HUNTINGTON'S DISEASE

John C. Mazziotta

TABLE OF CONTENTS

I. CLINICAL AND PATHOLOGICAL FEATURES

Huntington's disease is a fatal, hyperkinetic movement disorder characterized by chorea, dementia, and psychiatric symptoms.[12] The disease is inherited in an autosomal dominant fashion and the defective gene has been localized to the short arm of chromosome 4 through the use of molecular biological approaches.[3,4] The age of onset varies widely, but typically occurs during the third and fourth decades of life.

The early clinical symptoms include disorders of ocular motility (altered saccades and pursuits, diminished fixation and impaired optokinetic nystagmus), loss of fine motor control, and diminished rapid alternating movement.[5] This progresses to chorea which becomes more severe as the disease advances. In the late stages of the disease, typically 10 to 15 years after onset, chorea is gradually replaced by dystonia and hypokinetic rigidity. Dysphagia is typical of the terminal phases of the illness.[6] The average life span after diagnosis is 15 to 20 years.

Dementia, personality disorders, and physiatric symptoms occur in Huntington's disease and typically are more disabling to the patient than are the motor aspects of the disorder. Frequently, patients and their family members will indicate that psychological, psychiatric, or personality changes preceded the onset of the involuntary movements.[2,7]

The brunt of the pathological changes in the brains of patients dying of Huntington's disease is in the striatum. Severe neuronal loss and gliosis typify the changes in this structure.[8] In the terminal phase, neurophathological changes also occur diffusely throughout the brain but most prominently in the globus pallidus, motor nuclei of the thalamus, and front cortex.[9] The striatal cell loss is selective and is most severe for the medium-sized spiny neurons.[7] Spared are the aspiny neurons which contain somatostatin and neuropeptide Y.[7,10] Of interest is the fact that abnormalities in dendritic processes have been observed in the striatum in patients with early disease.[11] The patterns of these changes are such that they begin in the dorsal medial caudate and spread toward the ventral lateral putamen.

The differential diagnosis of patients presenting with acquired chorea includes, along with Huntington's disease, chorea secondary to and following rheumatic fever (Sydenham's chorea), pregnancy (chorea gravidum), systemic lupus erythematosus, tardive dyskinesia, acanthocytosis, hyperthyroidism, drug effects (phenytoin or birth control pills), and benign hereditary chorea. Huntington's disease can usually be identified clinically by the presence of the triad of chorea, dementia, and autosomal dominant inheritance. Clinical situations where family history is unobtainable or prior neuroleptic use is an issue can prove to be the most dificult diagnostic situations.

II. STRUCTURAL IMAGING STUDIES

As early as 1936, pneumoencephalography was used to demonstrate the focal caudate atrophy known to exist pathologically in advanced Huntington's disease patients.[12] These pneumoencephalographic reports demonstrated the loss of the convex shape that the normal caudate nucleus produces in the frontal horn of the lateral ventricle (Figure 1). Atrophy of these nuclei result in a focal enlargement of the anterior horns of the lateral ventricles with an increased caudate to septum distance.[12,14] No correlations were identified between these ventricular enlargements and duration of illness, severity of chorea, or degree of cognitive deficits.[13,14]

The advent of X-ray CT provided a noninvasive means of identifying caudate and generalized cerebral atrophy in Huntington's disease patients during life (Figure 2). In the last decade a large number of reports have refined and quantified the focal and generalized atrophic changes associated with Huntington's disease through the use of X-ray CT.[15,26] Various indices were developed as a means of quantifying caudate changes. These, in general,

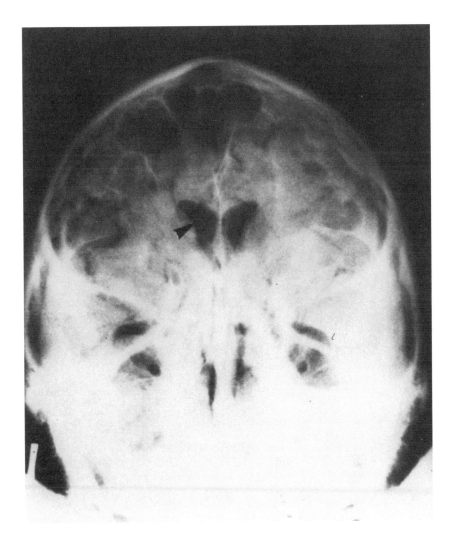

A

FIGURE 1. (A) A normal pneumoencephalogram (PEG) showing the characteristic indentation in the lateral ventricle due to the caudate nucleus (arrow). (B) A PEG of a 53-year-old man with advanced Huntington's disease, with ventricular dilation secondary to caudate nucleus atrophy. (From Hayden, M. R., *Huntington's Corea*, Springer-Verlag, New York, 1981. With permission.)

have referenced the distance of the medial surfaces of the two caudate nuclei (bicaudate diameter [CC]) to various other structures identifiable on X-ray CT images. These reference structures have included the width of the frontal horns (FH) or the outer table of the skull (OTcc) at the same angle, level and position as the bicaudate measurement.[15,17,19,21-24,26,27] Some reports have used the maximal internal diameter of the skull as the reference value.[15,17,26] The intercaudate distance (in either absolute terms or referenced to other brain dimensions) increases with disease progression as one would expect from knowledge of the relentless atrophy of the striatum with advancing disease.[16,19] There appears to be a good correlation between the overall functional capacity of the patient and the absolute or relative intercaudate distance.[15,16,18] Normal subjects have bicaudate distances in the range of 12.5 to 15mm.[23,17] Symptomatic Huntington's disease patients have values in excess of 21mm.[15,17,23,26] FH/CC ratios are typically greater than 2.3 in controls while symptomatic Huntington's disease patients have values ≤2.0.[15,17,19,21-23,26,27]

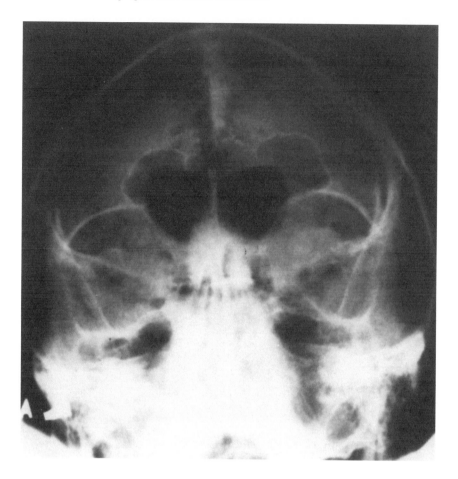

B

While differences in the tomographic angle and level used for patient scanning can affect these measured values and ratios, the characteristic ventricular shape and the large differences in values between normal controls and advanced Huntington's patients usually results in confirmatory diagnostic information being provided by X-ray CT. However, patients with early symptoms and indivduals who are offspring of symptomatic patients (at risk individuals) have normal X-ray CT studies.[15,17,19,22] While easily distinguishable clinically, patients with obstructive hydrocephalus can have flattening of the caudate nuclei and absolute or relative bicaudate indices similar to patients with symptomatic Huntington's disease.[26]

X-ray CT has been useful in defining the generalized cerebral atrophy which occurs in advanced Huntington's disease. Various reports have indicated generalized cortical atrophy and, in some cases, atrophy of the brain stem and cerebellum which is more typical of juvenile cases but can also be seen in adult subjects.[24,25] Finally, X-ray CT studies have been useful in identifying structural lesions that produce chorea not associated with Huntington's disease. Such structural lesions include cerebral infarction and unilateral or bilateral subdural hematomas.[28,29,30,72]

III. MAGNETIC RESONANCE IMAGING

Magnetic resonance imaging (MRI) studies of symptomatic Huntington's disease patients using low field magnets have duplicated the experience noted above with X-ray CT. Namely,

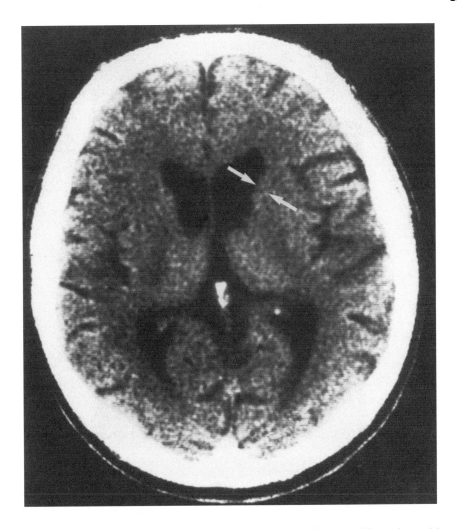

FIGURE 2.   X-ray CT in Huntington's disease demonstrating marked atrophy of the caudate nuclei and mild generalized atrophy of the cerebrum.

these studies have demonstrated striatal atrophy.[31-36] In a study of 13 choreic and 7 rigid Huntington's patients using spin echo pulse sequences by Sax et al.[34,37] both groups had evidence of caudate atrophy but the rigid patients selectively had an increase in signal intensity in the putamen.

MRI imaging with high field magnets (1.5 tesla) have provided additional information on Huntington's disease. While caudate atrophy is still identifiable, low signal intensity on T_2 weighted images has been seen in the globus pallidus and the striatum.[31,32] Studies by Drayer et al.[31] indicate a decrease in signal intensity in the striatum early in the disease and an increase in signal intensity in the same structure in the late stages of the disorder (Figure 3 and Plate 5*). Proposed as an explanation for this phenomenon is that iron, early in the disease, causes loss of signal intensity but late-stage gliosis compensates and overwhelms this earlier effect and results in a relative increase in signal intensity. These authors indicated that signal intensity was also reduced in T_2 weighted images for the substantia nigra, dentate nuclei of the cerebellum, and red nuclei of the midbrain.[31] Initial spectroscopic nuclear magnetic resonance (NMR) information from tissue obtained from post-mortem Huntington's

* Plate 5 appears after page 168.

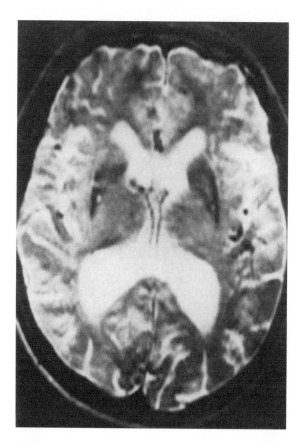

FIGURE 3. T$_2$-weighted (TR 2500 ms, TE 80 ms) MR image. Abnormal enlargement of the lateral ventricles with abnormally prominent hypointensity in the caudate and putamen compared to the globus pallidus suggesting excessive iron accumulation in the striatum in this 42-year old male with typical Huntington's disease.

disease brains has demonstrated a two- to threefold increase in phosphoethanolamine from tissue obtained from Huntington's disease brains and studied at 4.7 and 14.1 tesla.[38]

IV. METABOLIC AND HEMODYNAMIC IMAGING

At present there are no systematic evaluations of Huntington's disease patients using SPECT. PET, however, has been used to study an increasing number of symptomatic Huntington's disease patients since the initial PET study reported by Kuhl and co-workers[39] in 1982 (Figure 4). The findings in that report have been substantiated and refined by subsequent studies. In general glucose metabolism was reduced in the striatum of symptomatic Huntington's disease patients irrespective of whether striatal atrophy was grossly detectable by X-ray CT.[39-46,27] Only a few studies of blood flow and oxygen utilization have been performed in Huntington's disease patients but these indicate a matched reduction in these variables comparable to that seen for glucose metabolism.[47,48] SPECT studies of cerebral perfusion also indicated reduced values in the striatum.[49,50] The finding of reduced striatal metabolism seems to occur whether the symptoms are predominantly motoric or psychiatric.[27,39,40,42,51] Of note is the fact that reduced striatal glucose utilization occurs even in subjects with little or no atrophy demonstrated on X-ray CT. Thus, glucose hypometablism is not a reflection of a reduction in the size of the structure and secondary partial volume effects.[52]

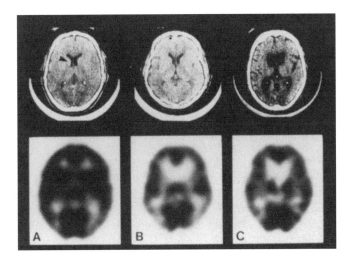

FIGURE 4. Atrophy and glucose metabolism in Huntington's disease demonstrated by X-ray CT and PET. All PET images were obtained using FDG. (A) Normal individual demonstrating the structural and metabolic appearance of the normal caudate nucleus (arrow) and putamen. (B) Patient with early clinical Huntington's disease, demonstrating the normal structural appearance of the caudate nucleus on X-ray CT but profound hypometabolism for glucose in PET study. (C) Patient with late Huntington's disease, demonstrating both structural (cortical and subcortical atrophy) in X-ray CT image and functional abnormalities (PET) of the caudate and putamen, bilaterally. Such studies demonstrate that the functional (as measured by glucose metabolism) abnormalities of the basal ganglia in patients with early HD precede structural cell loss sufficient to produce changes in X-ray CT. (From Kuhl, D. E. et al., *Ann. Neurol,,* 12, 425, 1982. With permission.)

In general, the reduction in striatal glucose metabolism has not been correlated with clinical signs, symptoms or their duration.[39,42] Young and co-workers[40] did find a correlation between caudate metabolic rate and patients' total functional capacity, learning and memory abilities, and general motor abnormalities with the exception of dystonia.[40] These investigators indicated that, like the sequence of histopathology changes in Huntington's disease, changes in putamenal metabolism were not as sensitive or early as changes in caudate metabolism.[11,40] They did, however, demonstrate that putamenal metabolism was better correlated to motor symptoms than was caudate metabolism. A number of reports have indicated that there is a trend, or in fact, a significant increase in thalamic metabolism in symptomatic Huntington's disease patients. It is postulated that this increase in thalamic metabolism may result from disinhibition of pallidal-thalamic circuits that are under striatal control.[53] This hypothesis will have to await imaging instruments with higher spatial resolution that will allow for specific examination of the metabolic activity of the globus pallidus and motor nuclei of the thalamus.

Cortical metabolism in symptomatic Huntington's disease patients has, in general, been normal.[39,40] However, a decrease in frontal cortical glucose or oxygen metabolism has been reported particularly in patients with disease durations in excess of 8 years.[39,48]

Thus, striatal hypometablism appears to be a sensitive indicator of functional change in symptomatic Huntington's disease patients. This is true whether the patient has primarily motoric or psychiatric symptoms at onset and also includes both the rigid and the choreic groups.[27,29-43,51] Striatal hypometabolism is not specific for Huntington's disease since it is also seen in chorea-acanthocytosis, benign hereditary chorea, and Lesch-Nyhan syndrome (Table 1).[54-56] Similarly, non-Huntingtonian chorea may occur without reductions in striatal

TABLE 1
Striatal Glucose Metabolism and Chorea

Magnitude vs. normals	Disorders
Decrease	Benign hereditary chorea (55), Huntington's Disease (27,39,40,42), Lesch-Nyhan Syndrome (57), Chorea Acanthocytosis (54), Wilson's disease
No change	Systemic lupus erythematosus (58)
Increase	Tardive dyskinesia (59,60)

metabolism or perfusion. Examples of the latter situation have been reported with chorea secondary to systemic lupus erythematosus.[58] Finally, choreiform movements are seen in tardive dyskinesia despite the fact that these subjects have elevated glucose utilization in the lenticular nuclei.[59,60]

V. PRE- AND POSTSYNAPTIC DOPAMINERGIC IMAGING STUDIES

Presynaptic dopaminergic function has been evaluated with PET and fluorine-18 labeled levodopa (fluorodopa), but because of the limited number of patients studied, these results should be considered preliminary.[48,60] Striatal fluorodopa uptake and retention was no different from controls when evaluated in symptomatic choreic Huntington's disease patients. The single patient reported by Stoessl et al.[61] with rigid juvenile Huntington's disease had a reduction in putamenal fluorodopa uptake with normal values for the caudate.

A limited amount of data is available from PET studies which evaluate postsynaptic D_2 dopamine receptors using carbon-11 labeled N-methylspiperone (MSP).[48,62-64] These preliminary studies demonstrate reductions in the apparent number of this receptor class in the striatum in Huntington's disease patients. These *in vivo* dopamine studies fit well with the known striatal pathology of Huntington's disease. Since nigrostriatal pathways are intact, presynaptic synthesis of dopamine from levodopa and its storage should be unimpaired. This has been substantiated by the finding of normal or even elevated levels of dopamine in the striatum at post-morten examination.[7,1,65] However, loss of intrinsic striatal neurons, presumably having dopaminergic receptors, would result in a decrease in this receptor population following the death of striatal cells. This is also in keeping with post-mortem studies.[66] Plate 6* demonstrates a single patient with symptomatic Huntington's disease who was evaluated for striatal perfusion, metabolism, and both pre- and postsynaptic dopaminergic integrity.

VI. METABOLIC EVALUATION OF PRESYMPTOMATIC (AT RISK) SUBJECTS

Because of the consistent finding of striatal hypometabolism in even the earliest symptomatic Huntington's disease patients, the possibility of finding striatal hypometabolism in patients with the Huntington's disease gene prior to the onset of symptoms has been investigated.[27,44-46,48,67-69] In the original UCLA study, just over one third (6/15) of the asymptomatic at risk individuals had caudate hypometabolism that was more than two standard deviations below that of control subjects.[39] In a subsequent study from the same institution a similar fraction (18/58) of at risk subjects were found to have reductions in caudate glucose metabolism that were outside the 95% confidence limits for inclusion in the control group (Figure 5).[27] It is presumed that these individuals with reductions in caudate glucose me-

---

* Plate 6 appears after page 168.

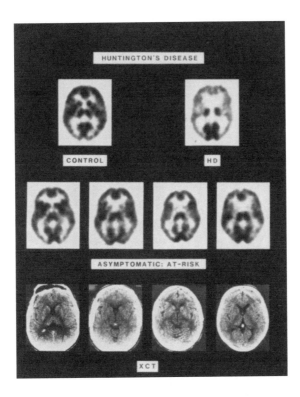

FIGURE 5. Position emission tomography and X-ray computed tomography (XCT) in subjects at risk for Huntington's Disease. The upper-left image demonstrates the typical, normal appearance of glucose metabolism at a tomographic level that passes through the heads of the caudate nuclei, the thalamus, and the visual cortex in a control subject. The upper-right image is from a symptomatic patient with Huntington's disease. Note the marked reduction in metabolism in the caudate nuclei. The middle and bottom rows of images are from four subjects, all of whom are asymptomatic (chorea-free) but at risk for Huntington's disease. CT studies (bottom row) were normal for all four subjects. The metabolic activity of the caudate nuclei, as determined by PET (middle row), demonstrates graded changes ranging from a normal appearance (left-most image) to one that closely resembles that seen in symptomatic patients (right-most image). Glucose metabolism in the caudate nuclei for these at risk subjects is indicate by the letters A, B, C, and D (from left to right) in Figure 6A. All PET studies were performed with the use of NeuroECAT device. (From Mazziotta, J. C. et al., *N. Engl. J. Med.*, 316, 357, 1987. With permission.)

tabolism in the absence of clinical symptoms, carry the HD gene and will eventually develop symptomatic Huntington's disease.[27] Of these 18 individuals, 4 have, in fact, developed clinical symptoms. None of the 40 individuals in the presumed normal group have, as yet, gone on to develop clinical Huntington's disease (Figure 6A).

In a similar and confirmatory report, Hayden et al.[46] evaluated 13 at risk individuals picked from four large families and found about $1/3$ (4/13) had caudate hypometabolism (Figure 6B).[44,46] In contrast to these results is a report by Young and co-workers indicating the caudate glucose metabolism was normal, both qualitatively and quantitatively in 29 at risk subjects whose mean age was 28 ± 5 years.[46] They concluded that measures of glucose metabolism from PET follow, rather than precede clinical symptoms.[45,68]

Of note is the fact that the study which found no metabolic abnormalities employed an at risk group whose mean age was considerably younger than the mean age of subjects in other studies.[27,44,46] If the rate of decline in caudate glucose metabolism decreases as a

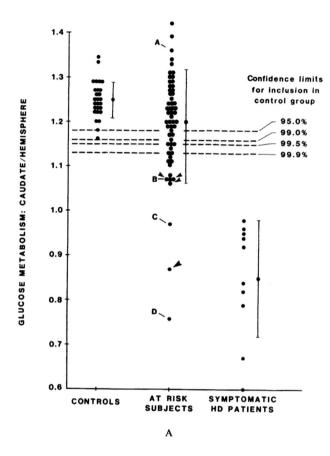

A

FIGURE 6.   (A) Caudate glucose metabolism expressed as a ratio of the
caudate to the hemispheric metabolic rate (cd/hem) in symptomatic patients
with Huntington's disease, person at risk for the disease, and normal
controls. In A, error bars indicate ± 1 SD. Notice the complete separation
of values for the control and symptomatic Huntington's disease groups.
Although the mean value for the at risk group is similar to that for the
controls, it is clear that values for a number of subjects fell well outside
the control distribution for this ratio and in fact overlapped with values
for persons in the symptomatic Huntington's disease group (i.e., the distribution of values for the at risk group is skewed unidirectional toward
lower values). A threshold for the cd/hem metabolic ratio of 1.15 separates
persons at risk into two subgroups in such a way that those above this
threshold have a 99.5% confidence limit of being included in the control
distribution. The labels A,B,C, and D indicate the cd/hem metabolic values
for the four at risk subjects whose PET studies are shown in Figure 5 (from
left to right). Arrowheads indicate at risk subjects who were studied in an
asymptomatic state but in whom clinical symptoms of Huntington's disease
developed approximately 2 to 4 years after their PET evaluation. (From
Mazziotta, J. C. et al., *N. Eng. J. Med.*, 316, 357, 1987. With permission.)
(B) Standardized right caudate and thalamic values for control, at risk and
symptomatic Huntington's disease patients along with regression line for
the normal controls. The graph shows separation of symptomatic patients
from controls and also identifies 4/14 at risk subjects whose values are <2
SEPs from controls. SEP, standard error of prediction; r, correlation between the thalamic and caudate values; M, slope of the regression line; b,
y-intercept of the regression line; n, number of subjects. (From Clark, C.
M. et al., *J. Cereb. Blood Flow Metab.*, 6, 756, 1986. With permission.)

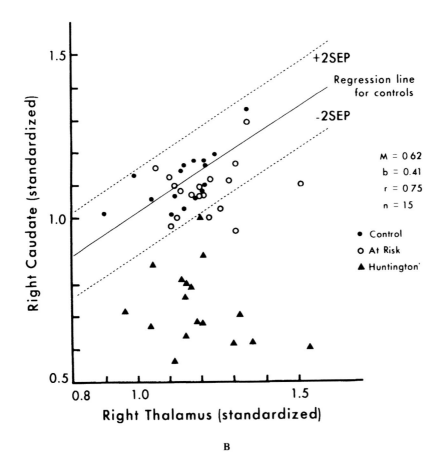

B

function of age of onset, glucose metabolism studies of at risk groups having a younger age will have fewer Huntington's disease gene carriers with caudate hypometabolism. Thus, a biological explanation for the disparate results exist. Also of note is the fact that the variance in the control data of the negative study is substantially larger than that reported in either of the positive studies and this would tend to mask positive findings.[27,44-46,70]

PET results of glucose metabolism have been compared to genetic linkage marker studies as depicted in Figure 7.[4,46,67] While the majority of outcomes match between PET and genetic data, the disparate results are of interest. Subjects who have a high probability (>90%) of having the Huntington's disease gene, by linkage marker criteria, but who have normal caudate glucose metabolism may represent false positive genetic results due to recombination, false negative results due to delay in development of caudate hypometabolism or a combination of the two. Those who have caudate hypometabolism and a low probability for having the Huntington's disease gene may be false negative genetic results due to recombination, false positive PET results due to choosing too low a threshold for defining caudate hypometabolism or combinations of the two.

These latter issues will be elucidated by studying larger numbers of subjects with the two methodologies and by following at risk individuals to the point of development of clinical symptoms. The value of PET in Huntington's disease is emphasized by the facts that, in our experience, all symptomatic Huntington's disease patients studied to date have had caudate hypometabolism, all previously asymptomatic at risk individuals who have developed clinical symptoms of Huntington's disease have had, in the presymptomatic state, caudate hypometabolism 1 to 4 years prior to symptom onset, and no at risk individual with

		G8 Marker	
		+	-
P	+	4	4
E			
T	-	5	10

		D4S43 Marker	
		+	-
P	+	5	2
E			
T	-	5	9

FIGURE 7.   Comparison of PET results of caudate glucose metabolism with genetic linkage studies using the original probe (G8) and a second probe (D4S43) which is closer to the HD gene. The (+) indicates a high probability (>90%) of having the HD gene or abnormal caudate glucose metabolism. The (−) symbol indicates the converse. The use of a marker closer to the HD gene resulted in two subjects being re-classified as having ambiguous results (one that was gene and PET (−), one that was PET (+) and gene (−) eliminating them from the comparison. An additional subject moved from the PET (+), gene (−) category to PET (+), gene (+). Thus, improvements in the accuracy of the genetic probes should reduce erroneous results and improve concordance between PET and genetic tests. The continued high rate of PET (−), gene (+) subjects is taken as evidenced for a period of time when caudate metabolism is normal in HD gene carriers.

presumed normal caudate metabolism has yet been reported to have developed clinical symptoms.

Thus, glucose metabolism and other physiologic variables may be useful in identifying gene carriers and confirming the diagnosis of Huntington's disease when family history, clinical data, or genetic informativeness is lacking. Finally, the opportunity to monitor the rate of change of glucose metabolism noninvasively and objectively in symptomatic or presymptomatic Huntington's disease subjects provides a unique opportunity to monitor experimental therapies for this disorder. The best candidate for experimental therapy to delay the onset of symptoms in Huntington's disease is a subject with the abnormal gene who is presymptomatic. Identification of such an individual can now occur through the combined use of linkage marker studies and PET. Knowledge about the rate of change of glucose metabolism or other physiological variables in the striatum could be used as a base line from which to compare experimental therapies aimed at slowing the rate of degeneration in this structure. Such information could indicate whether a given experimental therapy was beneficial, deleterious, or had no effect on the pathophysiological course of the disease.[27]

VII. FUTURE PROSPECTS

The identification of spared striatal neuronal populations and their evaluation in controlled experimental environments (e.g., tissue culture), provides an opportunity to develop selective probes for early pathophysiological changes in Huntington's disease through PET or SPECT.[7,71] Markers of the N-methyl-D-aspartate receptors are currently in a developmental phase and will provide a valuable link between such basic science research and clinical observations.[71]

Post-mortem studies of patients dying from Huntington's disease have demonstrated increased GABA and benzodiazepine receptors in the globus pallidus with decreased muscarinic receptors in that structure.[73] All these receptor types are reduced in the striatum.[73] Thus, the combined use of probes such as those for the measurement of protein synthesis, acetylcholine (e.g., ^{11}C-scopolamine), benzodiazepine/GABA (e.g., ^{11}C-flunitrazepam) and NMDA[74] receptor ligands will be important new neuroimaging tools for the study of Huntington's disease. Of equal importance will be the continued comparisons of at risk individuals whose PET data can be compared to clinical outcome and genetic linkage marker results. The deposition of ferromagnetic ions and the spectroscopic identification of biochemical striatal abnormalities via MRI may also prove to be valuable tools in understanding the pathophysiology of Huntington's disease, its genetic expression in the brain, and avenues towards its treatment or prevention.

ACKNOWLEDGMENTS

The author wishes to acknowledge the generous participation of all investigators who shared their results and illustrations. In addition, special thanks to Maureen Chang and Maggie Marquez in the preparation of the manuscript and to Lee Griswold for the preparation of illustrative materials. This work was supported in part by DOE cooperative agreement #DE-FC03-87ER60615, NIMH grant R01-MH-37916, NIH grants R01-6M-248388 and P01-NS-15654, and a grant from the Hereditary Disease Foundation.

REFERENCES

1. **Hayden, M. R.** *Huntington's Chorea*, Springer-Verlag, New York, 1981.
2. **Martin, J.,** Huntington's disease: new approaches to an old problem, *Neurology*, 34, 1059, 1984.
3. **Conneally, P. M.,** Huntington's disease: genetics and epi-demiology, *Am. J. Hum. Genet.*, 36, 506, 1984.
4. **Gusella, J. F., Wexler, N. S., Conneally, P. M., Naylor, S. L., Anderson, M. R., Sakaguchi, A. Y., Young, A. B., Shoulson, I., Bonilla, E. and Martin, J. B.,** A polymorphic DNA market genetically linked to Huntington's disease, *Nature*, 30, 234, 1983.
5. **Young, A. B., Shoulson, I., Penney, J. B., Starosta-Rubeinstein, S., Gomez, F., Travers, H., Ramos-Arroyo, M. A., Snodgrass, R., Bonilla, E., Moreno, H., and Wexler, N. S.,** Huntington's disease in Venezuela, *Neurology*, 36, 244, 1986.
6. **Shoulson, I.,** Huntington's disease, in *Diseases of the Nervous System*, Asbury, A. K., McKhann, G. M., and McDonald, W. I., Eds., W. B. Saunders, Philadelphia, 1986, 1258.
7. **Martin J. B. and Gusella, J. F.** Huntington's disease: pathognesis and management, *N. Eng. J. Med.*, 315, 1267, 1986.
8. **Vonsattel, J. P., Myers, R. H., Stevens, T. J. Ferrante, R. J., Bird, E. D., and Richardson, E. P.** Neuropathological classification of Huntington's disease, *J. Neuropathol. Exp. Neuro.*, 44, 559, 1985.
9. **Adams, J. H., Corsellis, J. A. N., and Duchen, L. W.,** (Eds., *Neuropathology*, John Wiley & Sons, New York, 1984.
10. **Ferrante, R. J., Kowall, N. W., Beal, M. F., Richardson, E. P., Bird, E. D., and Martin, J. B.,** Selective sparing of a class of striatal neurons in Huntington's disease, *Science*, 230, 561, 1985.

11. **Graveland, G. A., Williams, R. S., and DiFiglia, M.,** Evidence for degenerative and regenerative changes in neostriatal spiny neurons in Huntington's disease, *Science,* 227, 770, 1985.

12. **Goodhart, S. P., Balser, B. H., and Bieber, I.,** Encephalographic studies in cases of extrapyramidal disease, *Arch. Neurol. Psych.,* 35, 240, 1936.

13. **Blinderman, E. E., Weidner, W., and Markham, C. H.** The pneumoencephalogram in Huntington's chorea, *Neurology,* 11, 601, 1964.

14. **Gath, I. and Vinja, B.,** Pneumoencephalographic findings in Huntington's chorea, *Neurology,* 18, 991, 1968.

15. **Stober, T., Wussow, W., and Schimrigk, K.,** Bicaudate diameter—the most specific and simple CT parameter in the diagnosis of Huntington's disease, *Neuroradiology,* 26, 25, 1984.

16. **Shoulson, I.,** Huntington's disease: functional capacity in patients treated with neuroleptic and antidepressant drugs, *Neurology,* 31, 1333, 1981.

17. **Oepen, G. and Osterlag, C. H.,** Diagnostic value of CT in patients with Huntington's chorea and their offspring, *J. Neuroradiology,* 225, 189, 1981.

18. **Sax, D. S., O'Donnell, B., Butters, N., Menzer, L., Montgomery, K., and Kayne, H. L.,** Computed tomographic, neurologic, and neuropsychological correlates of Huntington's disease, *Int. J. Neurosci.,* 18, 21, 1983.

19. **Sax, D. S. and Menzer, L.,** Computerized tomography in Huntington's disease (abstr.), *Neurology,* 2, 388, 1977.

20. **Terrance, C. F. and Rao, G.,** Neuropathologic correlation of computerized tomography in Huntington's disease, *South Med. J.,* 73, 817, 1980.

21. **Terrence, C. F., Delaney, J. F., and Alberts, M. C.,** Computed tomography for Huntington's disease, *Neuroradiology,* 13, 173, 1977.

22. **Neophytides, A. N., DiChiro, G., Barron, S. A., and Chase, T. N.,** Computed axial tomography in Huntington's disease and persons at risk for Huntington's disease, *Adv. Neurol.,* 23, 185, 1979.

23. **Barr, A. N., Heinze, W. J., Dobben, G. D., Valvassori, G. E., and Sugar, O.,** Bicaudate index in computerized tomography of Huntington's disease and cerebral atrophy, *Neurology,* 28, 1196, 1978.

24. **Hattori, H., Takao, T., Ito, M., Nakano, S., Okuno, T., and Mikawa, H.,** Cerebellum and brain stem atrophy in a child with Huntington's disease, *Comp. Radiol.,* 8, 53, 1984.

25. **Bianco, F., Bozzao, L., Rizzo, P. A., and Morocutti, C.,** Cerebellar atrophy in Huntington's disease, *Acta Neurol. (Napoli),* 36, 425, 1981.

26. **Lang, C.** Is direct CT caudatometry superior to indirect parameters in confirming Huntington's disease, *Neuroradiology,* 27, 161, 1985.

27. **Mazziotta, J. C., Phelps, M. E., Pahl, J. J., Huang, S. C., Baxter, L. R., Riege, W. H., Hoffman, J. M., Kuhl, D. E., Lanto, A. B., Wapenski, J. A., and Markham, C. H.,** Reduced cerebral glucose metabolism in asymptomatic subjects at risk for Huntington's disease, *N. Eng. J. Med.,* 316, 357, 1987.

28. **Kotagal, S., Shuter, E., and Horenstein, S.,** Chorea as a manifestation of bilateral subdural hematoma in an elderly man, *Arch. Neurol.,* 38, 195, 1981.

29. **Bean, S. C. and Ladisch, S.,** Chorea associate with a subdural hematoma in a child with leukemia, *J. Pediatr.,* 90, 225, 1977.

30. **Gilmore, P. C. and Brenner, R. P.,** Chorea: a late complication of subdural hematoma, *Neurology,* 29, 1044, 1979.

31. **Drayer, B. P.,** Magnetic resonance imaging and brain iron: implications in the diagnosis and pathochemistry of movement disorders and dementia, *BNI Q.,* 3, 15, 1987.

32. **Kozachuk, W., Salanga, V., Conomy, J., and Smith, A.,** MRI (magnetic resonance imaging) in Huntington's disease, *Neurology,* 36 (Suppl. 1), 310, 1986.

33. **Simmons, J. T., Pastakia, B., Chase, T. N., and Schults, C. W.,** Magnetic resonance imaging in Huntington's disease, *AJNR,* 7, 25, 1986.

34. **Sax, D. S. Buonanno, F. S., Kramer, C., Miatto, O., Kistler, J. P., Martin, J. B., and Brady, T. J.,** Proton nuclear magnetic resonance imaging in Huntington's disease, *Ann. Neurol.,* 18, 142, 1985.

35. **Lukes, S. A., Aminoff, M. J., Crooks, L., Kaufman, L., Mills, C., and Newton, T. H.,** Nuclear magnetic resonance imaging in movement disorders, *Ann. Neurol.* 13, 690, 1983.

36. **Bydder, G. M. Stein, R. E., Young, I. R., Hall, A. S., Thomas, D. J., Marshall, J., Pallis, C. A., and Legg, N. J.,** Clinical NMR imaging of the brain: 140 cases, *AJNR,* 139, 215, 1982.

37. **Sax, D. S. and Buonanno, S.,** Putaminal changes in spin-echo magnetic resonance imaging signal in bradykinetic/rigid forms of Huntington's disease, *Neurology,* 36 (Suppl. 1), 311, 1986.

38. **Pettegrew, J. W., Kopp, S. J., Dadok, J., Minshew, N. J., Feliksik, J. M., and Glonek, T.,** Chemical characterization of a prominent phosphorylmonoester resonance in animal, Huntington, and Alzheimer Brain: phosphorus 31 and hydrogen 1 nuclear magnetic resonance analysis at 4.1 and 14.1 tesla, *Ann. Neurol.,* 16, 136, 1984.

39. **Kuhl, D. E., Phelps, M. E., Markham, C. H., Metter, E. J., Riege, W. H., and Winter, J.** Cerebral metabolism and atrophy in Huntington's disease determined by 18-FDG and computed tomographic scan, *Ann. Neurol.,* 12, 425, 1982.

40. **Young, A. B., Penney, J. B., Starosta-Rubenstein, S., Markel, D. S., Berent, S., Giordani, B., Ehrenkaufer, R., Jewett, D., and Hichwa, R.,** PET scan investigations of Huntington's disease: cerebral metabolic correlates of neurologic features and functional decline, *Ann. Neurol.,* 20, 296, 1986.

41. **Stober, T., Beil, C., Thielen, T., Emser, W., Pawlik, G., and Heiss, W. D.,** Isoniazid therapy in Huntington's disease: clinico-electrophysiologic-metabolic correlation, *Neurology,* 36 (Suppl. 1) 311, 1986.

42. **Hayden, M. R., Martin, W. R. W., Stoessl, A. J., Clark, C., Hollenberg, S., Adam, M. J., Ammann, W., Harrop, R., Rogers, J., Ruth, T., Sayre, C., and Pate, B. D.,** Positron emission tomography in the early diagnosis of Huntington's disease, *Neurology,* 36, 888, 1986.

43. **Young, A. B., Penney, J. B., Markel, D. S. Starosta-Rubenstein, S., Rothley, J., and Betley, A.,** Glucose metabolism in juvenile Huntington's disease: comparison with adult onset cases (abstr.), *Neurology,* 38, 360, 1988.

44. **Clark, C. M., Hayden, M. R., Stoessl, A. J., and Martin, W. R. W.,** Regression model for predicting dissociations of regional cerebral glucose metabolism in individuals at risk for Huntington's disease, *J. Cereb. Blood Flow Metab.,* 6, 756, 1986.

45. **Young, A. B., Penney, J. B., Starosta-Rubenstein, S., Markel, D., Berent, S., Rothley, J., Betley, A., and Hichwa, R.,** Normal caudate glucose metabolism in persons at risk for Huntington's disease, *Arch. Neurol.,* 44, 254, 1987.

46. **Hayden, M., Hewitt, B. S. C., Stoessl, A. J., Clark, C., Ammann, W., and Martin, W. R. W.,** The combined use of positron emission tomography and DNA polymorphisms for preclinical detection of Huntington's disease, *Neurology,* 37, 1441, 1987.

47. **Mazziotta, J. C., Wapenski, J., Phelps, M. E., Riege, W. H., Baxter, L. R., Fullerton, A., Kuhl, D. E., Selin, C., and Sumida, R.,** Cerebral glucose utilization and blood flow in Huntington's disease: symptomatic and at risk subjects, *J. Cereb. Blood Flow Metab.,* 5 (Suppl. 1), S25, 1985.

48. **Leenders, K. L., Frackowiak, R. S. J., Quinn, N., and Marsden, C. D.,** Brain energy metabolism and dopaminergic function in Huntington's disease measured *in vivo* using positron emission tomography, *Movement Disorders,* 1, 69, 1986.

49. **Smith, F. W., Besson, J. A. O., Gemmell. H. G., and Sharp, P. F.** The use of technetium-99m-HM-PAO in the assessment of patients with dementia and other neuropsychiatric conditions, *J. Cereb. Blood Flow Metab.,* 8, S116, 1988.

50. **Lassen, N. A.,** Single photon emission computed tomography, in *Adv. Clin. Neuroimaging,* Mazziotta, J. C. and Gilman, S., Eds., F. A. Davis, Philadelphia, in press.

51. **Garnett, E. S., Firnau, G., Nahmias, C., Carbotte, R. and Bartolucci, G.,** Reduced striatal glucose consumption and prolonged reaction time are early features in HD, *J. Neurol. Sci.,* 65, 231, 1984.

52. **Mazziotta, J. C., Phelps, M. E., Plummer, D., and Kuhl, D. E.,** Quantitation in positron emission computed tomography. V. Physical-anatomical effects, *J. Comput. Assist. Tomogr.,* 5, 734, 1981.

53. **Penney, J. B. and Young, A. B.** Speculations on the functional anatomy of basal ganglia disorders, *Annu. Rev. Neurosci.,* 6, 73, 1983.

54. **Phillips, P. C., Brin, M. F., Fahn, S., Greene, P. E., Sidtis, J. J., Ragass, J., Krol, G., Moeller, J. R., Sergi, M. L., and Rottenberg, D. A.** Abnormal regional cerebral glucose metabolism in choreoacanthocytosis: an F-18-fluoro-deoxyglucose positron emission tomographic study, *Neurology,* 37 (Suppl. 1), 211, 1987.

55. **Martin, W. R. W., Hayden, M. R., Suchowersky, O., Beckman, J., Adam, M., Ammann, W., Bergstrom, M., Harrop, R., Rogers, J., Ruth, T., Sayre, C., and Pate, B. D.** Striatal metabolism in Huntington's disease and in benign herediatary chorea, *Ann. Neurol.,* 16, 126, 1984.

56. **Suchowersky, O., Hayden, M. R., Martin, W. R. W., Stoessl, A. J., Hildebrand, A. M., and Pate, B. D.,** Cerebral metabolism of glucose in benign hereditary chorea, *Movement Disorders,* 1, 33, 1986.

57. **Palella, T. D., Hichwa, R. D., Ehrenkaufer, R. L., Rothley, J. M., McQuillan, M. A., Young, A. B., and Kelley, W. N.,** 18-F Fluorodeoxyglucose PET scanning in HPRT deficiency, *Am. J. Hum. Genet.,* 37, A70, 1981.

58. **Guttman, M., Lang, A. E., Garnett, E. S., Nahmias, C., Firnau, G., Tyndel, F. J., and Gordon, A. S.,** Cerebral glucose metabolism in SLE chorea: further evidence that striatal hypometabolism is not a correlate of chorea, *Movement Disorders,* 2(3) 201, 1987.

59. **Pahl, J. J., Mazziotta, J. C. Cummings, J., Bartzokis, G., Marder, S., Schwab, R., Sumida, R., Kuhl, D. E., Baxter, L. R. and Phelps, M. E,** Positron emission tomography in tardive dyskinesia and Huntington's disease: LCMRGlc in two patient populations with chorea (abstr.), *J. Cereb. Blood Flow Metab,* 7 (Suppl. 1), S373, 1987.

60. **Pahl, J. P., Mazziotta, J. C., Bartzokis, G., Cummings, J., Altschuler, L., Mintz, J., Marder, S. M., and Phelps, M. E.,** Positron emission tomography in tardive dyskinesia, *Arch. Gen. Psychol.,* submitted.

61. **Stoessl, A. J., Martin, W. R. W., Hayden, M. R., Adam, M. J., and Ruth, T. J.,** Dopamine in Huntington's disease: studies using positron emission tomography (abstr.), *Neurology,* 36 (Suppl. 1), 310, 1986.

62. **Wong, D. F., Links, J. M., Wagner, H. N., Folstein, S. E., Suneja, S., Dannals, R. F., Ravert, H. T., Wilson, A. A., Tune, L. E., Pearlson, G., Folstein, M. F., Bice, A., and Kuhar, M. J.,** Dopamine and serotonin receptors measured *in vivo* in Huntington's disease with C-11 N-methylspiperone PET imaging, *J. Nucl. Med.*, 26, 107, 1985.

63. **Hagglund, J., Aquilonius, S. M., Eckernas, S. A., Hartvig, P., Lundquist, H., Gullberg, P., and Langstrom, B.,** Dopamine receptor properties in Parkinson's disease and Huntington's chorea evaluated by positron emission tomography using C-11 N-methylspiperone, *Acta Neurol. Scand.*, 75, 87, 1987.

64. **Leenders, K. L., Frackowiak, R. S. J., Quinn, N. and Marsden, C. D.** Brain energy metabolism and dopaminergic function in Huntington's disease measured *in vivo* using positron emission tomography, *Movement Disorders*, 1, 69, 1986.

65. **Bird, E. D.,** Chemical pathology of Huntington's disease, *Annu. Rev. Pharmacol. Toxicol.*, 20, 533, 1980.

66. **Reisine, T. D., Fields, J. Z., Bird, E. D., Spokes, E., and Yamamura, H. I.,** Characterization of brain dopaminergic receptors in Huntington's disease, *Commun. Psycho-Pharmacol.*, 2, 79, 1978.

67. **Mazziotta, J. C., Pahl, J. J., Phelps, M. E., Baxter, L. R., Riege, W. H., Hoffman, J. M., Huang, S. C., Gusella, J., Hyslop, P., Schwab, R., Selin, C., Sumida, R., Kuhl, D. E., Wapenski, J., Conneally, M., and Markham, C. H.,** Presymptomatic evaluation of subjects at risk for Huntington's disease (HD): PET and DNA polymorphism studies (abstr.), *J. Cereb. Blood Flow Metab.*, 7 (Suppl. 1), S366, 1987.

68. **Young, A. B., Penney, J. B., Markel, D. S., Hollingsworth, Z., Teener, J., and Stern, J.** Genetic linkage analysis, glucose metabolism and neurological examination: comparison in persons at risk for Huntington's disease (abstr.), *Neurology*, 38, 359, 1988.

69. **Garnett, E. S., Firnau, G., Nahmias, C., Carbotte, R., and Bartolucci, G.,** Reduced striatal glucose consumption and prolonged reaction time are early features in Huntington's disease, *J. Neurol. Sci.*, 65, 231, 1984.

70. **Mazziotta, J. C., Phelps, M. E., Pahl, J. J., Huang, S. C., Baxter, L. R., Hoffman, J. M., Markham, C. H., Riege, W. H., and Lanto, A. B.** Studies of persons at risk for Huntington's disease, *N. Eng. J. Med.*, 317, 382, 1987.

71. **Koh, J. Y., Peters, S., and Choi, D. W.,** Neurons containing NADPH-diaphorase are selectively resistant to quinolinate toxicity, *Science*, 234, 73, 1986.

72. **Saris, S.,** Corea caused by caudate infarction, *Arch. Neurol.*, 40, 590, 1983.

73. **Penney, J. B. and Young, A. B.,** Quantitative autoradiography of neurotransmitter receptors in Huntington's disease, *Neurology*, 32, 1391, 1982.

74. **Young, A. D., Greenamyer, J. T., Hollingsworth, Z., Albin, R., D'Amato, C., Shoulson, I., and Penney, J. B.,** NMDA receptor losses in putamen from patients with Huntington's disease, *Science*, 241, 981, 1988.

Chapter 11

CLINICAL MANAGEMENT OF HUNTINGTON'S DISEASE: THE ROLE OF PET AND DNA LINKAGE STUDIES

Michael R. Hayden and Walter Ammann

TABLE OF CONTENTS

I. INTRODUCTION

The abnormalities seen with structural and functional imaging studies in Huntington's disease (HD) have been discussed in the preceding chapter. This chapter will discuss the clinical diagnosis and the potential role to be played by the combination of functional imaging and DNA studies in the management of symptomatic patients with and asymptomatic individuals at risk for HD.

II. THE CLINICAL PHENOTYPE

The diagnosis of HD depends on establishing a positive family history and on a detailed clinical assessment. The cardinal clinical features, involuntary movements associated with cognitive impairment, are almost always present in patients with established disease. The clinical diagnosis, however, can be much less clear in patients in the early stages of illness where the broad spectrum of clinical manifestations may result in misdiagnosis.[1,2]

The disease frequently presents with subtle mental changes. These alterations take the form of a change in personality with irritability, irascibility, impulsiveness, and depression as predominant features. Frank psychosis may herald the onset of HD.

Before the onset of involuntary movements, significant alterations in voluntary movements are frequently seen. Rapid alternative movements of the hands may be impaired. Some patients have dysrhythmic speech. A characteristic early sign is difficulty in maintaining constant pressure when squeezing two of the examiner's fingers for a constant period (the milkmaid's sign). Most patients are unable to maintain tongue protrusion without the advent of choreiform movements. Tandem walking often evokes a mild ataxia with abnormal movements which are not present at rest. Objective physical findings may be minimal, but disturbances in functional ability are often present, the most common being jerkiness, clumsiness, or mild incoordination. Lack of smoothness of eye movements and saccades are other early signs.

Chorea eventually becomes apparent in most patients and progresses inexorably. The face, trunk, and extremities are usually affected. Facial movements are often seen and produce a typical appearance with pouting of the lips, twitching of the cheeks, and irregular elevation of the eyebrows. When sitting, constant movement of the hands and legs is common. The legs are alternately crossed and uncrossed. In contrast to other choreiform movement disorders, the chorea in Huntington's disease is generally slower and more athetoid.

Increased deep tendon reflexes occur at the outset in at least 50% of persons. Other signs of pyramidal dysfunction become more prominent with time. Increased tone becomes frequent, and hypertonicity may predominate. There is a progressive evolution toward a rigid state. Slowness of speech occurs early, and eventually disorganization of speech and finally mutism supervene. Dysphagia is a late sign and occurs in patients with either predominant chorea or rigidity. Dystonic features are a common feature of advanced Huntington's disease.

III. GENETICS

Huntingon's disease is inherited as an autosomal dominant trait. The gene is fully penetrant and, therefore, all persons who inherit the mutant gene will manifest signs and symptoms if they live long enough. A polymorphic DNA marker has been described that is closely linked to the HD gene.[3] This marker has been mapped to the tip of the short arm of chromosome 4 (4p16), which indicates the approximate location of the gene for HD.[4,5] More recently, other genetic markers (D4S62, D4S95) in the region of the HD gene have also been described.[6,7]

The discovery of the linked marker has resulted in the development of pilot programs

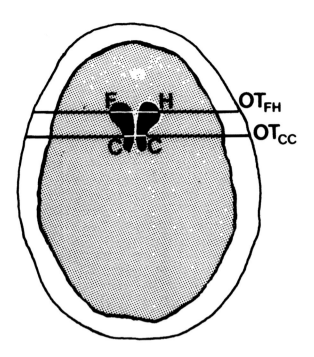

FIGURE 1. Computed tomography measurements used for assessing caudate nucleus size. FH is the largest frontal horn span; CC, the bicaudate diameter, is the shortest transverse distance between medial borders of the caudate nuclei; OT_{FH} and OT_{CC} are the distance between the outer tables of the skull at the level of the FH and CC lines, respectively. (From Hayden, M. R., *Huntington's Chorea*, Springer-Verlag, New York, 1981. With permission.)

for predictive testing of HD.[8,9] For the DNA test to be useful, however, numerous relatives including affected and unaffected persons must be tested. Using a combination of three DNA probes, persons will only rarely be excluded by virtue of limitations of the technology. The major obstacle to the implementation of routine DNA testing for HD is the unavailability of DNA from crucial family relatives.[10]

IV. PATHOLOGY

The characteristic pathologic finding in HD is widespread neuronal loss affecting mainly the caudate and putamen.[11] Within the striatum, the gamma-aminobutyric acid (GABA) and the cholinergic spiny neurons are selectively vulnerable while the type II aspiny neurons containing somatostatin, neuropeptide Y, and NADPH-diaphorase are spared.[12] As neuronal loss progresses, caudate atrophy develops. A sensitive *in vivo* measure of caudate nucleus atrophy is the ratio between the greatest distance between the frontal horns and the shortest distance between the heads of the caudate nuclei on X-ray computed tomography.[13] (Figure 1) This ratio (FH/CC) must be assessed with regard to age with which there is a significant inverse relationship.[14] (Figure 2) Caudate nucleus atrophy usually postdates the clinical onset of the disease. In the earliest phase of HD, the FH/CC ratio is most often normal.

V. POSITRON EMISSION TOMOGRAPHY IN THE DIAGNOSIS OF HUNTINGTON'S DISEASE

Pioneer studies of regional cerebral glucose utilization (CMRGlu) with positron emission tomography (PET) in HD were performed by Kuhl et al.[15] They found a significant decrease

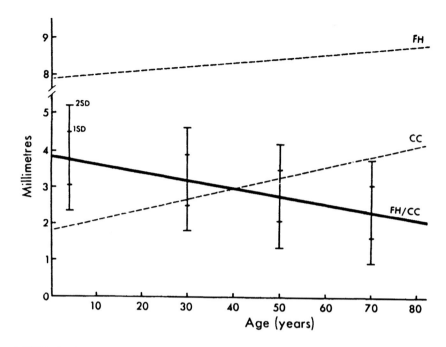

FIGURE 2.   The FH/CC ratio shows an inverse relationship with age. (From Hayden, M. R. et al., *Neurology,* 36, 888, 1986. With permission.)

in relative CMRGlu in the caudate nuclei of patients with established HD. We initially studied ten patients with early HD who had no significant caudate nucleus atrophy and had not received any medication. Of the ten patients, six had caudate metabolism which was 3 SD below the mean control value while the remaining four patients had values between 2 and 3 SD below the control mean.[14]

We have now measured CMRGlu with PET in 19 persons with early HD (less than 5 year duration) and no significant caudate nucleus atrophy, and 13 persons with HD of greater than 5 years duration. The results are summarized in Tables 1 and 2 and Figures 3, 4, and 5. In our conrols, a decrease of CMRGlu in all regions of the brain in subjects greater than 45 years of age as compared to subjects less than 45 years of age was evident, although this decrease did not reach statistical significance (Table 1).

Of 32 patients with clinically diagnosed HD, 31 had caudate metabolism and caudate/thalamic and caudate/global metabolic ratios more than 2 SD below mean control values. One patient had caudate metabolism 2 SD below the age-matched control mean but had caudate/thalamic ratios close to and caudate/global ratios well below 3 SD below the age-matched control mean (Figures' 3, 4, 5). This patient had no chorea but had mild clumsiness with alternating hand movements associated with slight slowness of pursuit eye movements on examination.

In the patients with early HD, 8 of 19 had absolute caudate metabolic rates between 2 and 3 SD below the mean of age-matched control values while 11 had caudate metabolism at lease 3 SD below the control mean. One patient had CMRGlu equivalent to 2 SD below the age-matched control mean as noted previously. Similarly 5 of 19 patients had caudate/thalamic rations between 2 and 3 SD below the age-matched control mean with 13 patients having values more than 3 SD below the control mean. One patient had a caudate/thalamic ratio between 1 and 2 SD of controls. Caudate/global ratios showed still less overlap with only 4 of 19 patients with early HD having a caudate/global ratio between 2 and 3 SD below

TABLE 1
Mean CMRGlu in Different Subject Groups

Subject Groups		Age (Year)	Regional glucose metabolism (mg/100 g/min)				
			Caudate	Thalamus	Global	Caudate/ thalamus	Caudate/ global
Normals	Mean	26.3	7.57	7.38	6.74	1.03	1.12
(N = 13)	SD	5.8	0.84	0.75	0.70	0.09	0.04
Normals	Mean	63.4	6.75	6.91	5.81	0.99	1.15
(N = 13)	SD	11.0	0.77	1.13	0.43	0.09	0.07
Early HD[a]	Mean	43.0	4.79	6.91	5.71	0.71	0.85
(N = 19)	SD	10.0	0.71	1.32	0.95	0.11	0.11
Late HD[b]	Mean	49.9	3.72	5.85	4.70	0.63	0.79
(N = 13)	SD	18.2	0.91	0.81	0.90	0.14	0.15
AD	Mean	65.9	5.72	6.02	4.76	0.95	1.20
(N = 28)	SD	9.0	0.92	1.03	0.66	0.09	0.13
PD	Mean	69.4	4.56	4.50	3.93	1.03	1.17
(N = 5)	SD	7.3	1.07	1.24	0.99	0.08	0.10
Depression	Mean	26.2	6.93	6.63	6.05	1.05	1.14
(N = 5)	SD	4.0	0.64	0.94	0.57	0.10	0.04

Note: HD = Huntington's Disease; AD = Alzheimer's Disease; PD = Parkinson's Disease

[a] Duration of symptoms less than 5 years.
[b] Duration of symptoms more than 5 years.

TABLE 2
Metabolic Changes in Symptomatic HD and Normal Controls

	Caudate CMRGlu		Caudate/thalamic metabolic ratio		Caudate/global metabolic ratio	
	Early HD	Late HD	Early HD	Late HD	Early HD	Late HD
Values 1—2 SD < controls	1	0	0	1	0	0
Values 2—3 SD < controls	8	1	6	1	1	1
Values <3 SD of controls	11	12	14	11	19	12

the control mean and the remaining 15 having values more than 3 SD below the control mean (Table 3).

Our findings show the importance of calculating the relative metabolic rates of glucose utilization as well as absolute rates. The caudate/whole slice ratio appears to have the greatest value in separating HD from controls followed by the caudate/thalamic and absolute caudate CMRGlu. All patients with HD had at least two of these three measurements of caudate metabolism which were 2 SD or more below the mean of age-matched controls.

VI. HOW SPECIFIC ARE THE PET FINDINGS TO HUNTINGTON'S DISEASE?

The demonstration of striatal hypometabolism of glucose is not only seen in HD. Similar findings hae been found in persons with benign hereditary chorea,[16] the Lesch-Nyhan syndrome,[17] and choreacanthocytosis.[18] In contrast, patients with systemic lupus erythematosus and chorea have normal striatal metabolism showing that striatal hypometabolism is not an invariant accompaniment of chorea.[19] Furthermore, some persons with tardive dyskinesia have striatal hypermetabolism.[20]

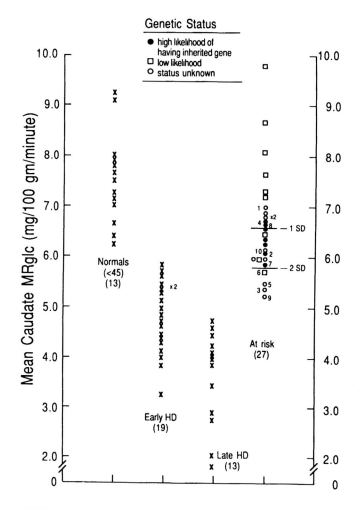

FIGURE 3.   Absolute caudate glucose metabolism in normals (age <45 years; n = 13), patients with early HD (clinical manifestations for <5 years; n = 19) and late HD (clinical manifestations for >5 years; n = 13), and those at risk for HD (n = 27). The genetic status of at risk individuals is shown. −1SD and −2SD represent levels compared to the mean of control values.

The progression of the disease and associated clinical features readily differentiates HD from these disorders. A clearly established family history of HD, preferably confirmed by autopsy studies, is therefore crucial prior to interpretation of PET studies. However, even if there is an established family history of HD, it is important to know whether other common neurological or psychiatric disorders which may occur incidently in families with HD can be confused with HD on PET investigation. This is particularly important when trying to develop appropriate guidelines for the use of PET in persons at risk for HD. Disorders which have occasionally been misdiagnosed as HD include Alzheimer's disease (AD), Parkinson's disease (PD), and depression.

We compared the PET results obtained in our first 21 affected HD patients, 26 persons at risk for HD by virtue of having an affected parent, 28 persons with clinically diagnosed AD, 5 patients with PD, 5 patients with depression, and 26 normal age-matched controls. Regions of interest used in this study were the left and right caudate nuclei, the left and right thalamic nuclei and the left and right inferior parietal regions. The inferior parietal

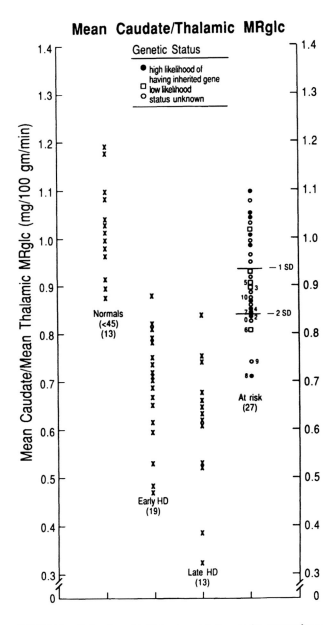

FIGURE 4. Ratio of caudate/thalamic metabolism in the same patients shown in Figures 3 and 5. In at risk patient 6, the abnormal caudate metabolism is thought to provide evidence for recombination between the marker and the HD gene itself (i.e., a "false negative" result on DNA analysis).

region was chosen as an additional discriminating parameter to aid in the differentiation of HD from AD. Global (whole slice) metabolism was also measured.

Our findings show that 8 of 28 AD patients had absolute caudate CMRGlu (Figure 6) which was more than 2 SD below the age-matched control mean. Similarly 3 of 6 PD patients had abnormal caudate CMRGlu. However, in both AD and PD, the siginficant decrease in local caudate CMRGlu is part of a global decrease in cerebral glucose metabolism, so that the use of relative rates of CMRGlu provides much improved discrimination between HD and AD on the one hand and HD and PD on the other. Only two patients with clearly

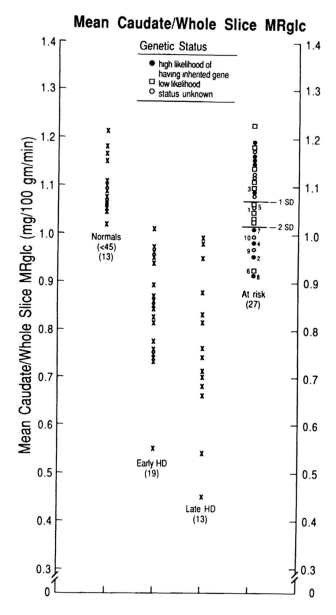

FIGURE 5.   Ratio of caudate/whole slice metabolism in the same patients shown in Figures 3 and 4.

TABLE 3
Persons At Risk with Abnormal PET Results

	Caudate CMRGlu	Caudate/thalamus metabolic ratio	Caudate/global metabolic ratio
Patient number with values less than 2 SD of controls	3,5,9,6	6,8,9	3,4,6,7,8,9,10

Note: Numbers refer to patient numbers as seen in Figures 3, 4, and 5.

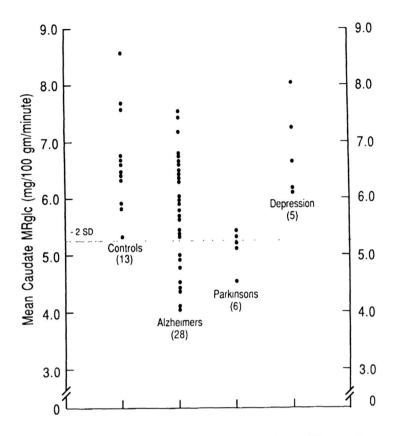

FIGURE 6. Absolute caudate glucose metabolism in controls (n = 13), and patients with Alzheimer's disease (n = 28), Parkinson's disease (n = 6), and depression (n = 5).

established AD had an abnormal caudate/global metabolic ratio; no patients with either AD or PD had abnormal (i.e., more than 2 SD below the mean) caudate/thalamic ratios (Figures 7 and 8).

These findings show that absolute caudate CMRGlu when used in isolation is inadequate in the differentiation of HD from Alzheimer's and Parkinson's diseases. The most useful indices for diagnosis and differentiation of HD from the other disorders remain the relative metabolic rates as expressed by caudate/thalamic and caudate/global ratio.

VII. STUDIES OF PERSONS AT RISK FOR HUNTINGTON'S DISEASE

The first step toward assessment of a test for preclinical detection of HD is to examine its role in the diagnosis and differentiation of HD from other disorders. As described above, the most sensitive parameters for an abnormal scan are the relative metabolic rates of glucose in the caudate. We have now examined 27 at risk persons by PET. All persons were clinically evaluated by two qualified examiners who found no clinical abnormalities. In particular, none of these persons had chorea, eye movements were normal, and there was no impairment of voluntary movement. Formal neuropsychological and neuroophthalmological examinations were not performed. Abnormal values were defined as those which were more than 2 SD below the age-matched control mean. Seven persons at risk had a normal caudate/global CMRGlu while four persons had abnormal absolute caudate metabolism (Figure 5) and three persons had abnormal caudate; thalamic ratios (Figure 4).[21]

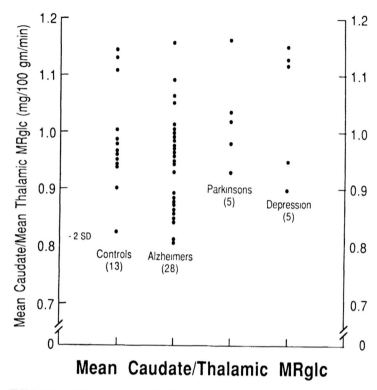

FIGURE 7.   Ratio of caudate/thalamic metabolism in the same patients shown in Figures 6 and 8.

The important question to be answered is what is the significance of these results and what can we reasonably tell an at risk person who wishes to know the scan results. Clearly, great caution must be maintained before PET studies can be recommended as a generally applicable useful service for at risk persons. Stringent criteria for assignment of an abnormal result must be applied. Currently, we regard at least two indices of caudate glucose metabolism more than 2 SD below the mean as abnormal in the presence of a positive family history of HD with no signs or symptoms of any other disease, as highly suggestive of the presence of the HD gene. Three persons (numbers 6, 8, and 9 on Figures 4 and 5) fell into this category. However, we are developing and expanding a previously reported prediction model [22] that will combine all the data and provide a probability estimate as to whether the results in a given individual are more compatible with HD or with normality.

VIII. THE COMBINATION OF TWO TECHNOLOGIES: PET AND DNA LINKAGE STUDIES IN HUNTINGTON'S DISEASE

The finding of a human DNA-linked polymorphic marker for HD has made it possible to divide the at risk population into those who are likely to be presymptomatic heterozygotes for the disorder and those unlikely to have inherited the abnormal gene. The use of linked DNA markers in such studies is limited by errors due to recombination and due to some proportion of affected persons not being heterozygous for the DNA marker. The combination of linked markers for predictive testing has significantly reduced these limitations. Furthermore, using a combination of probes, none of the 50 control individuals were homozygous for all the markers. The most significant current limitations to predictive testing using linked DNA markers is the absence of blood from crucial relatives, as such samples are necessary to determine which phase of the marker segregates with the mutant gene for HD.

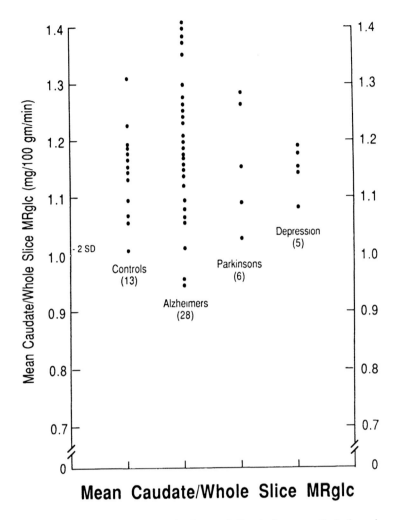

FIGURE 8. Ratio of caudate/whole slice metabolism in the same patients shown in Figures 6 and 7.

We have examined and reported on results in four large families with HD with numerous affected and at risk subjects available so that informative DNA analysis was likely.[21] The correlations between PET and DNA results in 13 at risk subjects are shown in Table 4. An abnormal PET result is defined by caudate/thalamic and/or caudate/global metabolic ratios more than 2 SD below age-matched control values. This is, in most instances, associated with an absolute caudate CMRGlu which is more than 2 SD below an age matched control value.

It is not surprising that metabolic changes precede clinical signs in some persons at risk for HD. In other genetic disorders causing neurological dysfunction, clinical changes are often preceded by changes detected by special investigations. For example, EMG abnormalities may precede the clinical signs in persons with hereditary motor sensory neuropathy. At the present time, the temporal pattern of changes of caudate metabolism in persons at risk is unknown. Repeated studies which document the natural history of changes in CMRGlu in persons at risk for HD together with detailed clinical assessment will help determine the expected interval between the first abnormal findings on PET and the clinical onset of the disease.

There is not complete agreement, however, on the finding that metabolic changes precede

TABLE 4
Correlations Between PET and DNA Results in Asymptomatic At Risk Subjects

	Normal PET study	Abnormal PET study	Total
DNA results indicating >90% probability of developing HD	5	3	8
DNA results indicating >79% probability of not developing HD	4	1	5
Total	9	4	13

clinical onset in HD. Mazziotta and co-workers at UCLA have shown reduced caudate to whole slice ratios in 18 of 58 subjects at risk for HD.[23] In our study 7 of 27 persons had similarly abnormal caudate metabolism. In contrast, Young et al. at the University of Michigan have not found any variance from normal values in their study of 29 persons at risk for HD.[24]

There are numerous possible explanations for these apparent discrepancies.[25] The method of analysis of the data between the first two groups on the one hand and the latter group on the other were different. The variation of PET results was greater in the Michigan study such that at least one patient with early HD had relative caudate metabolism within 2 SD of the age-matched control mean whereas no persons with HD in the UBC or UCLA studies had normal relative caudate metabolism. It could be argued that the persons included in the at risk group at UBC and UCLA already had subtle clinical findings. In our study, detailed neurological examination was targeted towards detecting early changes of HD. Disturbances of voluntary movements, included eye movements, complex movements of facial muscles, alternating movements of the hands and tandem walking were carefully assessed. Formal neuropsychological evaluation was not routinely undertaken. Based on this assessment, subjects in the at risk group did not have any such signs such that one was able to make or strongly suspect a diagnosis of HD. The mean age of the Michigan group was younger than that in the other two groups; the normal findings may reflect that the persons in that group were further away from the age of onset of clinical symptoms.

A normal PET scan for someone at risk does not indicate that they will never develop HD in the future. One can, however, clearly state that at the present time, no measurable metabolic changes indicative of HD are evident. For some at risk persons who fear that they may already be showing symptoms, a normal PET scan may provide considerable relief.

The finding that PET changes are present prior to clinical onset in some patients allows one to develop a model for the pathogenesis of HD (Figure 9). In all individuals, there is a decrease in caudate metabolism with age. In persons who have inherited the disease, the process appears to be hastened prematurely due to the effects of the gene product. When the metabolic rates have reached a critical level, clinical symptoms appear. What is unclear is the shape of the curve of glucose metabolism rates prior to clinical onset. However, the finding of normal glucose metabolism in some persons who have a high likelihood of having inherited the gene suggests that the effect of the gene product is to alter caudate function closer to the clinical onset of the disease.

IX. FUTURE NEEDS AND DIRECTIONS

The finding that metabolic changes precede structural cell loss in HD offers the hope that treatment directed appropriately at the metabolic defect might halt further cell loss and possibly restore some cells facing imminent death. In other words, it may be possible to intervene when a deviation from the expected curve for glucose metabolic rates in the caudate appears. Ideally, at risk persons who are found to have a high risk of developing HD on the basis of DNA studies could have PET scans at well-spaced intervals. When significant

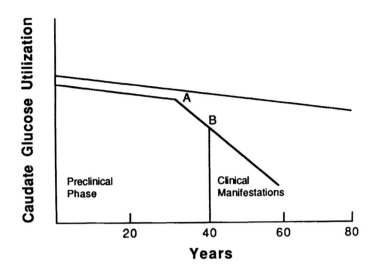

FIGURE 9. Proposed relationship between caudate metabolism, age, and the development of clinically overt HD. The upper line shows a slow decrease in caudate metabolism occuring as a function of age. The lower line shows the caudate metabolism in an asymptomatic gene carrier. That patient studied before point A will have normal caudate metabolism. The same individual studied between points A and B will have decreased caudate metabolism but remain asymptomatic. At point B, the threshold for the development of clinical symptoms is crossed.

changes in caudate CMRGlu occur, appropriate pharmacological interventions could be started. Furthermore, patients with HD could be monitored for failure of the expected reduction of caudate metabolism which might provide evidence for the efficacy of a particular pharmacological intervention. Clearly, what is needed is knowledge concerning the normal variation in caudate metabolism and the expected pattern of decline in persons affected with HD and in subjects at risk as they get closer to the clinical onset. Once this information is at hand, determination of cerebral glucose metabolism should provide a direct, noninvasive method for determining the efficacy of drug therapy in HD.

REFERENCES

1. **Hayden, M. R.**, *Huntington's Chorea*, Springer-Verlag, New York, 1981.
2. **Martin, J. B. and Gusella, J. F.**, Huntington's disease, pathogenesis and management, *N. Engl. J. Med.*, 315, 1267, 1986.
3. **Gusella, J. F., Wexler, N. S., Conneally, P. M., Naylor, S. G., Anderson, M. R., Sakaguchi, A. Y., Young, A. B., Shoulson, I., Bonilla, E., and Martin, J. B.**, A polymorphic marker genetically linked to Huntington's disease, *Nature*, 30, 234, 1983.
4. **Wong, H. D., Greenberg, C. R., Hewitt, J., Kalousek, D., and Hayden, M. R.**, Subregional assignment of the linked marker G8 (D4S10) for Huntington disease to choromosome 4p161-163, *Am. J. Hum. Genet.*, 39, 392, 1986.
5. **Gusella, J. F., Tanzi, R. E., Bader, P. J., Phelan, M. C., Stevenson, R., Hayden, M. R., Hoffman, K. J., Faryniarz, A. G., and Gibbons, K.**, Deletion of Huntington's disease linked G8 (D4S10) locus in Wolf-Hirschorn Syndrome, *Nature*, 318, 75, 1985.
6. **Hayden, M. R., Hewitt, J., Wasmuth, J. J., Langlois, S., Kastelein, J. J., Haines, J., Smith, B., Conneally, M., Hilbert, C., and Allard, D.**, A polymorphic marker which represents a conserved expressed sequence in the region of the Huntington disease gene, *Am. J. Hum. Genet.*, 42, 125, 1988.

7. **Wasmuth, J. J., Hewitt, J., Smith, B., Allard, D., Haines, J. L., Skarecky, D., Partlow, E., and Hayden, M. R.**, A highly polymorphic locus very tightly linked to the Huntington's disease gene, *Nature,* 332, 734, 1988.

8. **Fox, S., Bloch, M., Fahy, M., and Hayden, M. R.**, Predictive testing for Huntington disease. I. Description of a pilot project in British Columbia, *Am. J. Med. Genet.,* 32, 211, 1989.

9. **Meissen, G. J., Myers, R. H., Mastromauro, L. A., Koroshetz, W. J., Klinger, K. W., Farrer, L. A., Watkins, P. A., Gusella, J. F., Bird, E. D., and Martin, J. B.**, Predictive testing for Huntington disease with use of a linked DNA marker, *N. Engl. J. Med.,* 318, 533, 1988.

10. **Hayden, M. R., Allard, D., Haines, J., Hilbert, C., Robbins, C., Hewitt, J., Wasmuth, J. J., Fox, S., and Bloch, M.**, Improved predictive testing for Huntington disease using three linked DNA markers, *Am. J. Hum. Genet.,* 43, 689, 1988.

11. **Vonsattel, J. R., Myers, R. H., Stevens, T. J., Ferante, R. J., Bird, E. D., and Richardson, E. P.**, Neuropathological classification of Huntington's disease, *J. Neuropathol. Exp. Neurol.,* 44, 559, 1985.

12. **Ferrante, R. J., Kowall, N. W., Beal, M. F., Richardson, E. P., Bird, E., and Martin, J. B.**, Selective sparing of a class of striatal neurons in Huntington's disease, *Science,* 230, 561, 1985.

13. **Stober, T., Wussow, W., and Schimrigk, K.**, Bicaudate diameter—the most specific and simple CT parameter in the diagnosis of Huntington's disease, *Neuroradiology,* 26, 25, 1984.

15. **Kuhl, D. E., Phelps, M. E., Markham, C. W., Metter, E. J., Reige, W. H., and Winter, J.**, Cerebral metabolism and atrophy in Huntington's disease determined by FDG and computed tomagraphy scan, *Ann. Neurol,.* 12, 425, 1982.

14. **Hayden, M. R., Martin, W. R. W., Stoessl, A. J., and Clark, C.**, Positron emission tomography in the early diagnosis of Huntington's disease, *Neurology,* 36, 888, 1986.

16. **Suchowersky, O., Hayden, M. R., Martin, W. R. W., Stoessl, A. J., Hilderbrand, A. H., and Pate, B. D.**, Cerebral metabolism of glucose in benign herediary chorea, *Movement Disorders,* 1, 33, 1986.

17. **Palella, T. D., Hichwa, R. D., Ehrenkaufer, R. L., Rothley, J. M., McQuillan, M. A., Young, A. B., and Kelley, W. N.**, ^{18}F-Fluorodeoxyglucose PET scanning in HPRT deficiency, *Am. J. Hum. Genet.,* 37, A70, 1985.

18. **Phillips, P. C., Brin, M. F., Fahn, S., Greene, P. E., Sidtis, J. J., Ragassa, J., Krol, G., Moeller, J. R., Sergi, M. L., and Rottenberg, D. A.**, Abnormal regional cerebral glucose metabolism in choreoacanthocytosis. An F-18 fluorodeoxyglucose positron emission tomographic study, *Neurology,* 37, 211, 1987.

19. **Guttman, M., Lang, A. E., Garnett, E. S., Nahmias, C., Firnau, G., Tyndel, F. J., and Gordon, A. S.**, Cerebral glucose metabolism in SLE chorea: further evidence that striatal hypometabolism is not a correlate of chorea, *Movement Disorders,* 2, 201, 1987.

20. **Pahl, J. J., Mazziotta, J. C., Cummings, J., Bartzokis, G., Marder, S., Schwab, R., Sumida, R., Kuhl, D. E., Baxter, L. R., and Phelps, M. E.**, Positron emission tomography in tardive dyskinesia and Huntington's disease: LCMRGlu in two patient populations with chorea, *J. Cereb. Blood Flow Metab.,* 7, 5373, 1987.

21. **Hayden, M. R., Hewitt, J. Stoessl, A. J., Clark, C., Ammann, W. and Martin, W. R. W.**, The combined use of positron emission tomography and DNA polymorphisms for preclinical detection of Huntington's disease, *Neurology,* 37, 1441, 1987.

22. **Clark, C. M., Hayden, M. R., Stoessl, A. J., and Martin, W. R. W.**, A regression model for predicting dissociation of regional cerebral glucose metabolism in individuals at risk for Huntington's disease, *J. Cereb. Blood Flow Metab.,* 6, 756, 1986.

23. **Mazziotta, J. C., Phelps, M. E., Pahl, J. J., Huang, S. C., Baxter, L. R., Riege, W., Hoffman, J. M., Kuhl, D. E., Lanto, A. B., Wapenski, J. A., and Markham, C. H.**, Reduced cerebral glucose metabolism in asymptomatic subjects at risk for Huntington's disease, *N. Engl. J. Med.,* 316, 357, 1987.

24. **Young, A. B., Penney, J. B., Starosta-Rubinstein, S., Maskel, D., Berent, S., Rothley, J., Betley, A., and Hichwa, R.**, Normal caudate glucose metabolism in persons at risk for Huntington's disease, *Arch. Neurol.,* 44, 254, 1987.

Chapter 12

DYSTONIA

W. R. Wayne Martin

TABLE OF CONTENTS

I. INTRODUCTION

In contrast to many of the other movement disorders discussed in this volume, the underlying pathophysiology of dystonia remains an enigma. With the development of imaging techniques such as positron emission tomography (PET), it has become possible to assess functional abnormalities in areas of the brain which appear normal with structural imaging. The demonstration of a functional substrate for the often devastating clinical abnormalities seen in dystonia would represent a major advance to our understanding of brain function in general as well as to our understanding of this group of disorders.

Dystonia is a syndrome of sustained muscle contractions, frequently causing twisting and repetitive movements.[1] A dystonic posture results if the sustained contraction is prolonged. When dystonic movements are slow and continuous, they merge into athetosis. Some neurologists prefer to use the term "athetotic dystonia" to cover the full spectrum of athetosis merging into dystonia. Dystonic movements can be present in virtually any part of the body, when that part is "at rest" or when it is engaged in voluntary motor activity. Idiopathic dystonia commonly begins with a specific *action dystonia*, i.e, abnormal involuntary movements appearing with a special motor action and not present at rest. With progression, the dystonic movements may be present while the affected limb is at rest; eventually, sustained dystonic posturing becomes evident. Dystonia may be confined to one part of the body (*focal dystonia*), may involve two or three adjacent regions (*segmental dystonia*), or may involve multiple muscle groups throughout the body (*generalized dystonia*). Idiopathic generalized dystonia is synonymous with dystonia musculorum deformans. Dystonia affecting one half of the body is called *hemidystonia*.

The term dystonia has come to include not only the abnormal involuntary movements but also, to some extent, the diseases that produce them. Many patients are considered to have primary (or idiopathic) dystonia in which there is no underlying structural or metabolic abnormality. The primary dystonias are either sporadic or familial. Secondary (or symptomatic) dystonia may occur as a result of central nervous system impairment from an identifiable cause. There are numerous causes of secondary dystonia including inherited metabolic disorders such as Wilson's disease, Hallervorden-Spatz disease, GM1 gangliosidosis, focal brain injury such as that related to perinatal trauma, brain tumor or vascular disease, and drug-induced dystonia which may be due to levodopa or neuroleptics. The causes of secondary dystonia have recently been reviewed by Calne and Lang.[2]

In patients with primary dystonia, conventional neuropathological examination of the central nervous system usually reveals no abnormalities. Similarly, no reproducible neurochemical abnormalities have been found. Although *in vivo* studies of morphology have shown abnormalities in the basal ganglia in many forms of secondary dystonia,[3] there is no convincing evidence of structural changes detectable by either X-ray computed tomography (CT) or magnetic resonance imaging (MRI) in idiopathic dystonia. Nevertheless, basal ganglia dysfunction is thought to be involved in the pathophysiology of the primary dystonias because of the clear association between basal ganglia pathology and secondary dystonia. Confirmation of this hypothesis as well as elucidation of the neurotransmitter systems involved is potentially possible through the application of functional imaging techniques in carefully selected patients with these disorders.

II. CEREBRAL METABOLISM AND HEMODYNAMICS

A. PRIMARY DYSTONIA

The local cerebral metabolic rate for glucose (CMRGlu) is closely related to regional neuronal activity. The measurement of local CMRGlu with PET has been applied to patients with idiopathic dystonia in attempts to define loci of abnormal brain function.[4,5] In both of these reports, patients who had relatively asymmetric clinical involvement were selected for study to take advantage of the sensitivity of the PET technique for detecting metabolic asymmetries. Gilman and colleagues[4] reported no abnormalities in three patients with mild to moderate unilateral or asymmetric dystonia involving primarily the distal portions of the extremities. However, two patients with severe asymmetrical dystonia involving axial musculature had significant asymmetries of CMRGlu but affecting different regions. One had higher local CMRGlu in the caudate contralateral to the more involved limbs; the other had significant cerebellar asymmetry but symmetric basal ganglia. These authors postulate that the cerebellar asymmetry is due to altered cerebellar input either from muscle spindle afferents or from brainstem structures such as vestibular, reticular, locus coeruleus, or raphe nuclei. Chase and colleagues,[5] in a partial analysis of CMRGlu measurements in six subjects, found the most consistent abnormality to be that of relative lenticular hypermetabolism contralateral to the side of predominant dystonic symptoms.

Although these results are preliminary, they are consistent with the hypothesis of basal ganglia involvement in the generation of dystonic movements. One potential source of error to be considered in these studies is the relationship to head positioning. An asymmetric head position within the PET gantry can readily lead to an artifactual asymmetry of metabolic activity in small structures such as the basal ganglia.[6]

The measurement of regional CMRGlu has also been applied to the study of idiopathic torticollis, a form of focal dystonia characterized by abnormal movements and postures in the neck.[7] In 16 patients, no consistent metabolic abnormality was detected in the regions analyzed (caudate nuclei, lenticular nuclei, and thalamus). There was evidence, however, of a bilateral breakdown of the normal relationships between thalamus and basal ganglia when a correlational analysis was applied to the data.[7,8] In this initial study, normal controls studied at rest were compared to patients with torticollis in whom head movement was left uninhibited during the first 20 min after administration of fluorodeoxyglucose (FDG), i.e., during the time when most FDG is taken up and phosphorylated. In order to examine the possible contribution of proprioceptive input in the torticollis group, Stoessl and colleagues subsequently reported an extension of the original study with the addition of a second control group.[9] The second control group consisted of normal individuals who were asked to rotate the head during the uptake period in order to simulate the postural abnormality of torticollis. In this second control group, there was also disruption of normal inter-regional metabolic relationships associated with voluntary movement but the pattern of cortical-subcortical correlations differed substantially from that seen in both the resting control group and in the torticollis group. These findings led to the suggestion that in torticollis there exists a functional abnormality in cortical-subcortical connections and in subcortical interconnections rather than pathology in a specific structure.

B SECONDARY DYSTONIA

The presence of a unilateral hyperkinetic movement disorder suggests a structural abnormality in the region of the basal ganglia.[3] Perlmutter and Raichle have reported a patient with posttraumatic paroxysmal hemidystonia unassociated with other neurological abnormalities and with normal CT scan and cerebral angiography.[10] Abnormal function was demonstrated with PET in the contralateral basal ganglia where local oxygen extraction and metabolism were decreased while blood flow and volume were increased. In spite of the normal structural studies, the PET findings provide unequivocal evidence of a localized functional abnormality in this patient with a pure paroxysmal dystonia.

C. SENSORY ACTIVATION AND CEREBRAL BLOOD FLOW

The functional integrity of the somatosensory system in normal individuals has been tested with stimulus paradigms that give large, reproducible increases in regional cerebral blood flow (rCBF) in somatosensory cortex.[11] The increase in rCBF is thought to be secondary to increased neuronal activity. This is supported by the demonstration that visual stimulus rate determines regional blood flow in striate cortex.[12]

A vibrotactile sensory stimulation paradigm has been utilized in patients with predominantly unilateral dystonia in conjunction with the measurement of rCBF with PET.[13] In normal controls, the stimulation produced a readily reproducible 25 ± 5% increase in rCBF in somatosensory cortex. The response to vibration in dystonic patients, although still present, was significantly decreased on both sides. These preliminary results suggest an abnormality in the processing of sensory input in dystonia.

III. DOPAMINERGIC FUNCTION

A. PRESYNAPTIC FUNCTION
1. Focal Dystonia

Although no structural or biochemical pathophysiology has been defined for primary dystonia, there is evidence that structural lesions involving the striatum or its connections may be associated with secondary dystonia.[14,15] Fross and colleagues have reported the association of dystonia with structural lesions restricted to the putamen and suggest that this is the critical structure involved in the development of the movement disorder.[16] These authors reported a patient who developed dystonic movements in the left hand and foot following infarction of the contralateral putamen. A 6-fluorodopa PET study showed normal accumulation of radioactivity in the caudate, but markedly decreased activity in the putamen. Leenders et al. reported a bilateral decrease in striatal 6-fluorodopa derived radioactivity in two patients with marked torticollis but did not attempt to separate caudate from putamen.[17]

The loss of dopaminergic input to the putamen with relative sparing of caudate input is similar to the situation seen in Parkinson's disease as described elsewhere in this volume. While in Parkinson's disease this is thought to represent loss of dopaminergic input to intact striatal neurons, in a patient with focal putamenal infarction there is not only destruction of dopaminergic input, but also a loss of neurons intrinsic to the putamen. This allows speculation that the motor manifestations of parkinsonism derive from putamenal output released from nigral modulation, whereas dystonia results from a loss of putamenal influence on other structures.

2. Dystonia-Parkinsonism

A hereditary form of dystonia characterized by juvenile onset and a dramatic response to levodopa has been reported.[18,19] This is often associated with diurnal variation in the severity of symptoms and with signs of parkinsonism. The dramatic response of these patients to levodopa, as well as the single reported autopsy study[20] all point toward impairment of function of presynaptic nigrostriatal nerve endings in this disorder. 6-FD/PET studies in this group of patients, however, have given mixed results. Martin and colleagues reported that only two of four patients studied had definitely abnormal findings.[21] Interestingly, both abnormal patients had relatively late onset of the disease (ages 19 and 36) whereas the other two patients had very early onset (age 5). An example of these findings is illustrated in Figure 1. In the group of patients reported by Lang and colleagues, one, with onset at age 4, had generalized dystonia with marked diurnal variation and levodopa responsiveness.[22] This patient had marked reduction in radioactivity in the putamen on the left side in spite of the absence of parkinsonian signs. A second patient, clinically similar except for the presence of parkinsonism, had an entirely normal 6-FD scan. Leenders et al. reported two patients with idiopathic hemidystonia and hemiparkinsonism, both of whom had decreased radioactivity in the striatum contralateral to the affected limbs.[16]

These findings suggest that even this clinically distinct entity seems to be heterogeneous

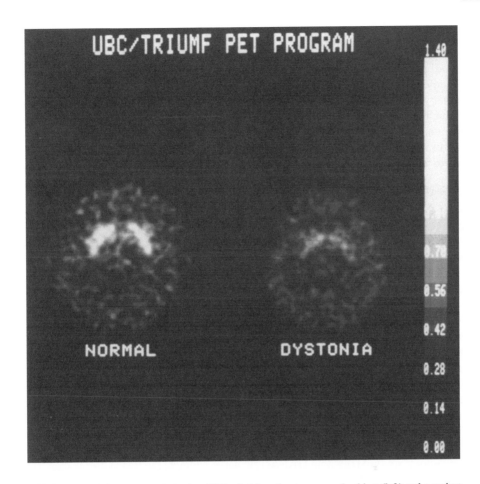

FIGURE 1. Images obtained following 6-FD administration to a normal subject (left) and a patient with levodopa-responsive dystonia-parkinsonism (right). Reduced uptake of radioactivity is evident bilaterally in the striata of the dystonic patient. Both images are at the same axial level through the basal ganglia and represent 30 min of emission data acquired during the second hour after tracer administration. Figures on the grey scale refer to radioactivity concentration in arbitrary units.

with marked presynaptic dopaminergic dysfunction in some patients but normal function in others. Although one would anticipate that nigrostriatal impairment would correlate with levodopa responsiveness, this appears not to be the case. These observations, however, provide no information concerning the functional activity of dopamine receptors. The measurement of receptor kinetics with PET may help explain the disparity between presynaptic integrity of the dopamine system and the therapeutic response to levodopa.

B. POSTSYNAPTIC RECEPTORS

Preliminary results concerning the imaging of striatal dopamine receptor binding with ^{11}C-methylspiperone and PET have been reported in four patients with hemidystonia, three of whom had associated hemiparkinsonism.[16] Increased binding was noted in the contralateral striatum in only one patient. The authors speculated that this increase might explain the development of dyskinesias in this patient secondary to levodopa treatment.

IV. CONCLUSIONS

Dystonia is a perplexing disorder to unravel. Although advances in the neurochemistry and neuropharmacology of other movement disorders have provided an improved understanding of basal ganglia function, the pathophysiology of dystonia remains obscure. The introduction of functional imaging techniques to the study of dystonia has not yet yielded major insights, but those studies are in their infancy. Only small numbers of patients have been studied and virtually all of the results referred to in this chapter must be considered preliminary. At the present time, the only PET methods which have been reported even in small numbers of dystonic patients are those for the measurement of CMRGlu, a relatively nonspecific indicator of neuronal function, and for the imaging of pre- and postsynaptic aspects of dopaminergic function. Numerous other neurotransmitter systems, however, are known to be involved in basal ganglia function (see Chapter 2) and may be relevant to dystonia.

As described previously in this chapter, evidence exists which suggests that a destructive lesion of the putamen can produce dystonia, possibly through abnormal activity of pallidal projection neurons resulting from decreased (or absent) striatal influence. The critical abnormality in idiopathic dystonia in the absence of a structural lesion in the putamen may be a functional impairment in striatopallidal projections. Although this hypothesis can be tested with the traditional methodology of neurotransmitter/neuroreceptor measurements or by newer immunohistochemical techniques, these methods have the disadvantage of relying on post-mortem tissue. The ability to detect specific neuronal markers *in vivo* with high resolution functional imaging techniques should provide information relating to this hypothesis provided appropriate radioligands are chosen. For example, the functional integrity of the striatopallidal GABA system could be studied with ligands which bind to presynaptic GABAergic nerve endings or to postsynaptic GABA receptors in the pallidum.

In order to investigate these possibilities, innovative radiolabeled ligands must be developed, based on specific hypotheses of impaired neuronal function. Biochemical principles in radiopharmaceutical design have been reviewed recently.[23] Several routes might be considered in attempts to develop a marker for GABAergic neurons based on the mechanisms of intraneuronal synthesis and reuptake. GABA is synthesized from glutamate by glutamic acid decarboxylase (GAD) within GABAergic nerve endings; the transmitter is then trapped within presynaptic vesicles and, after relase into the synaptic cleft, is taken up again into the presynaptic neuron by a high-affinity uptake system.[24] One method by which these neurons could be labeled is with a positron-emitting lipophilic glutamate analog which is a substrate for GAD. Alternatively, the high-affinity reuptake site might be labeled. These routes are analogous to existing methods to study dopaminergic pathways with 6-fluorodopa and with nomifensine.

It is this process of hypothesis-directed radiopharmaceutical development in conjunction with careful PET measurements of regional radioactivity and appropriate tracer kinetic models which may well be of great help in unraveling the pathophysiology of clinical problems such as dystonia. Successful application of these methods will require the dedicated collaboration of multidisciplinary groups which include the clinical neurologist, the basic neuropharmocologist, the radiochemist, and the PET scientist.

REFERENCES

1. **Fahn, S.**, Concept and classification of dystonia, in *Advances in Neurology,* Vol. 50, Fahn, S. Marsden, C. D., and Calne, D. B., Eds., Raven Press, New York, 1988, 1.
2. **Calne, D. B. and Lang, A. E.**, Secondary dystonia, in *Advances in Neurology,* Vol. 50, Fahn, S., Marsden, C. C., and Calne, D. B., Eds., Raven Press, New York, 1988, 9
3. **Martin, W. R. W. and Li, D. K. B.**, Disorders of the basal ganglia, in *Clinical Neuroimaging,* Theodore, W. H., Ed., Alan R. Liss, New York, 1988, 165.

4. **Gilman, S., Junck, L., Young, A. B., Hichwa, R. D., Market, D. S., Koeppe, R. A., and Ehrenkaufer, R. L. E.,** Cerebral metabolic activity in idiopathic dystonia studied with positron emission tomography, in *Advances in Neurology,* Vol. 50, Fahn, S., Marsden, C. D., and Calne, D. B., Eds., Raven Press, New York, 1988, 231.

5. **Chase, T. N. Tamminga, C. A., and Burrows, H.,** Positron emission tomographic studies of regional cerebral glucose metabolism in idiopathic dystonia, in *Advances in Neurology,* Vol. 50, Fahn, S., Marsden, C. D., and Calne, D. B., Eds., Raven Press, New York, 1988, 237.

6. **Martin, W. R. W., Beckman, J. H., Calne, D. B., Adam, M. J., Harrop, R., Rogers, J. G., Ruth, T. J., Sayre, C. I., and Pate, B. D.,** Cerebral glucose metabolism in Parkinson's disease, *Can. J. Neurol. Sci.,* 11 (Suppl.), 169, 1984.

7. **Stoessl, A. J., Martin, W. R. W., Clark, C., Adam, M. J., Ammann, W., Beckman, J. H., Bergstrom, M., Harrop, R., Rogers, J. G., Sayre, C. I., Pate, B. D., and Calne, D. B.,** PET studies of cerebral glucose metabolism in idiopathic torticollis, *Neurology,* 36, 653, 1986.

8. **Clark, C. M., Kessler, R., Buchsbaum, M. S., Margolin, R. A., and Holcomb, H. H.,** Correlational methods for determining regional coupling of cerebral glucose metabolism: a pilot study, *Biol. Psychiatry,* 19, 663, 1984.

9. **Stoessl, A. J., Martin, W. R. W., Clark, C. M., Pate, B. D., and Calne, D. B.,** Glucose metabolic relations in torticollis and voluntary head rotation, *Neurology,* 37 (Suppl. 1), 123, 1987.

10. **Perlmutter, J. S. and Raichle, M. E.,** Pure hemidystonia with basal ganglia abnormalities on positron emission tomography, *Ann. Neurol.,* 15, 228, 1984.

11. **Fox, P. T. and Raichle, M. E.,** Focal physiological uncoupling of cerebral blood flow and oxidative metabolism during somatosensory stimulation in human subjects, *Proc. Natl. Acad. Sci. U.S.A.,* 83, 1140, 1986.

12. **Fox, P. T. and Raichle, M. E.,** Stimulus rate determines regional brain blood flow in striate cortex, *Ann. Neurol.,* 17, 303, 1985.

13. **Tempel, L. W. and Perlmutter, J. S.,** Abnormal cerebral blood flow response to vibrotractile stimulation in dystonics, *Neurology,* 38 (Suppl. 1), 131, 1988.

14. **Marsden, C. D., Obeso, J. A. Zarranz, J. A., and Lang, A. E.,** The anatomical basis of symptomatic hemidystonia, *Brain,* 108, 463, 1985.

15. **Pettigrew, L. C. and Jankovic, J.,** Hemidystonia; a report of 22 patients and a review of the literature, *J. Neurol. Neurosurg. Psychiatry,* 48, 650, 1985.

16. **Fross, R. D., Martin, W. R. W., Li, D., Stoessl, A. J., Adam, M. J., Ruth, T. J., Pate, B. D., Burton, K., and Calne, D. B.,** Lesions of the putamen: their relevance to dystonia, *Neurology,* 37, 1125, 1987.

17. **Leenders, K. L., Quinn, N., Frackowiak, R. S. J., and Marsden, C. D.,** Brain dopaminergic system studied in patients with dystonia using postitron emission tomography, in *Advances in Neurology,* Vol. 50, Fahn, S., Marsden, C. D., and Calne, D. B., Eds., Raven Press, New York, 1988, 243.

18. **Segawa, M., Hosaka, A., Miyagawa, R., Nomura, Y., and Imai, H.,** Hereditary progressive dystonia with marked diurnal fluctuation, in *Advances in Neurology,* Vol. 14, Eldridge, R. and Fahn, S., Eds., Ravens Press, New York, 1976, 215.

19. **Nygaard, T. G. and Duvoisin, R. C.,** Hereditary dystonia-parkinsonism syndrome of juvenile onset, *Neurology,* 36, 1424, 1986.

20. **Yokochi, M., Narabayashi, H., Iizuka, R., and Nagatsu, T.,** Juvenile parkinsonism: some clinical, pharmacological, and neuropathological aspects, in *Advances in Neurology,* Vol. 40, Hassler, R. G. and Christ, J. F., Eds., Raven Press, New York, 1984, 407.

21. **Martin, W. R. W., Stoessl, A. J., Palmer, M., Adam, M. J., Ruth, T. J., Grierson, J. R., Pate, B. D., and Calne, D. B.,** PET scanning in dystonia, in *Advances in Neurology,* Vol. 50, Fahn, S., Marsden, C. D., and Calne, D. B., Eds., Raven Press, New York, 1988, 223.

22. **Lang, A. E., Garnett, E. S., Firnau, G., Nahmias, C., and Talalla, A.,** Positron tomography in dystonia, in *Advances in Neurology,* Vol. 50, Fahn, S., Marsden, C. D., and Calne, D. B., Eds., Raven Press, New York, 1988, 249.

23. **Barrio, J. R.,** Biochemcial principles in radiopharmaceutical design and utilization, in *Positron Emission Tomography and Autoradiography: Principles and Applications for the Brain and Heart,* Phelps, M., Mazziotta, J., and Schelbert, H., Eds., Raven Press, New York, 1986, 451.

24. **McGeer, P. L., Eccles, Sir J. C., and McGeer, E. G.,** *Molecular Neurobiology of the Mammalian Brain,* Plenum Press, New York, 1978, chap. 7.

Chapter 13

DEMENTIA IN MOVEMENT DISORDERS

Norman L. Foster

TABLE OF CONTENTS

I. INTRODUCTION AND HISTORICAL CONTEXT

Dementia, a decline in cognitive abilities from a previous level of attainment, is a common symptom in disease causing movement disorders. However, this has not always been appreciated. Dementia was included in the original description of some movement disorders, but in others, the striking abnormality of movement caused more subtle changes in mental capacity to be overlooked. In some cases it was many years before the full extent of dementia was recognized. Even today, issues of intellectual and behavioral change are controversial and poorly understood as any topic in the movement disorders.

The initial descriptions of progressive supranuclear palsy (PSP), Huntington's disease, and Wilson's disease all included accounts of behavioral or intellectual abnormalities. Dementia was one of the cardinal features that permitted PSP to be recognized as a distinct disease process by Steele, Richardson, and Olszewski.[1] It was soon noticed that the dementia exhibited by patients with PSP was different from that seen in other diseases. The term "subcortical dementia" was coined to emphasize its special characteristics,[2] and it has received much attention as a prototype for dementias associated with movement disorders.

The first description of Huntington's disease also described significant cognitive changes. George Huntington stated that patients had "insanity with a tendency to suicide,[3] and by 1900 a quite complete description of the dementia associated with this disorder had already appeared.[4] Psychotic symptoms, and a variety of changes in affect and personality may be seen in patients with Huntington's disease, but progressive dementia is almost always present.[5]

Wilson's first report of progressive lenticular degeneration, or Wilson's disease, indicated that there were psychiatric symptoms in 8 of his initial 12 patients. It is now recognized that almost every patient with clinically manifest Wilson's disease suffers from dementia, affective disturbance, or some other abnormality in behavior at some time in their illness.[6]

On the other hand, dementia was not a widely recognized feature of Parkinson's disease until recently. Parkinson's essay on shaking palsy in 1812 specifically noted the preservation of mentation despite an inability to perform everyday activities adequately.[7] It was widely felt that apparent changes in cognition could be attributable to motor impairment. However, when effective treatments became available for Parkinson's disease, it was obvious that better motor performance did not always lead to an improvement in mental symptoms. In the 1970s, a series of studies convincingly demonstrated that patients with Parkinson's disease perform poorly on neuropsychometric tests, and that this poor performance could not be explained entirely by motor disability.[8-10] It is now appreciated that many patients with this disease are demented. Estimates of the prevalence of moderate to severe dementia in Parkinson's disease now commonly range from 20 to 40%.[11]

The frequency of dementia in olivopontocerebellar atrophy (OPCA) is uncertain. Many individual case reports include descriptions of dementia,[12] but larger series disagree as to whether dementia is common[13] or occurs at all.[14] No comprehensive survey of cognition in patients with this disease is available, so the discrepancy between these reports could be due to patient selection. Dementia may be limited to certain variants of this disease, or to particular kindreds with hereditary forms of this disorder.

The development of our understanding of dementias specific to movement disorders parallels the development of our understanding of dementia in general. First came the recognition that intellectual decline could be ascribed to a disease, and was not simply the result of aging or debility. Next, it was realized that all dementias were not alike. Finally, it became possible to identify differences that distinguished the dementias due to each specific disease.

For many years the term organic brain syndrome was widely used to describe the intellectual and behavioral changes that resulted from any medical or neurologic illness or from exposure to any drug or toxin. The implication of this terminology was that dementia due to any of these causes had identical clinical features. Indeed, the Diagnostic and Statistical Manual of Mental Disorders published by the American Psychiatric Association indicated until the late 1960s that any variability in the symptoms of patients with organic brain syndrome was due to premorbid experiences and personality.[15,16] Clinical observations, however, were inconsistent with this view. Certain characteristics seemed to be shared in common by individuals with dementia from the same cause, and these similarities were found in patients with quite different premorbid personalities and environments. Among the first distinctions made between dementias with different "organic" etiologies was the development of the concept of "subcortical" and "cortical" dementia.

II. THE CONCEPT OF "CORTICAL" AND "SUBCORTICAL" DEMENTIAS

Albert, Feldman, and Willis in 1974 coined the terms "subcortical" and "cortical" dementia to express the differences that they observed between the symptoms of patients having PSP and those with dementia due to diseases thought to have pathology that was restricted to the cerebral cortex.[2] Thus, PSP, which has pathology almost entirely restricted to subcortical structures, caused "subcortical" dementia, while Alzheimer's disease and Pick's disease caused "cortical" dementia. The concept of "subcortical" dementia was then expanded, first to include Huntington's disease,[5] and eventually extended to include all dementias associated with a movement disorder.[12]

Although this classification scheme had considerable heuristic value, the distinction between "cortical" and "subcortical" dementias was difficult to document. Language impairment, apraxia, and other deficits that were usually a result of damage to the cerebral cortex were presumed to be absent in "subcortical" dementia.[2] However, this was often not true.[17-19] Slowing of thought, comprehension, and verbalization were also felt to be characterisitc features of "subcortical" dementia, but these changes were difficult to demonstrate.[20] Thus, this classification became dependent largely upon clinical description.

The anatomic basis for the distinction between "subcortical" and "cortical" dementia also became less clear. The "cortical" dementia, Alzheimer's disease and Pick's disease, were found to cause significant neuronal loss in subcortical structures.[21-23] Likewise, in diseases with "subcortical" dementia, pathological changes in the cerebral cortex have been discovered.[24] Results of studies performed with positron emission tomography (PET) has also brought this nomenclature into question. First, subcortical structures such as the thalamus, caudate nucleus, and putamen have been found to be hypometabolic in "cortical" dementia caused by Alzheimer's disease.[25] Second, glucose metabolic rates in the cerebral cortex also decline in "subcortical" dementia due to PSP, Wilson's disease, and Parkinson's disease with dementia.[26-29] While the cerebral cortex appears to be unimpaired in Huntington's disease when studied by PET,[30,31] the simplistic division of dementia into two categories does not appear to be satisfactory.[32] As the clinicoanatomic justification for "subcortical" and "cortical" dementia became muddled, this classification scheme has lost its attractiveness.

III. TECHNICAL CONSIDERATIONS IN CLINCIAL AND IMAGING STUDIES

Recent improvements in neuropsychometric techniques and clinical research design have made it feasible to characterize the dementia typical of each specific disease. When making comparisons between patients with movement disorders and controls or other patient groups, care must be taken to assess the effect of physical impairment, disease severity, and social factors such as socioeconomic group and education. Well-characterized, standardized test procedures should be used to assess cognition. These steps are necessary to identify disease differences when the symptomatology is similar. For example, in one recent study, patients with PSP, Parkinson's disease, Alzheimer's disease, and normals were all matched for age, sex, education, handedness, and overall severity of dementia as indicated by a deterioration index derived from several widely used and standardize neuropsychometric tests. By demonstrating differences in performance on a battery of other psychometric tests, it was possible to distinguish the characteristics of patients in each of these groups, despite the fact that all were impaired in most tests relative to normals.[19]

Functional brain imaging has also enhanced the understanding of dementias associated with different kinds of movement disorders. These studies are especially fruitful when patients are well characterized by careful neurological, psychiatric, and neuropsychometric examinations. As in any other clinical study, correct interpretation of findings is dependent on patient selection. Results are only as accurate as the subjects' diagnosis. Consequently, whenever possible, pathologic confirmation of the clinical diagnosis should be sought.

Performing brain imaging in patients with movement disorders is difficult. Many individuals are taking medication that might alter results. In some case, discontinuing medication to obtain a scan could lead to serious complications,[33,34] and is unjustifiable. Hyperkinetic movement disorders can make steady head position impossible, and hypokinetic movement disorders can cause fixed postures that prevent appropriate, reproducible head positioning. Patients with movement disorders also may have limited tolerance for the immobility required to accomplish scanning.

These constraints are of even greater concern in patients with both a movement disorder and dementia. In demented patients, cooperation may be fleeting, and sensory deprivation used in some PET studies often increases the patient's disorientation and anxiety. The observation that moderate diazepam sedation does not affect relative regional metabolic rates in patients with Alzheimer's disease[35] offers hope that patients who might otherwise be unable to cooperate with scanning procedures can be studied. However, the applicability of this technique in disorders other than Alzheimer's disease has not yet been tested. As a result, most functional brain imaging has been performed in individuals with mild to moderate dementia or motor disability, and it has not been possible to examine the consequences of severe disease.

Obtaining truly informed consent in demented individuals may also be problematic. Involving other family members in the decision to perform a scan and documenting the wishes of the individual while he is still competent will help to resolve this issue. The naming of a durable power of attorney for patients also clarifies whether participation in research is appropriate for that individual.[36] Despite these difficulties, the application of neuroanatomic principles and clinicopathologic correlation to functional brain imaging studies has resulted in significant improvements in our understanding of movement disorders and their associated dementias.

IV. FUNCTIONAL IMAGING IN SPECIFIC DEMENTIAS

A. PROGRESSIVE SUPRANUCLEAR PALSY

Progressive supranuclear palsy is characterized by dementia, supranuclear palsy of gaze, axial dystonia, and bradykinesia.[1] Except possibly for the dementia, these symptons all appear to be accounted for by the extensive pathological changes seen in subcortical structures. The caudate nucleus, putamen, thalamus, and most brainstem nuclei suffer neuronal loss. PET has shown reductions in glucose metabolism in all of these regions (Table 1),[26] and altered dopamine receptor binding in the striatum.[37]

Despite being categorized by some as a "subcortical" dementia, it is recognized that many behavioral symptoms seen in patients with PSP are suggestive of frontal lobe dysfunction,[2] and this has been further substantiated by phychometric testing.[19,27,38] In fact,

TABLE 1

Regional Glucose Metabolic Rates (mg/100 g/min) in Progressive Supranuclear Palsy and Normal Control Subjects[a]

	Normal Controls (n = 21)	PSP (n = 14)	PSP/normal	p value
Cerebral cortex	6.08 ± 0.94	4.92 ± 0.52	0.81 ± 0.09	.0001
Cerebellar cortex	6.10 ± 0.90	5.52 ± 0.74	0.91 ± 0.12	.048
Cerebellar vermis	5.54 ± 0.87	5.33 ± 0.84	0.96 ± 0.15	.49
Brainstem	4.46 ± 0.67	3.81 ± 0.49	0.86 ± 0.11	.0024
Caudate	6.48 ± 0.91	5.04 ± 0.63	0.78 ± 0.10	.00005
Putamen	7.14 ± 1.09	5.60 ± 0.99	0.79 ± 0.14	.0002
Thalamus	6.69 ± 1.29	5.65 ± 1.15	0.84 ± 0.17	.018

[a] Values represent means ± standard deviations, p values are for a test of equality of means by the Behrens-Fisher t test, which is equivalent to a test that PSP/normal ratio is unity. From Foster, N. L. et al., *Ann. Neurol.*, 24, 399, 1988. With permission.

patients with PSP exhibit a variety of behavioral and intellectual changes that classically have been localized to the cerebral cortex. Apathy or depression, impaired judgment, and perseveration are all observed in patients with this disease. Cognitive disabilities, such as aphasia, word-finding difficulties, and visuospatial impairment, which are generally localized to regions outside of the frontal cortex, may also be observed.[38-41]

PET has provided further evidence that impairment of the cerebral cortex may account for some of the intellectual and behavioral changes observed in these patients. Significant declines in glucose metabolic rate occur throughout the cerebral cortex (Plate 7*).[26] This hypometabolism is most prominent in front regions, especially in superior frontal cortex and in regions just anterior to the central sulcus, which probably include supplemental motor cortex and frontal eye fields (Figure 1).[26,27] Because the cerebral cortex generally appears to be spared in PSP when examined by standard neuropathologic techniques,[1,42] deafferentation appears to be the most likely cause for this pattern of hypometabolism. However, careful morphometric studies of the cerebral cortex have not yet been performed and loss of some neurons in the cerebral cortex cannot be excluded.

Declines in the rates of cerebral cortical glucose metabolism in PSP correlate with changes in cognition. The average glucose metabolic rate in the cerebral cortex correlates with severity of intellectual decline as measured by the Wechsler Adult Intelligence Scale.[43] The regional distribution of glucose hypometabolism also corresponds to the impairments seen in PSP. Relative loss of skills, such as verbal fluency and memory, are reflected in differing rates of metabolism in various regions of the cerebral cortex.[44] Functional impairment of the frontal eye fields may contribute to the pronounced visuomotor abnormalities, and supplementary motor cortex dysfunction may contribute to the abnormalities in initiating movement often seen in these patients. Thus, the clinical symptomatology of PSP is consistent with the abnormalities in glucose metabolism seen by PET.

B. HUNTINGTON'S DISEASE

As Huntington's disease develops, progressive neuronal loss in the caudate nucleus, putamen, and, to a lesser extent, thalamus and cerebral cortex is accompanied by increasing cognitive impairment and diminished capacity to perform the activities of daily living. Huntington's disease causes cognitive impairment that proceeds in a regular fashion. Subjects with early Huntington's disease demonstrate declines in intellectual capacity, with memory and acquisition of new knowledge being particularly impaired. On the Wechsler Adult

* Plate 7 appears after page 168.

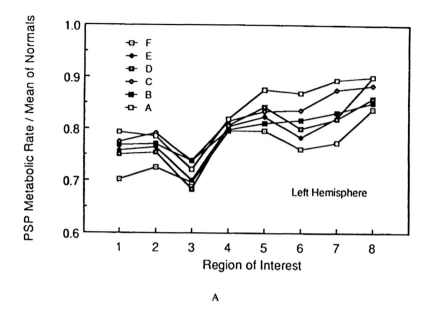

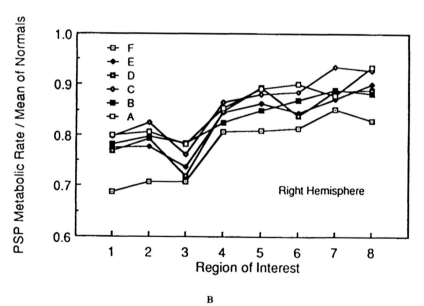

FIGURE 1. Regional cerebral cortical metabolic rates for glucose in the left hemisphere (A) and in the right hemisphere (B) in patients with progressive supranuclear palsy expressed as a ratio to the mean rate observed in the same region in normals. Horizontal sections compared are labeled from A, most inferior, to F, most superior. Regions of interest extend from the most anterior (1) to the most posterior (8). (From Foster, N. L. et al., *Ann. Neurol.*, 24, 399, 1988. With permission.)

Intelligence Scale (WAIS), performance IQ, particularly the digit symbol subtest, appears to be more affected than does verbal IQ. Decline in performance on the Wechsler Memory Score, especially the paired associate learning subtest, is also seen early.[45,46] As the disease progresses, these abnormalities worsen, but the discrepancy between performance and verbal IQ remains. The relatively selective deficits in perception and learning, especially perceptuomotor discrimination, have suggested to some predominantly frontal lobe damage.[46]

Because of the considerable impairment in memory,[47] others have suggested that functional impairment of the hippocampus could account for the dementia.[48] With further progression, a more severe dementia develops, which may appear similar to the dementia of Alzheimer's disease,[49] although there may continue to be a relative lack of aphasic symptoms.[45] At postmortem, atrophy of the cerebral cortex is apparent with neuronal loss primarily in the deeper cortical layers.[50]

Functional imaging reflects the pattern of neuropathological changes in the corpus striatum. Significant declines in glucose metabolism are seen in the caudate nucleus and putamen,[30,31,51] and these declines correlate with the severity of intellectual impairment. The general behavioral decline of patients with Huntington's disease can be evaluated using standardized rating scales, such as the total functional capacity of Shoulson and Fahn.[52] This scale assesses the patient's ability to be gainfully employed, to handle financial and domestic responsibilities, to perform activities of daily living, and to be cared for at home. Although motor impairments may play a significant role in the score achieved on this scale, dementia is probably a major factor accounting for declines in functional capacity. Using this scale, Young et al. found that indices of caudate metabolism correlated highly with the patient's overall functional capacity (Figure 2).[30]

Caudate metabolism also appears to be closely linked to performance on psychometric tests that deteriorate in early Huntington's disease.[53] Other abilities that remain less affected in early stages of the illness, such as vocabulary and verbal IQ, are not closely correlated. Glucose metabolic rate in the putamen also correlate with these measures, but thalamic metabolism does not (Table 2). Metabolic activity in subcortical structures is not related to performance in normals. Thus, functional impairment of the caudate nucleus and putamen appear to be responsible for the development of dementia in the early stages of Huntington's disease.

Despite the presence of intellectual impairment which is, in many ways, similar to that seen in other dementias, and despite documented neuronal loss in the cerebral cortex and thalamus,[50,54] positron emission tomography demonstrates no noticeable change in metabolism in these structures. To some extent, this may be due to the selection of patients who are in relatively early stages of their illness. For example, in one study patients were mostly in stages I and II of Huntington's disease, and none were in stages IV and V.[30] However, normal cerebral cortical metabolism has also been observed by others and appears to be a consistent finding.[31,51] It is not yet clear why damage to subcortical structures in Huntington's disease does not lead to hypometabolism of the cerebral cortex, as it does in other disorders with predominant subcortical pathology.

C. WILSON'S DISEASE

Four patients with Wilson's disease have been studied using FDG and PET.[28] A single patient who was neurologically normal showed a decrease in glucose metabolism only in the putamen. Global declines in glucose metabolism in the cerebral cortex were seen only in those with mild to moderately severe symptoms. In all cases, caudate metabolism appeared to be normal. There was no mention made of the type or severity of dementing symptoms in these patients and inadequate numbers were studied to permit any conclusions about the relationship between glucose metabolism and severity of dementia in Wilson's disease.

D. PARKINSON'S DISEASE

The pathology and clinical features of the dementia associated with Parkinson's disease are controversial. Some investigators have found that demented patients with Parkinson's disease have changes in the cerebral cortex to those seen in Alzheimer's disease. For example, Boller and co-workers compared clinical records and neuropathological specimens in 36 patients with autopsy-demonstrated idiopathic Parkinson's disease.[24] They found neuronal loss, senile plaques, and neurofibrillary tangles in the cerebral cortex that corresponded to

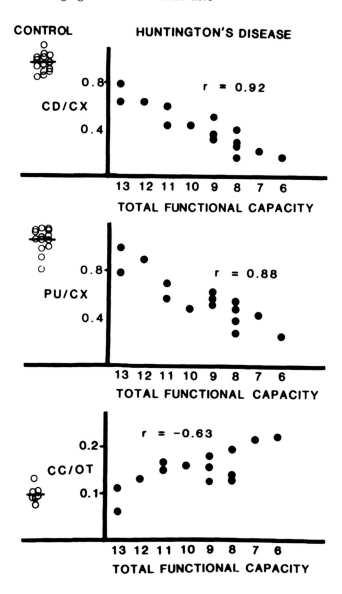

FIGURE 2. Plots of metabolic and computed tomographic (CT) data
in a group of controls (open circles) and Huntington's disease (HD)
patients (closed circles). There is a high degree of correlation between
functional capacity and both positron emission tomography (PET) and
CT measures. PET measures through caudate (top) distinguish the early
HD cases more accurately from the controls than do the putamen measures (middle). Numbers indicate the Spearman correlation coefficients
(r) of the data. (CD = caudate; PU = putamen; CX = cortex; CC =
intercaudate distance; OT = distance between outer tables of skull at
level of caudate) (From Young, A. B. et al., *Ann. Neurol.*, 20, 296,
1986. With permission.)

the severity of dementia documented before death. The weakness of this kind of retrospective
study of dementia, however, is that many patients with typical Alzheimer's disease eventually
develop parkinsonian signs. It is possible that this study could have been contaminated with
such individuals. Others, using a similar retrospective approach, have found that significant
intellectual decline in Parkinson's disease can occur without post-mortem evidence of in-

Table 2
Correlation Between Glucose Metabolism of Basal Ganglia and
Cognitive Performance in Patients With Huntington's Disease[a]

	Caudate		Putamen		Thalamus	
	r	p	r	p	r	p
Wechsler memory quotient	+.67	.008	+.50	ns	−.16	ns
Verbal memory (WMS)	+.73	.003	+.50	ns	+.05	ns
Visual memory (WMS)	−.04	ns	+.02	ns	−.53	ns
WAIS-R performance IQ	+.70	.01	+.66	.02	−.25	ns
Vocabulary (WAIS-R)	+.19	ns	+.30	ns	+18	ns

[a]   r values represent Pearson correlation coefficients, and p values are the probability that these correlations can be explained by chance. ns represents correlations with $p > 0.05$.

Adapted from Berent, S. et al., *Ann. Neurol.*, 23, 541, 1988. With permission.

Table 3
Glucose Metabolic Rates (mg/100 g/min) in the Basal Ganglia and
Thalamus in Normals and in Patients with Dementia due to Various
Movement Disorders[a]

	Normals (n = 21)	PSP (n = 14)	PD (n = 6)	HD (n = 14)
Caudate nuceleus	6.48 ± 0.91	5.04 ± 0.63*	4.01 ± 1.48*	3.66 ± 1.27*
Putamen	7.14 ± 1.09	5.60 ± 0.99*	5.52 ± 0.79*	5.22 ± 1.07*
Thalamus	6.69 ± 1.29	5.65 ± 1.15*	5.09 ± 0.59*	7.04 ± 1.82

Note: * = significantly different from normal by ANOVA, $p < 0.05$.

[a]   Values represent means ± standard deviations.

volvement of the cerebral cortex.[55] Further studies will be needed to resolve this disagreement.

Neuropsychological literature is also in conflict about the nature of the dementia in Parkinson's disease. Some have found cognitive impairment that appears to result from subcortical damage,[11] while others have noted impairment of visuospatial reasoning and language, consistent with dysfunction of the cerebral cortex.[17,18] Frontal lobe dysfunction has also been suggested.[19]

Functional brain imaging has not yet resolved these issues, but it has provided further evidence that similarities exist between Parkinson's disease complicated by dementia and Alzheimer's disease. There is a marked decline in metabolic rate throughout the cerebral cortex (Plate 8*). Despite CT studies demonstrating predominantly prefrontal atrophy,[56] these declines in glucose metabolism are most prominent in posterior temporoparietal association cortex similar to the pattern observed in Alzheimer's disease.[29] Significant declines in glucose metabolism are also observed in subcortical structures. These declines are most marked in the caudate nucleus, but are also significant in the putamen and thalamus (Table 3).

Changes in cognition reflect changes in cerebral cortical glucose metabolism in dementia associated with Parkinson's disease. Declines in glucose metabolic rates in the cerebral cortex are proportional to severity of dementia as indicatd by a clinical rating scale (Figure 3).[29] The longitudinal study of a patient with Parkinson's disease and dementia has also

---

* Plate 8 appears after page 168.

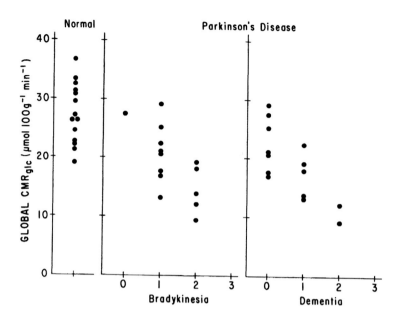

FIGURE 3.   Measures of global cerebral glucose utilization in 14 normal control subjects and 9 patients with Parkinson's disease. (A second study in 5 of the patients accounts for the 14 data points in the patient group.) Global cerebral metabolic rate for glucose (CMRGlc) was correlated inversely ($p < 0.01$) with the severity of bradykinesia and dementia. (From Kuhl, D. E. et al., *Ann. Neurol.*, 15, 419, 1984. With permission.)

demonstrated that declines in cerebral cortical metabolism and cognition occur in parallel (Figure 4).[29] Since post-mortem examinations have not yet been obtained in any patient with Parkinson's disease and dementia who has been scanned with PET, it is unclear whether this brain imaging pattern is indicative of Alzheimer-type pathology. Further studies will be needed to determine whether predominant posterior temporoparietal hypometabolism is a consistent feature of Parkinson's disease with dementia, regardless of the underlying pathology.

E. OLIVOPONTOCEREBELLAR ATROPHY

Despite numerous reports of dementia in OPCA, relatively little is known about the specific behavioral characteristics that may be typical in this disorder. Patients with OPCA show a distinctive pattern of glucose hypometabolism. Significant declines in metabolism are observed in the cerebellar vermis, cerebellar hemispheres, and brainstem with sparing of thalamic and cerebral cortex metabolism.[57-59] These changes are similar in both the sporadic and familial forms of the disease. However, PET studies have thus far been limited to individuals who do not demonstrate dementia.[14] As a result, no clear correlations can yet be drawn between the dementia of this disorder and changes in glucose metabolism as evidenced by PET.

V. COMPARISON OF IMAGING IN DEMENTIAS OF MOVEMENT DISORDERS

Functional brain imaging permits some general conclusions to be drawn about the nature of cerebral metabolic changes underlying the dementia associated with movement disorders. It is apparent from these studies that the cerebral metabolic activity seen in movement disorders is not all alike. Each disease causes a different pattern of hypometabolism which

PARKINSON'S DISEASE

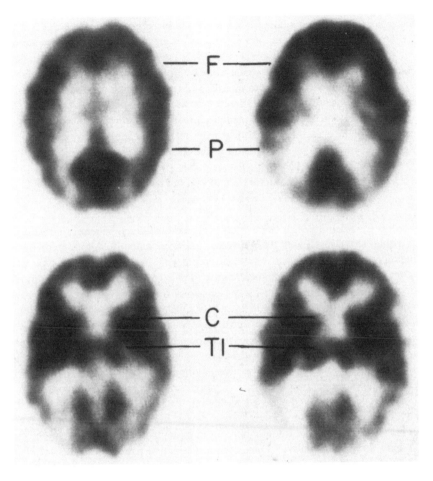

First Study   4 Years Later

FIGURE 4.   Over a 4-year period of increasing cognitive impairment, the cerebral metabolic pattern of this patient changed from a uniform reduction, commonly found in patients with Parkinson's disease, to marked hypometabolism of parietal cortex (P) accompanied by relative sparing of caudate (C) and thalamus (Tl) metabolism, a pattern typical of Alzheimer's disease. Note the relative prominence of frontal cortex (F) in comparison with parietal cortex metabolism. (From Kuhl, D. E. et al., *Ann. Neurol.*, 15, 419, 1984. With permission.

reflects the distribution of neuronal loss and neurochemical abnormalities produced by that disorder. Furthermore, the distribution of nueronal loss by itself does not account for the all of the functional impairment in glucose metabolism observed in these disorders. For example, in PSP the cerebral cortex demonstrates significant declines in cerebral cortical metabolism, despite the absence of neuronal damage in the cerebral cortex as demonstrated by conventional neuropathological techniques. On the other hand, in the case of Huntington's disease, where significant loss of cortical neurons has been described, no change in cerebral cortical metabolism is seen, at least in early stages of the disease.

In all of the movement disorders associated with dementia the basal ganglia are consistently involved (Table 3). Glucose metabolism in the caudate nucleus and putamen declines in patients with PSP, Parkinson's disease with dementia, and Huntington's disease when compared to normals. However, thalamus is only affected in those which also demonstrate cerebral cortical hypometabolism, namely PSP and Parkinson's disease with dementia. There are indications in Huntington's disease that declines in metabolism in the caudate nucleus and, to a lesser extent, in putamen are related to progression of cognitive impairment. In Parkinson's disease and PSP, dementia appears to be closely linked with the degree of hypometabolism observed in the cerebral cortex. However, the relative contributions of specific cortical and subcortical structures to the cognitive impairment seen in any of these disorders is still not understood. Further studies are needed in which PET results are carefully compared to clinical and pathological changes. Provocative studies in which medication, environment, or patient activity are modified during PET scanning may also improve our knowledge of the mechanisms of dementia in the movement disorders.

VI. FUNCTIONAL IMAGING IN THE DIFFERENTIAL DIAGNOSIS OF DEMENTIA

Movement disorders have distinctive clinical features which generally make it unlikely that they would be confused with other diseases causing dementia. Although the behavioral symptomatology of any of the movement disorders may be similar to that typical in Alzheimer's or Pick's disease, the supranuclear gaze of palsy of PSP, the choreiform movements of Huntington's disease, the Kayser-Fleischer rings of Wilson's disease, the bradykinesia and tremor of Parkinson's disease, or the ataxia of OPCA are unlikely to be mistaken. These physical signs along with a typical medical history and laboratory results do not require further confirmation by the performance of functional brain imaging. However, patients with an atypical clinical presentation, or in the late stages of dementia due to any cause, may pose a diagnostic dilemma that can be resolved by imaging. For example, patients with PSP may not have a supranuclear palsy of gaze as a prominent early feature,[60] and not uncommonly such individuals are initially diagnosed as having Parkinson's disease.[61] The patterns of glucose hypometabolism, however, are quite different in these two conditions. Likewise, if falling or ataxia is a prominent initial symptom in patients with PSP, an incorrect diagnosis of OPCA may be made initially.[26] Once again, distinctive patterns of glucose metabolism as demonstrated by PET can distinguish these conditions.

Recently it have been recognized that some patients with multiple infarcts develop supranuclear gaze palsy, dementia, and other symptoms similar to those seen in PSP.[62] Infarcts may be seen by conventional brain imaging techniques. However, since stroke causes larger abnormalities with PET than with CT,[63] PET may assist in arriving at the correct diagnosis in some cases. The typical pattern of patchy assymetric regions of hypometabolism seen in multi-infarct dementia[64,65] is quite distinct from the pattern seen in PSP (Figure 5).

Any patient developing prominent behavioral symptoms or intellectual decline may at first be considered to have Alzheimer's disease or Pick's disease. Yet both of these disorders cause distinctive patterns of cerebral glucose hypometabolism. PET may therefore be of diagnostic utility in demented patients whose motor abnormalities have been overlooked. Alzheimer's disease causes a decline in glucose throughout the cerebral cortex, in the putamen, thalamus, and caudate nucleus, but most prominently in the temporoparietal association areas (Plate 9*).[25,66,68] This pattern makes it clearly distinguishable from PSP.[69] Pick's disease also shows distinctive changes by PET. In this disorder, hypometabolism is seen predominantly in the frontal cortex.[70,71] Thus, among the movement disorders associated with dementia, confusion would only occur between Parkinson's disease and Alzheimer's disease or between Pick's disease and PSP if PET alone were relied upon for diagnosis. In

---

* Plate 9 appears after page 168.

MULTIPLE INFARCT DEMENTIA

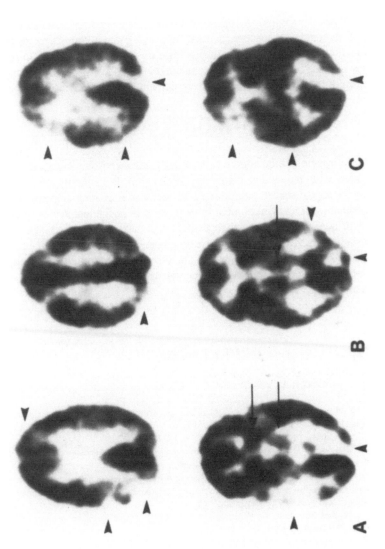

FIGURE 5. ¹⁸F-FDG scans of three patients with multiple infarct dementia. Upper images are approximately 8 cm and lower images 4 cm above the canthomeatal line. The ages of these subjects are A: 60 years, B: 62 years, C: 54 years. Scattered metabolic defects (arrowheads) are seen throughout the brain in each subject. Some lesions such as the occipital lobe infarct in patient C are seen in both images, while other lesions are seen only in a single image. (From Kuhl, D. E. et al., in Brain Imaging and Brain Function, vol. 63.)

the case of Pick's disease, glucose metabolism in subcortical structures has not yet been described, and therefore further experience may permit PSP and Pick's disease to be distinguished by PET.

In the late stages of dementia due to any cause, abilities become so limited that clinical examination alone may be of little help in distinguishing its cause. If historical information is unavailable, it may be impossible to distinguish these conditions during life. Positron emission tomography offers the hope that this may change. Because of technical considerations, few studies have been performed so far in patients with severe dementia. However, distinctive, localized neuropathological and neurochemical abnormalities persist in the brains of patients with all dementing disorders, even at autopsy. By applying different positron-emitting neurotransmitter precursors and receptor ligands, it should be possible to exploit known differences in these diseases. It thus appears likely that PET will become even more important in the future in recognizing when severe dementia has been caused by one of the movement disorders.

VII. SUMMARY

Functional brain imaging studies have substantially enhanced our understanding of the dementias associated with movement disorders. While PET is generally unnecessary for diagnosis of a movement disorder complicated by dementia, it may improve diagnostic accuracy in individuals with unusual clinical presentations or in the late stages of dementia. The development of new PET agents which exploit known biochemical and anatomic differences in these disorders will further improve diagnostic accuracy and will be useful in devising and monitoring new therapies. By imaginative application of PET techniques, the mechanisms underlying the development of dementia in patients with movement disorders may finally be unraveled.

REFERENCES

1. **Steele, J. C., Richardson, J. C., and Olszewski, J.,** Progressive supranuclear palsy, *Arch. Neurol.*, 10, 333, 1964.
2. **Albert, M. L., Feldman, R. G., and Willis, A. L.,** The "subcortical dementia" of progressive supranuclear palsy, *J. Neurol, Neurosurg. Psychiatry*, 37, 121, 1974.
3. **Huntingon, G.,** On chorea, *Med. Surg. Rep.*, 26, 317, 1872.
4. **Hallock, F. K.,** A case of Huntington's chorea with remarks upon the propriety of naming the disorder "dementia choreics", *J. Nerv. Ment. Dis.*, 25, 851, 1898.
5. **McHugh, P. R. and Folstein, M. F.,** Psychiatric syndromes of Huntington's chorea: a clinical and phenomenologic study, in *Psychiatric Aspects of Neurologic Disease*, Benson, D. F. and Blumer, D., Eds., Grune & Stratton, New York, 1975, 267.
6. **Scheinberg, I. H. and Sternlieb, I.,** Wilson's Disease, XXIII, *Major Problems in Internal Medicine*, W. B. Saunders, Philadelphia, 1984, 86.
7. **Parkinson, J.,** An essay on the shaking palsy, *Med. Classics*, 2, 964, 1938.
8. **Reitan, R. M. and Boll, T. J.,** Intellectual and cognitive functions in Parkinson's disease, *J. Consult. Clin. Psychol.*, 37, 364, 1971.
9. **Loranger, A. W., Goodell, H., McDowell, F. H., Lee, J. E., and Sweet, R. D.,** Intellectual impairment in Parkinson's syndrome, *Brain*, 95, 405, 1972.
10. **Riklan, M., Whelihan, W., and Cullinan, T.,** Levodopa and psychometric test performance in parkinsonism—5 years later, *Neurology*, 36, 173, 1976.
11. **Mortimer, J. A., Christensen, K. J., and Webster, D. D.,** Parkinsonia dementia, in *Neurobehavioral Disorders*, Volume 2, Series 2, Frederiks, J. A. M., Ed., Elsevier, Amsterdam, 1985, 371.
12. **Cummings, J. L. and Benson, D. F.,** *Dementia: A Clinical Approach*, Butterworths, Boston, 1983.
13. **Kish, S., Freedman, M., El-Awar, M., Leach, L., Oscar-Berman, M., and Schut, L.,** Neuropsychological deficits in olivopontocerebellar atrophy: implications for the cholinergic hypothesis of Alzheimer's dementia, *Ann. Neurol.*, 22, 121, 1987.

14. **Berent, S., Giordani, B., Gilman, S., Junck, L., Lehtinen, S., Markel, D., Boivin, M., Kluin, K., and Parks, R.**, A quantitative analysis of cognitive intellectual and emotional function in olivopontocerebellar atrophy, *Neurology*, 38 (Suppl. 1), 285, 1988.

15. *Diagnostic and Statistical Manual of Mental Disorders. DSM I*, 1st ed., American Psychiatric Association, Washington, D. C., 1952.

16. *Diagnostic and Statistical Manual of Mental Disorders. DSM II, 2nd ed.*, American Psychiatric Association, Washington, D. C., 1968.

17. **Bayles, K. A. and Stern, L. Z.**, Language impairment in Parkinson disease, *Int. Neuropsychol. Soc. Bull.*, September, 16, 1982.

18. **Boller, F., Passafiume, D., Keefe, N. C., Rogers, K., Morrow, L., and Kim, Y.**, Visuospatial impairment in Parkinson's disease: role of perceptual and motor factors, *Arch. Neurol.*, 41, 485, 1984.

19. **Pillon, B., Dubois, B., Lhermitte, F., and Agid, Y.**, Heterogeneity of cognitive impairment in progressive supranuclear palsy, Parkinson's disease, and Alzheimer's disease, *Neurology*, 36, 1179, 1986.

20. **Rafal, R. D., Posner, M. I., Walker, J. A., and Friedrich, F. J.**, Cognition and the basal ganglia. Separating mental and motor components of performance in Parkinson's disease, *Brain*, 107, 1083, 1984.

21. **Uhl, G. R., Hilt, D. C., Hedreen, J. C., Whitehouse, P. J., and Price, D. L.**, Pick's disease (lobar sclerosis): depletion of neurons in the nucleus basalis of Meynert, *Neurology*, 33, 1470, 1983.

22. **Whitehouse, P. J., Price, D. L., Clark, A. W., Coyle, J. T., and DeLong, M. R.**, Alzheimer disease: evidence for selective loss of cholinergic neurons in the nucleus basalis, *Ann. Neurol.*, 10, 122, 1981.

23. **Yamamoto, Y. and Hirano, A.**, Nucleus raphe dorsalis in Alzheimer's disease: neurofibrillary tangles and loss of large neurons, *Ann. Neurol.*, 17, 573, 1985.

24. **Boller, F., Mizutani, T., Roessmann, U., and Gambetti, P.**, Parkinson disease, dementia, and Alzheimer disease: clinicopathological correlations, *Ann. Neurol.*, 7, 329, 1980.

25. **Foster, N. L., Morin, E. M., Kuhl, D. E., and Gilman, S.**, Glucose metabolic activity in the basal ganglia and thalamus differs in progressive supranuclear palsy and Alzheimer's disease, *Neurology*, 38 (Suppl. 1), 369, 1988.

26. **Foster, N. L., Gilman, S., Berent, S., Morin, E. M., Brown, M. B., and Koeppe, R. A.**, Cerebral hypometabolism in progressive supranuclear palsy studied with positron emission tomography, *Ann. Neurol.*, 24, 399, 1988.

27. **D'Antona, R., Baron, J. C., Samson, Y., Serdaru, M., Viader, F., Agid, Y., and Cambier, J.**, Subcortical demential: frontal cortex hypometabolism detected by positron tomography in patients with progressive supranuclear palsy, *Brain*, 108, 785, 1985.

28. **Hawkins, R. A., Mazziotta, J. C., and Phelps, M. E.**, Wilson's disease studied with FDG and positron emission tomography, *Neurology*, 37, 1707, 1987.

29. **Kuhl, D. E., Metter, E. J., and Riege, W. H.**, Patterns of local cerebral glucose utilization determined in Parkinson's disease by the (18F) fluorodeoxyglucose method, *Ann. Neurol.*, 15, 419,1984.

30. **Young, A. B., Penney, J. B., Starosta-Rubinstein, S., Markel, D. S., Berent, S., Giordani, B., Ehrenkaufer, R., Jewett, D., and Hichwa, R.**, PET scan investigations of Huntington's disease: cerebral metabolic correlates of neurological features and functional decline, *Ann. Neurol.*, 20, 296, 1986.

31. **Kuhl, D. E., Phelps, M. E., Markham, C. H., Metter, E. J., Riege, W. H., and Winter, J.** Cerebral metabolism and atrophy in Huntington's disease determined by 18FDG and computed tomographic scan, *Ann. Neurol.*, 12, 425, 1982.

32. **Whitehouse, P. J.**, The concept of subcortical and cortical dementia: another look, *Ann. Neurol.*, 19, 1, 1986.

33. **Sechi, G., Tanda, F., and Mutani, R.**, Fatal hyperpyrexia after withdrawal of levodopa, *Neurology*, 34, 249, 1984.

34. **Mayeux, R., Stern, Y., Mulvey, K., and Cote, L.**, Reappraisal of temporary levodopa withdrawal ("drug holiday") in Parkinson's disease, *N. Engl. J. Med.*, 313, 724, 1985.

35. **Foster, N. L., VanDerSpek, A. F. L., Aldrich, M. S., Berent, S., Hichwa, R. H., Sackellares, J. C., Gilman, S., and Agranoff, B. W.**, The effect of diazepam sedation on cerebral glucose metabolism in Alzheimer's disease as measured using positron emission tomography, *J. Cereb. Blood Flow Metab.*, 7, 415, 1987.

36. **Fletcher, J. C., Dommel, F. W., and Cowell, D. D.**, Trial policy for the intramural programs of the National Institutes of Health: consent to research with impaired human subjects, *IRB: Rev. Hum. Subj. Res.*, 7, 1, 1985.

37. **Baron, J. C., Mazière, B., Loc'h, C., Cambon, H., Sgouropoulos, P., Bonnet, A. M., and Agia, Y.**, Loss of striatal (^{76}Br) bromospiperone binding sites demonstrated by positron tomography in progressive supranuclear palsy, *J. Cereb. Blood Flow Metab.*, 6, 131, 1986.

38. **Kimura, D., Barnet, H. J. M., and Burkhart, G.**, The psychological test pattern in progressive supranuclear palsy, *Neuropsychologia*, 19, 301 1981.

39. **Perkin, G. D., Lees, A. J., Stern, G. M., and Kocen, R. S.**, Problems in the diagnosis of progressive supranuclear palsy (Steele-Richardson-Olszewski syndrome), *Can. J. Neurol. Sci.*, 5, 167, 1978.

40. **Fisk, J. D., Goodale, M. A., Burkhart, G., and Barnet, H. J. M.** Progressive supranuclear palsy: the relationship between ocular motor dysfunction and psychological test performance, *Neurology*, 32, 698, 1982.

41. **Maher, E. R. and Lees, A. J.**, The clinical features and natural history of the Steele-Richardson-Olszewski syndrome (progressive supranuclear palsy), *Neurology*, 36, 1005, 1986.

42. **Jellinger, K.**, Progressive supranuclear palsy (subcortical argyrophilic dystrophy), *Acta Neuropath.*, 19, 347, 1971.

43. **Foster, N. L., Berent, S., Brown, M. B., Gilman, S., and Hichwa, R. D.**, Cerebral cortical metabolism reflects performance on the Wechsler adult intelligence scale, *Neurology*, 37 (Suppl. 1), 172, 1987.

44. **Berent, S. Foster, N. L., Gilman, S., Hichwa, R., and Lehtinen, S.**, Patterns of cortical 18F-FDG metabolism in Alzheimer's and progressive supranuclear palsy patients are related to the types of cognitivie impairments, *Neurology*, 37 (Suppl. 1), 172, 1987.

45. **Butters, N., Sax, D., Montgomery, K., and Tarlow, S.**, Comparison of the neuropsychological deficits associated with early and advanced Huntington's disease, *Arch. Neurol.*, 35, 585, 1978.

46. **Fedio, P., Cox, C. S., Neophytides, A., Canal-Frederick, G., and Chase, T. N.**, Neuropsychological profile of Huntington's disease: patients and those at risk, in *Huntington's Disease*, 23 Advances in Neurology, Chase, T. N., Wexler, N. S., and Barbeau, A., Eds., Raven Press, New York, 1979, 239.

47. **Caine, E. D., Ebert, M. H., and Weingartner, H.**, An outline for analysis of dementia. The memory disorder of Huntington's disease, *Neurology*, 27, 1087, 1977.

48. **Weingartner, H., Caine, E. D., and Ebert, M. H.**, Encoding processes, learning, and recall in Huntington's disease, in *Huntington's Disease*, 23, Advancees in Neurology, Chase T. N., Wexler, N. S., and Barbeau, A., Eds., Raven Press, New York, 1979, 215.

49. **Aminoff, M., Marshall, J., Smith, E. M., and Wyke, M. A.**, Pattern of intellectual impairment in Huntington's disease, *Psychol. Med.*, 5, 169, 1975.

50. **Hayden, M. R.** *Huntington's Chorea*, Springer-Verlag, New York, 1981.

51. **Hayden, M. R., Martin, W. R. W., Stoessl, A. J., Clark, C., Hollenberg, S., Adam, M. J., Ammann, W., Harrop, R., Rogers, J., Ruth, T., Sayre, C., and Pate, B. D.**, Positron emission tomography in the early diagnosis of Huntington's disease, *Neurology*, 36, 888, 1986.

52. **Shoulson, I. and Fahn, S.**, Huntington's disease: clinical care and evaluation, *Neurology*, 29, 1, 1979.

53. **Berent, S., Giordani, B., Lehtinen, S., Markel, D., Penney, J. B., Buchtel, H. A., Starosta-Rubinstein, S., Hichwa, R., and Young, A. B.**, Positron emission tomographic scan investigations of Huntington's disease: cerebral metabolic correlates of cognitive function, *Ann. Neurol.* 23, 541, 1988.

54. **Dom, R., Malford, M., and Baro, F.**, Neuropathology of Huntington's chorea: cytometric studies of the ventrobasal complex of the thalamus, *Neurology*, 26, 64, 1976.

55. **Chui, H. C., Mortimer, J. A., Slager, U., Zarow, C., Bondareff, W., and Webster, D. D.**, Pathologic correlates of dementia in Parkinson's disease, *Arch. Neurol.*, 43, 991, 1986.

56. **Adam, P., Fabre, N., Guell, A., Bessoles, G., Roulleau, J., and Bes, A.**, Cortical atrophy in Parkinson disease: correlation between clinical and CT findings with special emphasis on prefrontal atrophy, *AJNR*, 4, 442, 1983.

57. **Gilman, S., Markel, D. S., Koeppe, R. A., Junck, L., Kluin, K. J., Gebarski, S. S., and Hichwa, R. D.**, Cerebellar and brainstem hypometabolism in olivopontocerebellar atrophy detected with PET, *Ann. Neurol.*, 23, 223, 1988.

58. **Rosenthal, G., Gilman, S., Koeppe, R. A., Kluin, K. J., Markel, D. S., Junck, L., and Gebarski, S. S.**, Motor dysfunction in olivopontocerebellar atrophy is related to cerebral metabolic rate studied with positron emission tomography, *Ann. Neurol.*, 24, 414, 1988.

59. **Kluin, K. J., Gilman, S., Markel, D. S., Koeppe, R. A., Rosenthal, G., and Junck, L.**, Speech disorders in olivopontocerebellar atrophy with positron emission tomography findings, *Ann. Neurol.*, 23, 547, 1988.

60. **Nuwer, M. R.**, Progressive supranuclear palsy despite normal eye movements, *Ann. Neurol.*, 38, 784, 1981.

61. **Kristensen, M. O.**, Progressive supranuclear palsy—20 years later, *Acta Neurol. Scand.*, 71, 177, 1985.

62. **Dubinsky, R. M. and Jankovic, J.**, Progressive supranuclear palsy and a multi-infarct state, *Neurology*, 37, 570, 1987.

63. **Kuhl, D. E., Phelps, M. E., Kowell, A. P., Metter, E. J., Selin, C., and Winter, J.**, Effects of stroke on local cerebral metabolism and perfusion: mapping by emission computed tomography of 18FDG and 13NH3, *Ann. Neurol.*, 8, 47, 1980.

64. **Metter, E. J., Mazziotta, J. C., Itabashi, H. H., Mankovich, N. J., Phelps, M. E., and Kuhl, D. E.**, Comparison of glucose metabolism, x-ray CT, and post-mortem data in a patient with multiple cerebral infarcts, *Neurology*, 35, 1695, 1985.

65. **Kuhl, D. E., Metter, E. J., and Riege, W. H.**, Patterns of cerebral glucose utilization in depression, multiple infarct dementia, and Alzheimer's disease, in *Brain Imaging and Brain Function*, Vol. 63, Sokoloff, L., Ed., Raven Press, New York, 1985, 211.

66. Foster, N. L., Chase, T. N., Mansi, L., Brooks, R., Fedio, P., Patronas, N., and DiChiro, G., Cortical abnormalities in Alzheimer's disease, *Ann. Neurol.,* 16, 649, 1984.
67. Friedland, R. P., Budinger, T. F., Ganz, E., Yano, Y., Mathis, C. A., Koss, B., Ober, B., Huesman, R. H., and Derezo, S. E., Regional cerebral metabolic alterations in dementia of the Alzheimer type: positron emission tomography with 18-F-fluorodeoxyglucose, *J. Comput. Assist. Tomogr.,* 7, 590, 1983.
68. Duara, R., Grady, C., Haxby, J., Sundaram, M., Cutler, N. R., Heston, L., Moore, A., Schlageter, N., Larsen, S., and Rapoport, S. I., Positron emission tomography in Alzheimer's disease, *Neurology,* 36, 879, 1986.
69. Foster, N. L., Gilman, S., Berent, S., and Hichwa, R. D., Distinctive patterns of cerebral cortical glucose metabolism in progressive supranuclear palsy and Alzheimer's disease studied with positron emission tomography, *Neurology,* 36, (Suppl. 1), 338, 1986.
70. Friedland, R. P., Jagust, W. J., Ober, B. A., Dronkers, J. F., Koss, E., Simpson, G. V., Ellis, W. G., and Budinger, T. F., The pathophysiology of Pick's disease: a comprehensive case study, *Neurology,* 36 (Suppl. 1), 268, 1986.
71. Kamo, H., McGeer, P. L., Harrop, R., McGeer, E. G., Caine, D. B., Martin, W. R. W., and Pate, B. D., Positron emission tomography and histopathology in Pick's disease, *Neurology,* 37, 439, 1987.

Chapter 14

FUTURE DIRECTIONS FOR PET IN NEUROLOGY

Donald B. Calne

Any attempt to foresee future directions of medicine is fraught with uncertainty because of the inherently unpredictable way in which science evolves, and also because of the network of interrelationships that exists between different branches of scientific endeavor so that a development in one area can have profound implications for another. Over the last decade positron emission tomography (PET) of the brain has evolved as a unique technique for showing the distribution of radioisotopes *in vivo* with greater precision than was ever possible with the traditional methods of nuclear medicine. Both in-plane and axial resolution of images have improved from over 12 to 5 mm and 15 transverse slices of the brain can now be obtained routinely.

Images per se, however, have limited application, there being substantially greater potential use for observations based on quantification of the regional concentrations of substances that are of biological importance. This goal requires (1) the capacity to attach positron emitting labels to substances of biological significance; (2) the ability to quantify radioactivity in small structures with a PET imaging system; and, (3) the ability to generate mathematical models which describe the kinetics of these radiolabeled tracers. Substantial progress has been made in all these endeavors. Cerebral blood flow, oxygen consumption, and glucose metabolism can all be measured with considerable precision. Insofar as these indices of cellular metabolism reflect neuronal activity, we have a method for examining the localized activity of different regions in the living brain in varying states of normal and abnormal function. This capability has been exploited in several settings to elucidate normal physiology and pathophysiology.

If there is continued expansion of our capacity to label new compounds and to model their kinetics, what extension of the functional analysis of the brain can we expect? An encouraging start has been made in the quest to map pathways defined by their neurotransmitters or synaptic receptors. A large body of information is accruing on the accumulation of fluorodopa and/or its metabolites in the brain. This is likely to provide a measure of the ability of neurons to synthesize and store dopamine, which is in turn an index of the integrity of dopaminergic pathways. Similarly, ligands of the D_1 receptor (^{11}C-SCH 23390) and the D_2 receptor (^{11}C-raclopride) are now being employed in mapping studies of animal and human brains. Nonspecific binding has been measured with labeled inactive enantiomers; by subtracting such data from scans with the active enantiomer, greater accuracy of quantification of receptor binding kinetics has been achieved.

It is reasonable to expect that over the next decade PET tracers will be developed for other transmitters, such as acetylcholine, glutamate and GABA. Similarly, ligands for the various subtypes of receptors for these transmitters should allow more extended mapping of pathways defined by their utilization of neurohumoral agents. This mapping is not simply an anatomical exercise, but should play a major role in elucidating pathology, establishing clinicopathological correlations, and determining the nature and extent of wanted and unwanted drug actions. In this way, one may conceive of the major projections of the human brain becoming highlighted like a telephone exchange wiring diagram. Changes induced by physiological input, output, and cognitive function should become accessible to study in health and disease. In addition to detecting markers related to neuronal metabolism and transmission, PET is potentially a tool for delineating structural elements such as glia and blood vessels.

What type of problem may be approached if technical advances allow tracers and modeling to be developed in the ways that currently seem possible? Much depends on whether the resolution of PET can also be improved. Will we be able to study substantia nigra or the dentate nucleus? Certainly such enhanced detail would greatly expand the potential application of PET, but even without a major increase in resolution, one can speculate on the biological questions that may become accessible to study.

First and foremost, PET should enable us to gain critical insight into disease of the brain that is not accompanied by macroscopic or microscopic anatomic abnormality. Dystonia, schizophrenia, essential tremor, and idiopathic epilepsy exemplify the problem of identifying the origin and nature of a disturbance of function in the absence of a structural abnormality. PET should facilitate the early detection of lesions, which may still be subclinical, and studies on the nature and evolution of such lesions may contribute to our understanding of etiology. By enabling neural pathways to be characterized as normal or abnormal, the profile of functional changes in disorders of mental status such as depression and Alzheimer's disease should be elucidated and this in turn may allow a more rational approach to therapy. In the field of clinical pharmacology, the kinetics of therapeutic agents is accessible to study, together with the mechanism of central adverse reactions, such as involuntary movements, hallucinations, and confusion. It is not unreasonable to speculate that PET tracers may be developed to signal certain types of pathological tissue disturbance, such as inflammation, edema, or neoplastic infiltration, with greater sensitivity than that attainable by CT or MRI. If transplantation into the brain ever becomes a creditable form of treatment, PET has the potential for demonstrating viability and measuring functional activity of grafted tissue. It is quite possible that a detailed metabolic map of the consequences of stroke might provide guidance to prognosis and management. Further knowledge may be acquired on the cogent problem of deteriorating brain function in normal senescence.

The list of possible gains in our understanding and management of neurological disease is endless, but such speculation is of limited value because the natural history of technological development is characterized by unforeseeable steps which create new ranges of opportunity and new categories of questions. In this context the future of PET could be profoundly influenced by developments in therapy. If treatment became available to arrest or slow down the progress of, for example, Alzheimer's disease or Parkinson's disease, early diagnosis would suddenly assume major importance in management, and it may be that the best instrument for early detection would prove to be PET.

PET is an expensive development that requires a serious and sustained effort to formulate biological experiments that may be answered. The main danger to its future is the disrepute that would result from employing such a powerful tool for trivial, anecdotal, and uninterpretable scanning.

In conclusion, PET is a new technique for measuring regional brain chemistry that enables us to infer regional brain function. While much progress has been made in its short life time, its growth has been impeded by the problems deriving from any methodology that involves a large team of specialists in different fields. How should priorities be assigned? How much can be answered with images alone? How much more with kinetic modeling? What are the limits of radiation exposure with each tracer? How much animal testing is required before introducing new tracers into human subjects? Is PET solely a research tool, or does it have clinical applications? How does PET compare with single photon emission computed tomography and magnetic resonance spectroscopy? How many PET centers should there be? How should they be funded? Who should control them?

Some of these questions are scientific, some are ethical, some are economic, and some are political. All will have to be resolved over the next decade if PET is to fulfill its considerable potential for extending our understanding of brain function in health and disease which should, in turn, lead to more tangible benefits to health care by improving our ability to diagnose and treat neurological disease.

INDEX